Pediatric Gastrointestinal Diseases: Diagnosis and Management

Pediatric Gastrointestinal Diseases: Diagnosis and Management

Cristina Oana Marginean

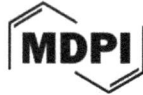

Basel • Beijing • Wuhan • Barcelona • Belgrade • Novi Sad • Cluj • Manchester

Cristina Oana Marginean
Pediatrics
"George Emil Palade"
University of Medicine,
Pharmacy, Science, and
Technology of Targu Mures
Targu Mures
Romania

Editorial Office
MDPI AG
Grosspeteranlage 5
4052 Basel, Switzerland

This is a reprint of articles from the Special Issue published online in the open access journal *Diagnostics* (ISSN 2075-4418) (available at: www.mdpi.com/journal/diagnostics/special_issues/pediatric_gastrointestinal_diseases).

For citation purposes, cite each article independently as indicated on the article page online and as indicated below:

Lastname, A.A.; Lastname, B.B. Article Title. *Journal Name* **Year**, *Volume Number*, Page Range.

ISBN 978-3-7258-1772-6 (Hbk)
ISBN 978-3-7258-1771-9 (PDF)
https://doi.org/10.3390/books978-3-7258-1771-9

© 2024 by the authors. Articles in this book are Open Access and distributed under the Creative Commons Attribution (CC BY) license. The book as a whole is distributed by MDPI under the terms and conditions of the Creative Commons Attribution-NonCommercial-NoDerivs (CC BY-NC-ND) license (https://creativecommons.org/licenses/by-nc-nd/4.0/).

Contents

Preface vii

Cristina Oana Mărginean
Multidisciplinarity and Trandisciplinarity in the Diagnosis and Treatment of Pediatric Gastrointestinal Diseases
Reprinted from: *Diagnostics* 2024, 14, 852, doi:10.3390/diagnostics14080852 1

Ancuta Lupu, Ingrith Crenguta Miron, Andrei Tudor Cernomaz, Cristina Gavrilovici, Vasile Valeriu Lupu and Iuliana Magdalena Starcea et al.
Epidemiological Characteristics of *Helicobacter pylori* Infection in Children in Northeast Romania
Reprinted from: *Diagnostics* 2023, 13, 408, doi:10.3390/diagnostics13030408 4

Maria Oana Săsăran, Cristina Oana Mărginean and Ana Maria Koller
Impact of *Helicobacter pylori* Infection upon the Evolution and Outcome of Pediatric Immune Thrombocytopenic Purpura: A Comprehensive Review
Reprinted from: *Diagnostics* 2023, 13, 3205, doi:10.3390/diagnostics13203205 16

Ancuta Lupu, Cristina Gavrilovici, Vasile Valeriu Lupu, Anca Lavinia Cianga, Andrei Tudor Cernomaz and Iuliana Magdalena Starcea et al.
Helicobacter pylori Infection in Children: A Possible Reason for Headache?
Reprinted from: *Diagnostics* 2023, 13, 1293, doi:10.3390/diagnostics13071293 31

Vasile Valeriu Lupu, Gabriela Stefanescu, Ana Maria Laura Buga, Lorenza Forna, Elena Tarca and Iuliana Magdalena Starcea et al.
Is There a Potential Link between Gastroesophageal Reflux Disease and Recurrent Respiratory Tract Infections in Children?
Reprinted from: *Diagnostics* 2023, 13, 2310, doi:10.3390/diagnostics13132310 42

Vasile Valeriu Lupu, Ingrith Miron, Ana Maria Laura Buga, Cristina Gavrilovici, Elena Tarca and Anca Adam Raileanu et al.
Iron Deficiency Anemia in Pediatric Gastroesophageal Reflux Disease
Reprinted from: *Diagnostics* 2022, 13, 63, doi:10.3390/diagnostics13010063 54

Jovan Jevtić, Nina Ristić, Vedrana Pavlović, Jovana Svorcan, Ivan Milovanovich and Milica Radusinović et al.
The Usefulness of the Eosinophilic Esophagitis Histology Scoring System in Predicting Response to Proton Pump Inhibitor Monotherapy in Children with Eosinophilic Esophagitis
Reprinted from: *Diagnostics* 2023, 13, 3445, doi:10.3390/diagnostics13223445 64

Dana-Teodora Anton-Păduraru, Alina Mariela Murgu, Laura Iulia Bozomitu, Dana Elena Mîndru, Codruța Olimpiada Iliescu Halițchi and Felicia Trofin et al.
Diagnosis and Management of Gastrointestinal Manifestations in Children with Cystic Fibrosis
Reprinted from: *Diagnostics* 2024, 14, 228, doi:10.3390/diagnostics14020228 76

Anca Cristina Drăgănescu, Victor Daniel Miron, Oana Săndulescu, Anuța Bilașco, Anca Streinu-Cercel and Roxana Gabriela Sandu et al.
Omicron in Infants—Respiratory or Digestive Disease?
Reprinted from: *Diagnostics* 2023, 13, 421, doi:10.3390/diagnostics13030421 100

Andreea Sălcudean, Andreea Georgiana Nan, Cristina Raluca Bodo, Marius Cătălin Cosma, Elena Gabriela Strete and Maria Melania Lica
Association between Childhood Onset Inflammatory Bowel Disease and Psychiatric Comorbidities in Adulthood
Reprinted from: *Diagnostics* **2023**, *13*, 1868, doi:10.3390/diagnostics13111868 . . . . **111**

Cristina Oana Mărginean, Lorena Elena Meliț, Reka Borka Balas, Anca Meda Văsieșiu and Tudor Fleșeriu
The Crosstalk between Vitamin D and Pediatric Digestive Disorders
Reprinted from: *Diagnostics* **2022**, *12*, 2328, doi:10.3390/diagnostics12102328 . . . . **126**

Preface

This Special Issue aims to emphasize the importance of multidisciplinary and transdisciplinary approaches in pediatric gastrointestinal diseases to provide the adequate management of these patients. The topics addressed within this article collection cover a vast majority of pediatric digestive pathology and include research articles, reviews or clinical case reports. The published articles aid in a better understanding of the pathogenesis and management controversies of pediatric gastrointestinal disorders, and enrich the literature. These articles reflect the progress in the field and the required future steps in pediatric gastroenterology.

Cristina Oana Marginean
Editor

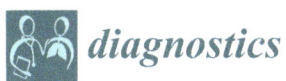

Editorial

Multidisciplinarity and Trandisciplinarity in the Diagnosis and Treatment of Pediatric Gastrointestinal Diseases

Cristina Oana Mărginean

Department of Pediatrics I, University of Medicine, Pharmacy, Sciences and Technology George Emil Palade of Târgu Mureș, 540136 Târgu Mureș, Romania; marginean.oana@gmail.com

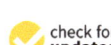

Citation: Mărginean, C.O. Multidisciplinarity and Trandisciplinarity in the Diagnosis and Treatment of Pediatric Gastrointestinal Diseases. *Diagnostics* **2024**, *14*, 852. https://doi.org/10.3390/diagnostics14080852

Received: 18 March 2024
Accepted: 18 April 2024
Published: 20 April 2024

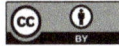

Copyright: © 2024 by the author. Licensee MDPI, Basel, Switzerland. This article is an open access article distributed under the terms and conditions of the Creative Commons Attribution (CC BY) license (https://creativecommons.org/licenses/by/4.0/).

It is an honor and a privilege to have helped bring this Special Issue titled "Multidisciplinarity and Trandisciplinarity in the Diagnosis and Treatment of Pediatric Gastrointestinal Diseases" to you.

The specialty of pediatric gastroenterology has experienced accelerated development in recent decades through its development as a subspecialty and later a specialty from its "mother" discipline, pediatrics. This occurred due to its tendency, in the recent years, to be more and more specialized in a smaller area and because of improvements in diagnosis and therapeutic techniques and skills associated with this discipline, such as ultrasound, endoscopy, echo-endoscopy, or endoscopic retrograde cholangiopancreatography [1]. Thus, pediatric gastro-entero-intestinal diseases are problems that require diagnosis and short- and long-term management for rare disorders and complex cases of more common disorders that affect the gastrointestinal tract; moreover, these diseases frequently need a multidisciplinary team in order to provide adequate management [2].

The purpose of this Special Issue is to allow researchers from around the world to report on the new insights into pediatric gastrointestinal diseases. Thus, we aim to include papers related to both the diagnosis and management of a wide spectrum of pediatric gastrointestinal diseases, such as celiac disease, acute and chronic diarrhea, inflammatory bowel disease, food allergies, nutritional disorders, gastritis, and other functional gastrointestinal disorders. Assessing and reporting novel information regarding different gastrointestinal disorders is highly important as it is a major concern of pediatricians in clinical practice. It is a well-documented fact that gastrointestinal diseases represent the most important cause of morbidity in pediatric patients. The proper diagnosis and management of these pathologies independently of their organic or functional etiology will create healthier adult populations, decreasing the costs related to health services and improving the care that might have to be individualized for each patient.

Therefore, an important topic in this area is pediatric gastroesophageal reflux disease (GERD), whose manifestations can be divided into esophageal and extraesophageal syndromes, with the latter including respiratory tract changes such as reflux cough syndrome, reflux laryngitis syndrome, asthma, wheezing, reflux dental erosion syndrome, pharyngitis, sinusitis, as well as irritability, failure to thrive, anemia, feeding refusal dystonic neck posturing (Sandifer syndrome), and other neurological symptoms that need an experienced gastroenterologist and a multidisciplinary team to carry out correct management [3].

Another challenge in pediatric gastrointestinal diseases is offered by eosinophilic esophagitis (EoE), an immune-mediated disease that produces esophageal dysfunction secondary to an increase in the eosinophil count, in the absence of other diseases, and needs histopathological confirmation (histology scoring system) [4,5]. EoE needs a correct diagnosis and an appropriate therapy to be selected to prevent complications [4], such as esophageal stenosis or perforation [6]. The treatment consists of proton pump inhibitors (PPIs), corticosteroids, and a dietary regimen (the elimination of foods) [4].

Of course, the most complex field that constantly transcends boundaries is represented by the *Helicobacter pylori* (*H. pylori*) infection—with high incidence in children, especially in teenagers—which is responsible for gastrointestinal complications (chronic active gastroenteritis, gastric and duodenal ulcers, gastric cancer), but which has also been incriminated as a key player in the development of extra-digestive conditions, including neurological, cardiac, metabolic, hematologic (immune thrombocytopenic purpura, anemia), ocular, and dermatological pathologies. The discovery of the modulatory effect of *H. pylori* upon the gut–brain axis and the gastric microenvironment suggested possible systemic effects of the infection [7,8]. Neurological manifestations include cognitive impairment, migraine, or Alzheimer's disease, which have been extensively studied, but without a clear pathophysiology of the process [9]. Nevertheless, *H. pylori* has been associated with a variety of innate as well as acquired autoimmune disorders [10].

Cystic fibrosis (CF), an autosomal recessive monogenic disease, is a multiorgan disorder affecting the respiratory tract, exocrine pancreas, intestine, hepatobiliary system, sweat glands, and myeloid cells [11,12]. It has a chronic, progressive, and potentially fatal course of development. The gene responsible for cystic fibrosis is the transmembrane conductance regulator (CFTR) protein, with multiple well-known and studied mutations, out of which F508del is the most frequent [11]. Although the respiratory symptoms dominate the clinical picture in CF, the gastrointestinal manifestations should be recognized and treated promptly as they can lead to exocrine pancreas involvement, distal intestinal obstruction syndrome (DIOS), and small intestinal bacterial overgrowth (SIBO), whose management is very important for the quality of life in patients with CF [11].

Some digestive chronic diseases, such as inflammatory bowel disease (IBD), can have an unpredictive evolution, and even become debilitating. The constant fatigability, short stature, growth delay, and delayed puberty that can accompany these conditions can impair an individual's mental and emotional wellbeing and place them at a higher risk for developing psychiatric conditions. Therefore, a quick diagnosis and a good management of these diseases can prevent psychiatric distress, which can later ensure prophylaxis of psychiatric disorders, later in adult life [13].

Several viruses with traditional tropism for the gastrointestinal mucosa have been regarded as major factors of gastroenteritis-associated morbidity and mortality, especially at a young age. Still, viral infections that usually cause respiratory tract infections can also determine digestive manifestations. Although the SARS-CoV-2 infection frequently produces respiratory symptoms, its Omicron variant poses 1.5-fold higher odds of determining loss of appetite in the infected individual and 1.6-fold more frequent digestive symptoms in infants between 7 and 9 months of age. Moreover, its frequent association with hepatic cytolysis has also been reported [14].

Through this Special Issue, we aimed to emphasize that multidisciplinarity and trandisciplinarity in pediatric gastrointestinal diseases are very useful for providing correct management of children affected by these diseases. The topics addressed within this collection of articles have covered the vast majority of pediatric digestive pathology and have included research articles, reviews, and clinical case reports. The articles were written by experts in their fields, with high expertise in clinical management of the disorders that involve crossing the borders between specialties. The published articles aided in providing a better understanding of the pathogenesis, outlined management controversies of pediatric gastrointestinal disorders, and enriched literature data. All these articles reflect the progress in the field and the future steps in pediatric gastroenterology should be undertaken. Editing this Special Issue was a great, delightful experience for me—a learning opportunity—and I hope for that it will prove similar for its audience.

Funding: This research received no external funding.

Institutional Review Board Statement: Not applicable.

Informed Consent Statement: Not applicable.

Conflicts of Interest: The author declares no conflicts of interest.

References

1. ESPGHAN Training Syllabus 2019 | ESPGHAN. Available online: http://www.espghan.org/knowledge-center/education/ESPGHAN_Training_Syllabus_2019 (accessed on 18 February 2024).
2. Paediatric Gastroenterology, Hepatology and Nutrition—Sub-Specialty. Available online: https://www.gmc-uk.org/-/media/documents/appendix-4i---pghan_pdf-86370658.pdf (accessed on 18 February 2024).
3. Rosen, R.; Vandenplas, Y.; Singendonk, M.; Cabana, M.; DiLorenzo, C.; Gottrand, F.; Gupta, S.; Langendam, M.; Staiano, A.; Thapar, N.; et al. Pediatric Gastroesophageal Reflux Clinical Practice Guidelines: Joint Recommendations of the North American Society for Pediatric Gastroenterology, Hepatology, and Nutrition and the European Society for Pediatric Gastroenterology, Hepatology, and Nutrition. *J. Pediatr. Gastroenterol. Nutr.* **2018**, *66*, 516–554. [CrossRef] [PubMed]
4. Dhar, A.; Haboubi, H.N.; Attwood, S.E.; Auth, M.K.H.; Dunn, J.M.; Sweis, R.; Morris, D.; Epstein, J.; Novelli, M.R.; Hunter, H.; et al. British Society of Gastroenterology (BSG) and British Society of Paediatric Gastroenterology, Hepatology and Nutrition (BSPGHAN) Joint Consensus Guidelines on the Diagnosis and Management of Eosinophilic Oesophagitis in Children and Adults. *Gut* **2022**, *71*, 1459–1487. [CrossRef] [PubMed]
5. Collins, M.H.; Martin, L.J.; Alexander, E.S.; Boyd, J.T.; Sheridan, R.; He, H.; Pentiuk, S.; Putnam, P.E.; Abonia, J.P.; Mukkada, V.A.; et al. Newly Developed and Validated Eosinophilic Esophagitis Histology Scoring System and Evidence That It Outperforms Peak Eosinophil Count for Disease Diagnosis and Monitoring. *Dis. Esophagus* **2017**, *30*, 1–8. [CrossRef] [PubMed]
6. Straumann, A.; Bussmann, C.; Zuber, M.; Vannini, S.; Simon, H.-U.; Schoepfer, A. Eosinophilic Esophagitis: Analysis of Food Impaction and Perforation in 251 Adolescent and Adult Patients. *Clin. Gastroenterol. Hepatol.* **2008**, *6*, 598–600. [CrossRef] [PubMed]
7. Baj, J.; Forma, A.; Sitarz, M.; Portincasa, P.; Garruti, G.; Krasowska, D.; Maciejewski, R. *Helicobacter Pylori* Virulence Factors-Mechanisms of Bacterial Pathogenicity in the Gastric Microenvironment. *Cells* **2020**, *10*, 27. [CrossRef] [PubMed]
8. Mayer, E.A.; Tillisch, K.; Bradesi, S. Review Article: Modulation of the Brain-Gut Axis as a Therapeutic Approach in Gastrointestinal Disease. *Aliment. Pharmacol. Ther.* **2006**, *24*, 919–933. [CrossRef] [PubMed]
9. Pellicano, R.; Ribaldone, D.G.; Fagoonee, S.; Astegiano, M.; Saracco, G.M.; Mégraud, F. A 2016 Panorama of Helicobacter Pylori Infection: Key Messages for Clinicians. *Panminerva Med.* **2016**, *58*, 304–317. [PubMed]
10. Wang, L.; Cao, Z.-M.; Zhang, L.-L.; Dai, X.; Liu, Z.; Zeng, Y.; Li, X.-Y.; Wu, Q.-J.; Lv, W. Helicobacter Pylori and Autoimmune Diseases: Involving Multiple Systems. *Front. Immunol.* **2022**, *13*, 833424. [CrossRef] [PubMed]
11. Fiorotto, R.; Strazzabosco, M. Pathophysiology of Cystic Fibrosis Liver Disease: A Channelopathy Leading to Alterations in Innate Immunity and in Microbiota. *Cell Mol. Gastroenterol. Hepatol.* **2019**, *8*, 197–207. [CrossRef] [PubMed]
12. Betapudi, B.; Aleem, A.; Kothadia, J.P. Cystic Fibrosis and Liver Disease. In *StatPearls*; StatPearls Publishing: Treasure Island, FL, USA, 2024.
13. Sălcudean, A.; Nan, A.G.; Bodo, C.R.; Cosma, M.C.; Strete, E.G.; Lica, M.M. Association between Childhood Onset Inflammatory Bowel Disease and Psychiatric Comorbidities in Adulthood. *Diagnostics* **2023**, *13*, 1868. [CrossRef] [PubMed]
14. Drăgănescu, A.C.; Miron, V.D.; Săndulescu, O.; Bilașco, A.; Streinu-Cercel, A.; Sandu, R.G.; Marinescu, A.; Gunșahin, D.; Hoffmann, K.I.; Horobeț, D.Ș.; et al. Omicron in Infants-Respiratory or Digestive Disease? *Diagnostics* **2023**, *13*, 421. [CrossRef] [PubMed]

Disclaimer/Publisher's Note: The statements, opinions and data contained in all publications are solely those of the individual author(s) and contributor(s) and not of MDPI and/or the editor(s). MDPI and/or the editor(s) disclaim responsibility for any injury to people or property resulting from any ideas, methods, instructions or products referred to in the content.

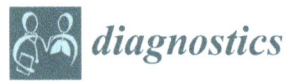

Article

Epidemiological Characteristics of *Helicobacter pylori* Infection in Children in Northeast Romania

Ancuta Lupu [1,†], Ingrith Crenguta Miron [1,†], Andrei Tudor Cernomaz [2,*], Cristina Gavrilovici [1,†], Vasile Valeriu Lupu [1,*], Iuliana Magdalena Starcea [1,*], Anca Lavinia Cianga [1,*], Bogdan Stana [1,†], Elena Tarca [3,†] and Silvia Fotea [4,†]

1 Pediatrics, "Grigore T. Popa" University of Medicine and Pharmacy, 700115 Iasi, Romania
2 3rd Medical Department, "Grigore T. Popa" University of Medicine and Pharmacy, 700115 Iasi, Romania
3 Pediatric Surgery, "Grigore T. Popa" University of Medicine and Pharmacy, 700115 Iasi, Romania
4 Medical Department, Faculty of Medicine and Pharmacy, "Dunarea de Jos" University of Galati, 800008 Galati, Romania
* Correspondence: a_cernomaz@yahoo.com (A.T.C.); valeriulupu@yahoo.com (V.V.L.); magdabirm@yahoo.com (I.M.S.); ancalaviniacianga@gmail.com (A.L.C.)
† These authors contributed equally to this work.

Abstract: (1) Background: Although gastritis has been associated with multiple etiologies, in pediatrics the main etiology is idiopathic. Many studies have reported mild-to-severe gastritis *Helicobacter pylori* (*H. pylori*) as an etiological factor. We evaluated the distribution of the infection with *H. pylori* by age, gender and place of living; (2) Methods: A retrospective study was conducted over a period of 3 years, over a cohort of 1757 patients of both sexes, aged between 1 and 18 years, admitted to a regional gastroenterology center in Iasi, Romania, with clinical signs of gastritis which underwent upper gastrointestinal endoscopy. The research was based on the analysis of data from patient observation charts and hospital discharge tickets, as well as endoscopy result registers; (3) Results: Out of the 1757 children, in 30.8% of cases the *H. pylori* infection was present. Out of them, 26.8% were males and 73.2% females. The average age of children with an *H. pylori* infection was higher (14.1 + 2.8 DS), compared with children without *H. pylori* (12.8 + 3.7 SD), an average difference of 1.3 years (95% confidence interval 0.96 to 1.66; $p < 0.001$). By place of living, children with *H. pylori* infection were from urban areas at 24.7% and from rural areas at 75.3%; (4) Conclusions: *H. pylori* infection incidence is still high in children, especially in teenagers, so extensive prevention and treatment programs are needed.

Keywords: gastritis; *H. pylori*; child; endoscopy; epidemiology

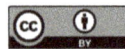

1. Introduction

Acute gastritis is a term that covers a wide spectrum of entities that induce inflammatory changes in the gastric mucosa. Some etiologies share the same general clinical presentation, but they differ histologically [1]. Some conditions (*Helicobacter pylori* (*H. pylori*), inflammatory bowel disease, allergic gastroenteritis) that injure the gastric mucosa can lead to inflammation. Thus, gastritis, as suggested by the suffix -itis, is characterized by the presence of inflammatory cells [2]. The inflammation of the gastric and/or duodenal mucosa is the end result of an imbalance between defensive and aggressive mucosal factors. The degree of inflammation and the presence of this imbalance may subsequently result in varying degrees of gastritis and/or ulceration of the mucosa [3].

Although gastritis has been associated with multiple etiologies, in pediatrics the main etiology is idiopathic. Many studies have reported mild-to-severe gastritis *H. pylori* as an etiological factor. [4].

H. pylori is a Gram-negative microaerophilic bacterium which colonizes the gastric mucosa generally in childhood and can determine chronic active gastritis, peptic ulcer disease, gastric cancer and mucosa-associated lymphoid tissue lymphoma later on during adulthood [5]. Its transmission route is still partially unclear, but the infections occur as a result of direct human-to-human transmission or environmental contamination [6]. The increased number of siblings, the education level of the parents, the water sources and garbage collection are also known to be representing important risk factors for the *H. pylori* infection among the pediatric population [7].

It is known that the rate of infection with *H. pylori* reaches a percentage of 50% of the total population and approximately one-third of all children around the world with a high prevalence in low-income countries and in the absence of sanitary conditions, the incidence of infection being severely influenced by the socioeconomic status [8]. In their review, Zabala et al. made an examination of the data from seven cohort studies and showed that the rate of the infection with *H. pylori* in healthy children under 5 years of age remained between 20% and 40% in high-income countries, whereas in the upper-middle income ones, the infection rates variated between 30% and 50%. These data suggest the importance of the country of birth concerning the prevalence of the infection [9]. Additionally, Venneman et al. found in their complex review that in Europe the *H. pylori* infection reached its highest rates in Eastern and Southern Europe which represent, as well, the regions with the highest stomach cancer incidence rates in the European Union [10]. Evidently, the clinical outcome of an *H. pylori* infection depends on multiple favorizing circumstances such as the virulence factors or the host gastric mucosal factors [11].

Clearly, the importance of an early diagnostic of the *H. pylori* infection is undeniable as it can prevent complications in adulthood and implicitly the apparition of gastric cancer [12].

In children, the guidelines recommend that the diagnosis of *H. pylori* infection be based on positive culture or gastritis with *H. pylori* on histopathology with at least one other positive test based on biopsy [13]. The authors of a recent study from Iraq regarding detection of *H. pylori* infection by invasive and non-invasive techniques in adults concluded markedly the role of real-time PCR as more sensitive and accurate than other diagnostic methods because it offers several advantages over culture [14].

Once diagnosed, an *H. pylori* infection has to be eradicated, but the efficacy of the regimen consisting of a standard triple therapy involving antibiotics as amoxicillin, clarithromycin and metronidazole along with a proton pump inhibitor seems to be decreasing lately due to *H. pylori*-resistant strains [15]. Thus, eradicating *H. pylori* infection is starting to become a challenge for all the pediatricians all around the world [16].

As for the epidemiological aspects of the treatment, the results of the EuroPed*HP* Registry 2013 to 2016 showed that the primary antibiotic resistance rates may vary significantly across the geographical regions and that they can also be correlated with the migrant status [17]. In the present study, we aimed to evaluate the cases' distribution based on sex, age and environmental sources of the *H. pylori* infection. Although its prevalence seems to decrease lately, *H. pylori* infection remains an important public health problem in Romania, and epidemiological studies on its impact among the pediatric population in our country are limited. We evaluated the data from a certain region of Romania, namely the northeast of the country, trying to identify the particularities of *H. pylori* infection among children in relation to their age, gender and environment of origin.

2. Materials and Methods

A retrospective study was carried out over a period of 3 years on a cohort of 1757 patients of both sexes, aged between 1 and 18 years, mainly hospitalized in the Gastroenterology Pediatric Clinic, but also in the other clinics of the Emergency Hospital for Children "St. Maria" in Iasi, Romania, with symptoms suggestive of gastritis or gastroduodenal ulcer such as upper abdominal pain, abdominal distension, dyspepsia, nausea or vomiting, in which superior digestive endoscopy (SDE) was performed. Some of them had a positive fecal *H. pylori* antigen in ambulatory. Our hospital is the only one in the northeast of

Romania where SDEs can be performed, so our results reflect the epidemiological situation of the pediatric population suffering from this disease in this area with great accuracy.

The main criterion for inclusion in the study was the definite diagnosis of the disease by performing SDE with biopsies taken from the gastric and/or duodenal mucosa. Intravenous sedation was given and standard upper gastrointestinal endoscopy, using the Olympus and Pentax video pediatric gastro-duodenoscopes, was performed to identify the macroscopic changes. General anesthesia in children aged below 10 years of age was used. We obtained 2 biopsies from the antrum, 2 biopsies from the corpus for the histopathological evaluation and 1 biopsy from antrum for the rapid urease test [18,19]. The gastritis was graded according to Houston-updated Sydney system: absent inflammation (Grade 0), mild inflammation (Grade 1), moderate inflammation (Grade 2) and severe inflammation (Grade 3).

During this period, 2042 SDEs were conducted, out of which we excluded 256 SDEs that were performed for verifying the response to therapy rather than for initial diagnosis purposes. Out of the 1786 children for which SDE was performed for diagnosis, we excluded another 29 children who did not have complete data in the observation files. The study was conducted on a final number of 1757 patients.

The research was based on the analysis of data from hospital discharge tickets, patient observation charts and endoscopy result registers. The data regarding the batch considered for the study were organized into a table structure containing a number of 90 category variables and 2 continuous variables. The processing of these data was performed using the SPSS 17.0 platform as well as Excel 2016 software. Chi Squared was calculated to asses association of independent values. Cox regression models adjusting for patient age, sex and area of origin were used characterize the relationship in pediatric patients with gastritis and the probability of testing HP-positive.

All patient's caregivers have given written informed consent and the "St. Mary" Children Emergency Hospital Ethics Committee's approval was obtained for publishing this study (31490/29 October 2021).

3. Results

We evaluated 1757 patients, out of which 1210 were females and 547 males, whereas 1114 of them originated from rural areas and 643 patients were from urban areas.

Of the 1757 children diagnosed in our study with various forms of gastritis and/or gastroduodenal ulcers, 542 of them (30.8%) had an associated *H. pylori* infection, while the other 1215 (69.2%) did not have the infection at the time of diagnosis. All 542 children were confirmed with *H. pylori* infection by endoscopy with biopsies, all of whom underwent rapid urease testing (RUT).

In the studied group, the average age of children who had an *H. pylori* infection was higher (14.1 ± 2.8 DS) than in those without an *H. pylori* infection (12.8 ± 3.7 DS) (Figures 1 and 2), the average difference being 1.3 years; confidence interval 95% 0.96–1.66; $p < 0.0001$ (Table 1).

In the studied batch, the female gender represented approximately two-thirds of the entire batch with a percentage of 68.9% (1210 female children), compared to one-third represented by the male gender with a percentage of 31.1% (547 children). The distribution of children with an *H. pylori* infection according to the gender variable revealed a frequency of 26.6% for boys and a frequency of 32.8% for girls (Figure 3). From the statistical analysis, it was concluded that there was a significant difference of this association (χ^2, $p = 0.009$) (Table 2). The possibility for females displaying gastritis with *H. pylori* is 1.34 times higher as compared to males (OR = 1.34).

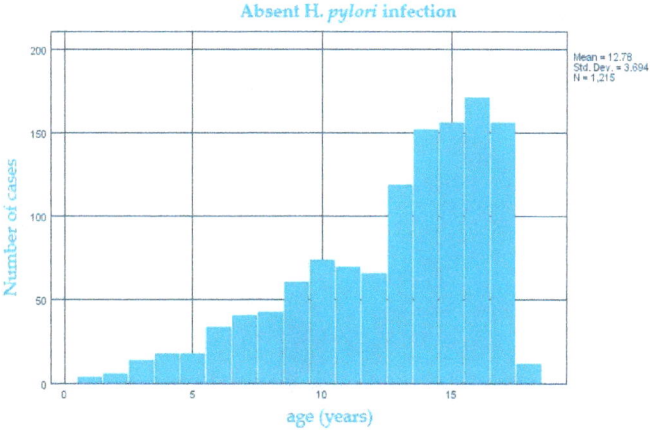

Figure 1. Structure of the group of patients without *H. pylori* infection by age (years).

Table 1. Average age of diagnosis of infection with *H. pylori*.

Age (Years)	Frequency Total	H. pylori Negative	H. pylori Positive	Pearson Chi Square	Likelihood Ratio	p Value
1	4 (0.2%)	4 (100%)	0			
2	6 (0.3%)	6 (100%)	0			
3	14 (0.8%)	14 (100%)	0			
4	22 (1.3%)	18 (81.8%)	4 (18.2%)			
5	23 (1.3%)	18 (78.3%)	5 (21.7%)			
6	39 (2.2%)	34 (87.2%)	5 (12.8%)			
7	49 (2.8%)	41 (83.7%)	8 (16.3%)			
8	49 (2.8%)	43 (87.8%)	6 (12.2%)			
9	74 (4.2%)	61 (82.4%)	13 (17.6%)	61.7	72.33	$p < 0.0001$
10	93 (5.3%)	74 (79.6%)	19 (20.4%)			
11	100 (5.7%)	70 (70%)	30 (30%)			
12	97 (5.5%)	66 (68%)	31 (32%)			
13	181 (10.3%)	119 (65.7%)	62 (34.3%)			
14	217 (12.4%)	152 (70%)	65 (30%)			
15	238 (13.5%)	157 (66%)	81 (34%)			
16	273 (15.5%)	171 (62.6%)	102 (37.4%)			
17	260 (14.8%)	152 (59.6%)	105 (40.4%)			
18	18 (1%)	12 (66.7%)	6 (33.3%)			
Total	1757 (100%)	1215 (69.2%)	542 (30.8%)			

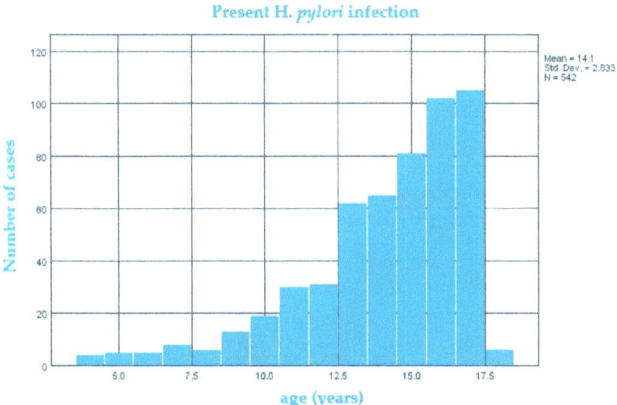

Figure 2. Structure of the group of patients with *H. pylori* infection by age (years).

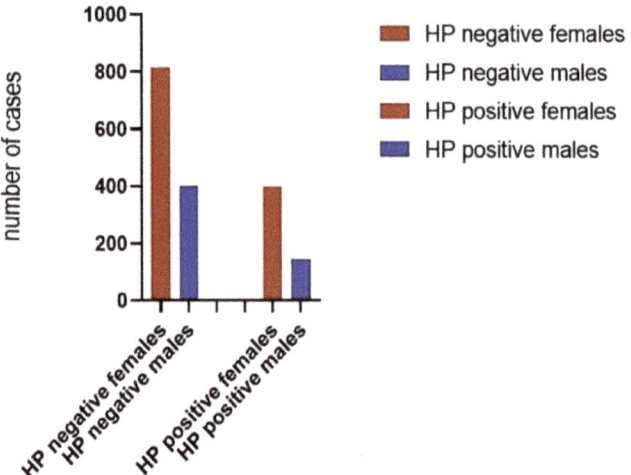

Figure 3. Structure of the batch of patients with or without *H. pylori* infection by gender.

Table 2. Estimated parameters in testing the association between *H. pylori* infection and the gender variable.

	Female	Male	Pearson Chi Square	Likelihood Ratio	*p* Value
HP positive	397 (32.81%)	145 (26.51%)			
HP negative	813 (67.19%)	402 (73.49%)	7.01	7.13	$p = 0.008$
Total	1210 (100%)	547 (100%)			

The first column represents females with *H. pylori* infection (32.81%) and without *H. pylori* infection (67.19%). The second column describes males with HP infection (26.51%) and without HP infection (73.49%). Chi Squared test of independence was performed and showed there was significant association between gender and *H. pylori* infection ($\chi^2 = 7.01$, $p = 0.008$).

We also evaluated the distribution of the *H. pylori* infection according to age within both genders and we noticed that the number of cases increases along with the median age of 13.6 years for females compared to 12.2 years for males, the average difference being 1.4 years. (Figures 4 and 5)

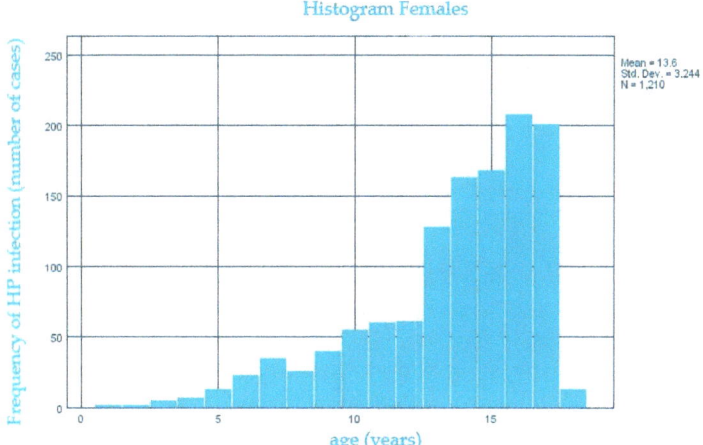

Figure 4. Distribution of *H. pylori* infection (number of cases) according to age (years) in females.

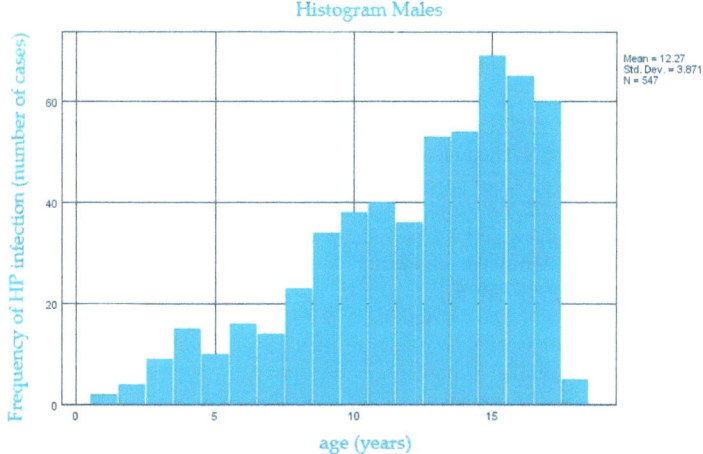

Figure 5. Distribution of *H. pylori* infection (number of cases) according to age (years) in males.

A direct comparison between the median age of debut of the *Helicobacter pylori* infection for males and females demonstrates similarities between both genders (Figure 6).

According to patients' backgrounds, out of the total number of 1757 patients, we observed that 1114 of them (63.4%) originated from the rural areas, whereas 643 of them originated from urban areas with a percentage of 36.6%. (Table 3). From the statistical analysis, it was concluded that there was a powerfully significant difference of this association (χ^2; $p < 0.0001$) (Table 3). The presence of gastritis with *H. pylori* in patients from rural environments is 2.2 times higher than in patients from urban environments (OR = 2.2).

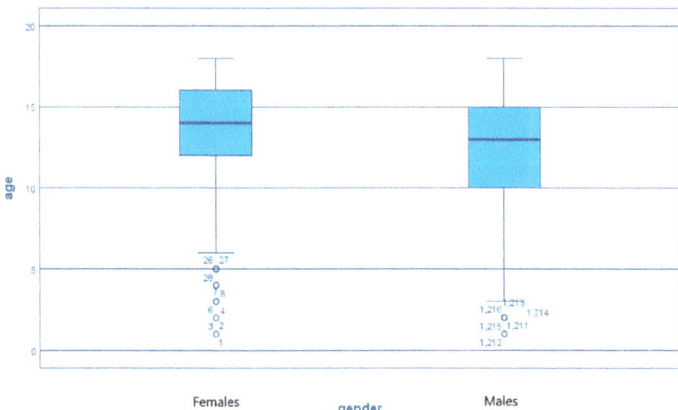

Figure 6. The distribution of age (years) within gender variables in *H. pylori* infection.

Table 3. Estimated parameters in testing the association between *H. pylori* infection and the origin variable.

	Rural (Number/Percentage)	Urban (Number/Percentage)	Pearson Chi Square	Likelihood Ratio	*p* Value
HP positive	408 (36.6%)	134 (20.8%)			
HP negative	706 (63.4%)	509 (79.2%)	47.62	49.38	$p < 0.0001$
Total	1114 (100%)	643 (100%)			

The first column represents patients originating from rural environment with *H. pylori* infection (36.6%) and without *H. pylori* infection (63.4%). The second column describes children originating from the urban areas with HP infection (20.8%) and without HP infection (79.2%). Chi Squared test of independence was performed and showed there was significant association between environment of origin and *H. pylori* infection (χ^2 = 47.62, p = 0.0001).

The distribution of children with an *H. pylori* infection according to the origin variable showed a frequency of 24.7% in the urban environment and a frequency of 75.3% in the rural environment (Figure 7).

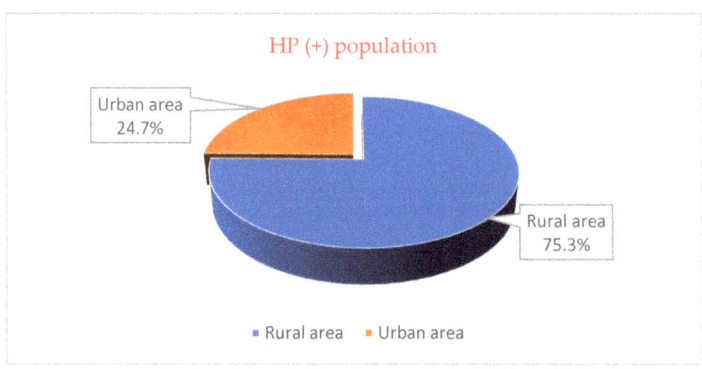

Figure 7. The structure of the group of patients according to the place of living for *H. pylori* present.

Logistic regression was used to characterize the relationship between age, gender and living conditions (stratified as urban/rural area) for pediatric gastritis patients and the probability of testing *H. pylori*-positive. The most parsimonious model included only age; the results from the model indicate an increased risk of *H. pylori* infection mirroring the aging process. A more complex model included age and living conditions with a similar log likelihood ratio suggesting an increased risk of *H. pylori* infection associated with rural living conditions—odds ratio ~2. A summary of the logistic regression results is shown in Table 4. Adding gender to a third model was considered but the result was not statistically significant ($p = 0.34$) (Wald).

Table 4. Logistic regression model including age, living conditions and *H. pylori* infection status for pediatric patient with gastritis.

	B	S.E.	Wald	df	Sig.	OR	95% CI for OR	
							Lower	Upper
Age (years)	0.11	0.02	44.25	1	0.000	1.12	1.08	1.16
Urban area			39.05	1	0.000			
Rural area	0.73	0.12	39.05	1	0.000	2.08	1.65	2.61
Constant	−2.84	.25	126.09	1	0.000	0.06		

B = beta coefficient; S.E. = standard error; df = degrees of freedom; Sig. = statistical significance; OR = odds ratio; CI = confidence interval.

4. Discussion

The results of our analysis confirm that almost one-third of the children enrolled in the study have a *H. pylori* infection but unfortunately, in the Romanian medical literature the data regarding this subject are not updated and comparisons are difficult to be made within our country's territory. However, at the national level, the prevalence of *H. pylori* infection seems to be decreasing lately.

Usually, an *H. pylori* infection is acquired during childhood and persists as chronic gastritis if the organism is not eradicated. With the progress of gastritis over the years, the gastric mucosa undergoes a series of changes that can lead to glandular atrophy, intestinal metaplasia and with increased risk of gastric dysplasia and carcinoma [1,20,21]. On the other hand, a recent study conducted in China identified an inverse relationship between *H. pylori* and asthma, indicating that this infection may represent a protective factor for asthma (OR 1.887–2.008, $p < 0.05$) [22]. This affirmation is supported by the results of a meta-analysis by Chen et al. who observed the same inverse association between the CagA(+) strains of *H. pylori* and the risk of childhood asthma (OR = 0.58; CI, 0.35–0.96, $p = 0.034$) [23].

In the United States, the prevalence of gastritis with *H. pylori* in children appears to be age-dependent. Below the age of 5, few cases are reported but prevalence increases with age, becoming the most common cause of gastritis in adolescents [1,2,24].

The authors of a recent systematic review and meta-analysis regarding global prevalence of pediatric *H. pylori* infection reported that this was present in 32.3% of children and it was higher in low-income and middle-income countries than in high-income countries (43.2% vs. 21.7%). Additionally, the prevalence of infection was higher in older children than in younger ones (41.6% in 13–18-year-olds; 33.9% in 7–12-year-olds; 26.0% in 0–6-year-olds). *H. pylori* infection in children was associated with lower economic status, more children, room sharing, no access to a sewage system, having parents infected with *H. pylori*, drinking non-treated water and adolescents [25].

It has been suggested that gastric pathology (gastritis and ulcer) has become more prevalent in Western countries in the nineteenth century due to a change in the epidemiology of the *H. pylori* infection [24]. Starting from this hypothesis, from environmental changes (which can cause changes in the gastritis pattern) and from current nutrition, we have studied some aspects of gastritis and ulcers in children.

The gastric pathology associated with *H. pylori* infection was more common among adolescents, with 17-year-olds registering the highest frequency with an average age of 14.1 ± 2.8 DS. This distribution could be explained by adolescents' diet consisting of fast food, carbonated juices, alcohol and coffee, which can exacerbate the symptoms of gastritis with *H. pylori* [25,26]. Their better compliance with digestive endoscopy with the possibility of clear diagnosis could also contribute to the deviation of the frequency to the adult age. There are studies that reported spontaneous elimination of the infection with age, thus explaining the lower prevalence of infection at age 10 [27]. Some authors also argue that the lower prevalence of infection in adolescence age could be explained by an increased attention to health problems in this age group and the use of antibiotics for other infectious diseases [28,29]. In our case, we cannot support these hypotheses, as the prevalence of infection increased in relation to age. The low prevalence at the age of 18 cannot be taken into account, given the lower number of children we have examined, since at this age most patients with similar symptoms resorted to adult gastroenterology exams.

In our study, the female sex was affected in 68.9% of cases (1210 girls out of a total of 1757) and 32.8% had the bacteria present. This may result from the fact that girls give more importance to the symptoms they have, thus increasing the addressability to the doctor. In contrast with our results, Ibrahim et al. show in their meta-analysis that the *H. pylori* infection was more frequent in males than in females (102 studies, OR = 1.06, 95%CI: 1.01, 1.12, I^2 = 43.7%) [30]. Other studies did not find statistical differences between females and males [31–33].

According to the place of living, our statistical analysis showed that there is a higher prevalence of *H. pylori* infection among the children originating from the rural environments with a percentage of 63.35% in northeast Romania. Our data are in agreement with the results obtained by Melit et al. in their study conducted on 137 patients from Romania where the *H. pylori* infection rate was more important in the rural environment than in the urban areas ($p = 0.0089$) [34]. However, our results are not entirely consistent with a similar analysis made recently in a center in the northwest part of Romania which proved that there were no statistically significant differences between the prevalence of *H. pylori* infection in the rural areas (42.29%) versus the urban environment (39.75%) ($p = 0.6$) [35].

The higher frequency of infection in the rural environment could be explained by the lower socio-economic level and by the larger families in this environment, which promotes the spread of the bacterium. Several studies have reported a higher prevalence of the infection in large families [36,37].

More than 50% of the world's population is infected with *H. pylori*, which is almost always acquired in the first 5 years of life [38]. In developed countries, the prevalence varies between 1.2% and 12.2% [39,40]. In developing countries, the prevalence is higher. In Indian children, the prevalence of *H. pylori* infection was reported to be 45% [41]. In Bolivia, seroprevalence at age 9 was 70% and in Alaska 69% [40,41].

In Romania, the authors of a retrospective study conducted in Cluj-Napoca, on 194 children, reported the general prevalence of *H. pylori* infection as 36.6% [42]. In another study in Romania, in Targu Mures, conducted on 1041 children aged from 2 to 18 years, the prevalence was similar, of 33.05% [43].

In our study, we found a prevalence of *H. pylori* infection of 30.85%, similar to that reported in the other Romanian studies. The prevalence of the bacteria was roughly the same over the three years of study.

Initially, the specific guidelines for eradicating *H. pylori* infection were limited to peptic ulcer, but in 1997, the "Digestive Health Initiative" (DHI) during the "International Update Conference on *H. pylori*" extended the recommendations for testing and treating *H. pylori* [44]. Thus, the recommendations for *H. pylori* treatment are as follows: in the presence of *H. pylori*-associated peptic ulcer, treating *H. pylori* infection in the absence of peptic ulcer in children with dyspeptic symptoms may be considered, a "test and treat" strategy is not recommended in children based on non-invasive methods, in children infected with *H. pylori* who have a first-degree relative with gastric cancer, treatment may be recommended and the monitoring of antibiotic resistance rates of *H. pylori* strains in children and adolescents is recommended in different countries and geographical areas [45].

For the diagnosis, we performed SDE with biopsies taken from the gastric and/or duodenal mucosa such as in the recommendation of the new guidelines. The guidelines recommended that the initial diagnosis of *H. pylori* infection should not be based on noninvasive tests. A positive bacterial culture or *H. pylori* gastritis on histopathology with at least one other positive test such as rapid urease test, or molecular-based assays (polymerase chain reaction or fluorescent in situ hybridization) are necessary [13].

H. pylori has been shown to be highly resistant to clarithromycin in both children and adults, which is why studies at all ages recommend testing for antimicrobial susceptibility in *H. pylori* using molecular biopsy-based techniques, such as real-time PCR [13,46]. In our center, this test is not available and we considered it a limitation for our study. This is added to the unavailable laboratory investigations due to the fluctuation of existing funds (the study of vacA and cagA strains of *H. pylori*, the analysis of *H. pylori* antigen from fecal samples throughout the study period) and the impossibility of long-term follow-up of patients due to their very large number, but also to the lack of cooperation on their part.

5. Conclusions

The infection rate with *H. pylori* is still high in children, especially in teenagers, so extensive prevention and treatment programs are needed. An early diagnosis can significantly minimize complications during adulthood and, undoubtedly, can present an important impact on the socio-economic status in Romania.

Author Contributions: Conceptualization, A.L. and V.V.L.; methodology, I.C.M. and E.T.; software, A.T.C.; formal analysis, A.T.C. and B.S.; investigation, A.L., A.L.C. and V.V.L.; data curation, A.T.C.; writing—original draft preparation, A.L., A.L.C., I.M.S. and V.V.L.; writing—review and editing, I.C.M., E.T., A.T.C., C.G., B.S. and S.F.; visualization, I.M.S. and B.S.; supervision, I.C.M. and C.G.; project administration, S.F. All authors have read and agreed to the published version of the manuscript.

Funding: This research received no external funding.

Institutional Review Board Statement: The study was conducted in accordance with the Declaration of Helsinki and approved by the Ethics Committee of the "St. Mary" Children Emergency Hospital, Iasi, Romania (31490/29 October 2021).

Informed Consent Statement: Informed consent was obtained from all subjects involved in the study.

Data Availability Statement: The data presented in this study are available on request from the corresponding author.

Conflicts of Interest: The authors declare no conflict of interest.

References

1. Sarah El-Nakeep, B.S. Anand Acute Gastritis. Medscape 2021. Available online: https://emedicine.medscape.com/article/175909-overview?reg=1 (accessed on 30 August 2022).
2. Dohil, R.D.; Hassall, E.; Jevon, G.; Dimmick, J. Gastritis and Gastropathy of Childhood. *J. Pediatr. Gastroenterol. Nutr.* **1999**, *29*, 378–394. [CrossRef]
3. Blecker, U.; Mehta, D.I.; Gold, B.D. Pediatric gastritis and peptic ulcer disease. *Indian J. Pediatr.* **1999**, *66*, 725–733. [CrossRef] [PubMed]
4. Gold, B.D.; Colletti, R.B.; Abbott, M.; Czinn, S.J.; Elitsur, Y.; Hassall, E.; Macarthur, C.; Snyder, J.; Sherman, P.M. Medical position statement: The north American society for pediatric gastroenterology and nutrition: *Helicobacter pylori* infection in children: Recommendations for diagnosis and treatment. *J. Pediatr. Gastroenterol. Nutr.* **2000**, *31*, 490–497. [CrossRef] [PubMed]
5. Malfertheiner, P.; Megraud, F.; O'Morain, C.A.; Gisbert, J.P.; Kuipers, E.J.; Axon, A.T.; Bazzoli, F.; Gasbarrini, A.; Atherton, J.; Graham, D.Y.; et al. European Helicobacter and Microbiota Study Group and Consensus panel. Management of *Helicobacter pylori* infection-the Maastricht V/Florence Consensus Report. *Gut* **2017**, *66*, 6–30. [CrossRef] [PubMed]
6. Rothenbacher, D.; Bode, G.; Berg, G.; Knayer, U.; Gonser, T.; Adler, G.; Brenner, H. *Helicobacter Pylori* among preschool children and their parents: Evidence of parent-child transmission. *J. Infect. Dis.* **1999**, *179*, 398–402. [CrossRef]

7. Jafri, W.; Yakoob, J.; Abid, S.; Siddiqui, S.; Awan, S.; Nizami, S.Q. Helicobacter pylori infection in children: Population-based age specific prevalence and risk factors in a developing country. *Acta Paediatr.* **2010**, *99*, 279–282.
8. Okuda, M.; Lin, Y.; Kikuchi, S. Helicobacter pylori Infection in Children and Adolescents. *Adv. Exp. Med. Biol.* **2019**, *1149*, 107–120.
9. Zabala Torrres, B.; Lucero, Y.; Lagomarcino, A.J.; Orellana-Manzano, A.; George, S.; Torres, J.P.; O'Ryan, M. Review: Prevalence and dynamics of Helicobacter pylori infection during childhood. *Helicobacter* **2017**, *22*, e12399. [CrossRef]
10. Venneman, K.; Huybrechts, I.; Gunter, M.J.; Vandendaele, L.; Herrero, R.; Van Herck, K. The epidemiology of Helicobacter pylori infection in Europe and the impact of lifestyle on its natural evolution toward stomach cancer after infection: A systematic review. *Helicobacter* **2018**, *23*, e12483. [CrossRef]
11. Sgouros, S.N.; Bergele, C. Clinical outcome of patients with Helicobacter pylori infection: The bug, the host, or the environment? *Postgrad. Med. J.* **2006**, *82*, 338–342. [CrossRef]
12. Mărginean, C.O.; Meliț, L.E.; Săsăran, M.O. Traditional and Modern Diagnostic Approaches in Diagnosing Pediatric Helicobacter pylori Infection. *Children* **2022**, *9*, 994. [CrossRef] [PubMed]
13. Jones, N.L.; Koletzko, S.; Goodman, K.; Bontems, P.; Cadranel, S.; Casswall, T.; Czinn, S.; Gold, B.D.; Guarner, J.; Elitsur, Y.; et al. Joint ESPGHAN/NASPGHAN Guidelines for the Management of Helicobacter pylori in Children and Adolescents (Update 2016). *J. Pediatr. Gastroenterol. Nutr.* **2017**, *64*, 991–1003. [CrossRef] [PubMed]
14. Hussein, R.A.; Al-Ouqaili, M.T.S.; Majeed, Y.H. Detection of Helicobacter Pylori infection by invasive and non-invasive techniques in patients with gastrointestinal diseases from Iraq: A validation study. *PLoS ONE* **2021**, *16*, e0256393. [CrossRef]
15. Agudo, S.; Alarcón, T.; Urruzuno, P.; Martínez, M.J.; López-Brea, M. Detection of Helicobacter pylori and Clarithro-mycin Resistance in Gastric Biopsies of Pediatric Patients by Using a Commercially Available Real-Time Polymerase Chain Reaction after NucliSens Semiautomated DNA Extraction. *Diagn. Microbiol. Infect. Dis.* **2010**, *67*, 213–219. [CrossRef] [PubMed]
16. Meliț, L.E.; Mărginean, C.O.; Săsăran, M.O. The Challenges of Eradicating Pediatric Helicobacter Pylori Infection in the Era of Probiotics. *Children* **2022**, *9*, 795. [CrossRef] [PubMed]
17. Kori, M.; Le Thi, T.G.; Werkstetter, K.; Sustmann, A.; Bontems, P.; Lopes, A.I.; Oleastro, M.; Iwanczak, B.; Kalach, N.; Misak, Z.; et al. Helicobacter pylori Infection in Pediatric Patients Living in Europe: Results of the EuroPedHP Registry 2013 to 2016. *J. Pediatr. Gastroenterol. Nutr.* **2020**, *71*, 476–483. [CrossRef] [PubMed]
18. Lupu, A.; Miron, I.C.; Cianga, A.L.; Cernomaz, A.T.; Lupu, V.V.; Munteanu, D.; Ghica, D.C.; Fotea, S. The Relationship between Anemia and Helicobacter Pylori Infection in Children. *Children* **2022**, *9*, 1324. [CrossRef] [PubMed]
19. Lupu, A.; Miron, I.C.; Cianga, A.L.; Cernomaz, A.T.; Lupu, V.V.; Gavrilovici, C.; Stârcea, I.M.; Tarca, E.; Ghica, D.C.; Fotea, S. The Prevalence of Liver Cytolysis in Children with Helicobacter pylori Infection. *Children* **2022**, *9*, 1498. [CrossRef]
20. Uemura, N.; Okamoto, S.; Yamamoto, S.; Matsumura, N.; Yamaguchi, S.; Yamakido, M.; Taniyama, K.; Sasaki, N.; Schlemper, R.J. Helicobacter pylori infection and the development of gastric cancer. *N. Engl. J. Med.* **2001**, *345*, 784–789. [CrossRef]
21. Asaka, M.; Sugiyama, T.; Nobuta, A.; Kato, M.; Takeda, H.; Graham, D.Y. Atrophic gastritis and intestinal metaplasia in Japan: Results of a large multicenter study. *Helicobacter* **2001**, *6*, 294–299. [CrossRef]
22. Wang, D.; Chen, Y.; Ding, Y.; Tu, J. Inverse association between Helicobacter pylori infection and childhood asthma in a physical examination population: A cross-sectional study in Chongqing, China. *BMC Pediatr.* **2022**, *22*, 615. [CrossRef] [PubMed]
23. Chen, Y.; Zhan, X.; Wang, D. Association between Helicobacter pylori and risk of childhood asthma: A meta-analysis of 18 observational studies. *J. Asthma* **2022**, *59*, 890–900. [CrossRef] [PubMed]
24. Snyder, J.D.; Hard, S.C.; Thorne, G.M.; Hirsch, B.Z.; Antonioli, D.A. Primary antral gastritis in young American children. Low prevalence of Helicobacter pylori infections. *Dig. Dis. Sci.* **1994**, *39*, 1859–1863. [CrossRef] [PubMed]
25. Yuan, C.; Adeloye, D.; Luk, T.T.; Huang, L.; He, Y.; Xu, Y.; Ye, X.; Yi, Q.; Song, P.; Rudan, I.; et al. The global prevalence of and factors associated with Helicobacter pylori infection in children: A systematic review and meta-analysis. *Lancet Child Adolesc. Health* **2022**, *6*, 185–194. [CrossRef] [PubMed]
26. Drăgan, F.; Lupu, V.V.; Pallag, A.; Barz, C.; Fodor, K. Rational consumption of nutrients at school-aged children. *IOP Conf. Ser. Mater. Sci. Eng.* **2017**, *200*, 012063. [CrossRef]
27. Rothenbacher, D.; Bode, G.; Brenner, H. Dynamics of Helicobacter pylori infection in early childhood in a high-risk group living in Germany: Loss of infection higher than acquisition. *Aliment. Pharmacol. Ther.* **2002**, *16*, 1663–1668. [CrossRef]
28. Hestvik, E.; Tylleskar, T.; Kaddu-Mulindwa, D.H.; Ndeezi, G.; Grahnquist, L.; Olafsdottir, E.; Tumwine, J.K. Helicobacter pylori in apparently healthy children aged 0-12 years in urban Kampala, Uganda: A community-based cross-sectional survey. *BMC Gastroenterol.* **2010**, *10*, 62. [CrossRef]
29. Broussard, C.S.; Goodman, K.J.; Phillips, C.V.; Smith, M.A.; Fischbach, L.A.; Day, R.S.; Aragaki, C.C. Antibiotics taken for other illnesses and spontaneous clearance of Helicobacter pylori infection in children. *Pharmacoepidemiol. Drug Saf.* **2009**, *18*, 722–729. [CrossRef]
30. Ibrahim, A.; Morais, S.; Ferro, A.; Lunet, N.; Peleteiro, B. Sex-differences in the prevalence of Helicobacter pylori infection in pediatric and adult populations: Systematic review and meta-analysis of 244 studies. *Dig. Liver Dis.* **2017**, *49*, 742–749. [CrossRef]
31. Torres, J.; Pérez-Pérez, G.; Goodman, K.J.; Atherton, J.C.; Gold, B.D.; Harris, P.R.; Madrazo-de la Garza, A.; Guarner, J.; Muñoz, O. A comprehensive review of the natural history of Helicobacter pylori infection in children. *Arch. Med. Res.* **2000**, *31*, 431–469. [CrossRef]

32. Malaty, H.M.; El-Kasabany, A.; Graham, D.Y.; Miller, C.C.; Reddy, S.G.; Srinivasan, S.R.; Yamaoka, Y.; Berenson, G.S. Age at acquisition of *Helicobacter pylori* infection: A follow-up study from infancy to adulthood. *Lancet* **2002**, *359*, 931–935. [CrossRef] [PubMed]
33. Soltani, J.; Amirzadeh, J.; Nahedi, S.; Shahsavari, S. Prevalence of *Helicobacter Pylori* Infection in Children, a Population-Based Cross-Sectional Study in West Iran. *Iran J. Pediatr.* **2013**, *23*, 13–18.
34. Meliț, L.E.; Mărginean, M.O.; Mocan, S.; Mărginean, C.O. The Usefulness of Inflammatory Biomarkers in Diagnosing Child and Adolescent's Gastritis: STROBE Compliant Article. *Medicine* **2019**, *98*, e16188. [CrossRef] [PubMed]
35. Corojan, A.L.; Dumitrașcu, D.L.; Ciobanca, P.; Leucuta, D.C. Prevalence of *Helicobacter pylori* infection among dyspeptic patients in Northwestern Romania: A decreasing epidemiological trend in the last 30 years. *Exp. Ther. Med.* **2020**, *20*, 3488–3492. [CrossRef]
36. Santos, I.S.; Boccio, J.; Santos, A.S.; Valle, N.C.; Halal, C.S.; Bachilli, M.C.; Lopes, R.D. Prevalence of *Helicobacter pylori* infection and associated factors among adults in Southern Brazil: A population-based cross-sectional study. *BMC Public Health* **2005**, *5*, 118. [CrossRef]
37. Ueda, M.; Kikuchi, S.; Kasugai, T.; Shunichi, T.; Miyake, C. *Helicobacter pylori* risk associated with childhood home environment. *Cancer Sci.* **2003**, *94*, 914–918. [CrossRef] [PubMed]
38. Suerbaum, S.; Michetti, P. *Helicobacter pylori* infection. *N. Engl. Med.* **2002**, *347*, 1175–1186. [CrossRef]
39. Mourad-Baars, P.E.; Verspaget, H.W.; Mertens, B.J.; Luisa Merain, M. Low prevalence of *Helicobacter pylori* infection in young children in the Netherlands. *Eur. J. Gastroenterol. Hepatol.* **2007**, *19*, 213–216. [CrossRef] [PubMed]
40. Rajindrajith, S.; Devanarayana, N.M.; de Silva, H.J. *Helicobacter Pylori* Infection in Children. *Saudi J. Gastroenterol.* **2009**, *15*, 86–94. [CrossRef]
41. Gold, B.J. *Helicobacter pylori* infection in children. *Curr. Prob. Pediatr.* **2001**, *31*, 247–266. [CrossRef]
42. Slăvescu, K.C.; Șarban, C.; Pîrvan, A.; Gheban, D.; Mărgescu, C.; Miu, N. Prevalența infecției cu *Helicobacter pylori* la copiii cu gastrită și ulcer gastro-duodenal în nord-vestul și centrul României. *Clujul Med.* **2012**, *85*, 456–461.
43. Mărginean, O.; Pitea, A.M.; Brînzaniuc, K. *Helicobacter pylori* Gastritis in Children—Assessment of Resistance to Treatment on the Casuistry of the Ist Pediatric Clinic Tîrgu Mures. *AMM* **2015**, *21*, 487–490.
44. Akiva, J.M.; Anand, B.S. Chronic Gastritis Treatment & Management. Medscape 2019/176156. Available online: https://emedicine.medscape.com/article/176156-treatmentlast (accessed on 30 August 2022).
45. Kalach, N.; Bontems, P.; Cadranel, S. Advances in the treatment of *Helicobacter pylori* infection in children. *Ann. Gastroenterol.* **2015**, *28*, 10–18. [PubMed]
46. Hussein, R.A.; Al-Ouqaili, M.T.S.; Majeed, Y.H. Detection of clarithromycin resistance and 23SrRNA point mutations in clinical isolates of *Helicobacter pylori* isolates: Phenotypic and molecular methods. *Saudi J. Biol. Sci.* **2022**, *29*, 513–520. [CrossRef]

Disclaimer/Publisher's Note: The statements, opinions and data contained in all publications are solely those of the individual author(s) and contributor(s) and not of MDPI and/or the editor(s). MDPI and/or the editor(s) disclaim responsibility for any injury to people or property resulting from any ideas, methods, instructions or products referred to in the content.

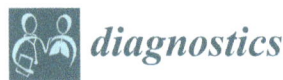

Review

Impact of *Helicobacter pylori* Infection upon the Evolution and Outcome of Pediatric Immune Thrombocytopenic Purpura: A Comprehensive Review

Maria Oana Săsăran [1], Cristina Oana Mărginean [2,*] and Ana Maria Koller [3]

1. Department of Pediatrics 3, University of Medicine, Pharmacy, Sciences and Technology George Emil Palade from Târgu Mureș, Gheorghe Marinescu Street No. 38, 540136 Târgu Mureș, Romania; oanam93@yahoo.com
2. Department of Pediatrics 1, University of Medicine, Pharmacy, Sciences and Technology George Emil Palade from Târgu Mureș, Gheorghe Marinescu Street No. 38, 540136 Târgu Mureș, Romania
3. Clinics of Pediatrics, Emergency County Clinical Hospital, Gheorghe Marinescu Street No. 50, 540136 Târgu Mureș, Romania; kolleranamaria@gmail.com
* Correspondence: marginean.oana@gmail.com

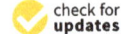

Citation: Săsăran, M.O.; Mărginean, C.O.; Koller, A.M. Impact of *Helicobacter pylori* Infection upon the Evolution and Outcome of Pediatric Immune Thrombocytopenic Purpura: A Comprehensive Review. *Diagnostics* **2023**, *13*, 3205. https://doi.org/10.3390/diagnostics13203205

Academic Editor: Paolo Aseni

Received: 24 August 2023
Revised: 8 October 2023
Accepted: 12 October 2023
Published: 13 October 2023

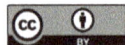

Copyright: © 2023 by the authors. Licensee MDPI, Basel, Switzerland. This article is an open access article distributed under the terms and conditions of the Creative Commons Attribution (CC BY) license (https://creativecommons.org/licenses/by/4.0/).

Abstract: In adults with immune thrombocytopenic purpura (ITP), the identification of *H. pylori* infection and its subsequent eradication proved to aid platelet recovery. Similar findings, at a smaller scale, were allegedly reported by some pediatric studies. This review's objective was to establish the influence of *H. pylori* infection and its eradication upon platelet count and recovery in pediatric ITP. Three databases, namely Pubmed, Scopus and Web of Science, were searched for pediatric studies which investigated a link between *H. pylori* infection and thrombocytopenia. The search results retrieved a number of 21 articles which complied to the inclusion and exclusion criteria. Some studies report lower platelet values among children with ITP and documented *H. pylori* infection, as well as an improve in platelet numbers after *H. pylori* treatment. However, results are controversial, as multiple authors failed to identify a higher prevalence of *H. pylori* among children with ITP or a lack of significant change in therapeutic outcome with the addition of an eradication regimen to standard treatment. The main limitations of current pediatric studies remain the small study samples and the short follow-up periods of the included subjects. Hence, the long-term impact of *H. pylori* in children with ITP is still uncertain.

Keywords: *Helicobacter pylori* infection; immune thrombocytopenic purpura; children

1. Introduction

Immune thrombocytopenic purpura (ITP) is defined as an isolated, transitory or persistent decrease in platelet count, under a diagnostic threshold of 100×10^9/L, mediated by an immune process. The term, "immune", is nowadays preferred to the old "idiopathic" label, in order to highlight a disorder of the immune system characterized by the coating of platelets with autoantibodies that act against platelet membrane antigens and inhibit megakaryocyte function [1,2]. Immunoglobulin G (IgG) antibodies bind to platelet membrane glycoproteins, which leads to the sequestration and phagocytosis of platelets within the spleen and can simultaneously impair platelet production [3,4]. The absence of a known cause or other underlying disorders responsible for the autoimmune thrombocytopenia suggests a diagnosis of primary ITP, whereas secondary ITP refers to each type of immune-mediated thrombocytopenia with the exception of primary ITP [2].

The result is a decrease in platelet numbers, which, depending on its severity, can lead to cutaneous hemorrhages such as petechiae and ecchymoses, mucosal bleedings including epistaxis or genito-urinary hemorrhages [5]. Severe bleeding complications, such as intracranial hemorrhage, occur with a general frequency of 1/800 at pediatric ages, in both newly onset and chronic ITP forms and are the main cause of long-term morbidity and mortality [5,6]. In spite of the potential severe outcome of ITP, which prompts for early recognition of the disease, its diagnosis still remains a challenge, as it involves exclusion of other causes of isolated thrombocytopenia [7].

In children, acute ITP prevails, usually develops a few weeks after a viral infection and has a self-limiting evolution in most cases, while chronic ITP develops in approximately 20% of the cases, especially in teenagers [8–11]. As pediatric ITP rarely becomes chronic, the incidence of ITP in children is estimated at 5 cases/100,000 children/year, significantly lower than the one in adults [12,13]. Recent data sustain the definition of chronic ITP as thrombocytopenia (<100,000/μL) which lasts for more than 12 months, whereas a 3–12-month interval of thrombocytopenia qualifies as persistent thrombocytopenia [2]. Risk factors for ITP chronicity include age at diagnosis, female sex and platelet count at the time of the diagnosis [14].

Primary ITP accounts for 80–90% of adult cases [3,15]. In similar fashion, around 20% of children cases can be attributed to secondary causes, according to a Spanish study [16]. *H. pylori* has been regarded as one of the potential causes of secondary ITP, but it is yet unclear whether treatment of this particular infection might be sufficient to improve platelet numbers [17,18]. There are several hypotheses that link *H. pylori* to ITP. Firstly, molecular mimicry plays a huge part. This is characterized by specific bacterial antibody production that cross-react with platelet glycoprotein antigens [19]. A specific cross-reactivity between platelet antigens and the cytotoxin-associated gene A (CagA) has also been described [20], together with a higher prevalence of CagA *H. pylori* positive strains among populations diagnosed with ITP [21]. Lewis (Le) antigens, expressed by particular *H. pylori* strains, adhere to platelets, which are consequently targeted by anti-Le antibodies in genetically susceptible patients. These also interfere with ITP pathogenesis through the same molecular mimicry-related processes [22]. Particular enhancement of platelet phagocytosis by the monocytes in *H. pylori* infected individuals seems to be involved in the development of secondary ITP as well [23]. Particular haplotypes such as HLA-DRB1*11,*14 and -DQB1*03 are more frequently encountered in ITP patients infected with *H. pylori*, whereas HLA -DRB1*03 is more rarely found within the same individuals [24]. Moreover, intestinal microbiota dysbiosis, which appears in the setting of *H. pylori* infection, has also been linked to ITP pathogenesis [25]. However, after *H. pylori* eradication, autoantibodies disappear after a period of one to two years, whereas a positive platelet response is seen in some studies after only one to two weeks, which suggests that other intricated mechanisms might play a role in the pathogenesis of ITP as well [26].

An association between *H. pylori* infection and ITP was proven for the first time in 1998, by Gasbarrini et al. [27]. Since then, the beneficial effect of *H. pylori* eradication over platelet numbers has been proved in adult patients with moderate ITP forms in studies with a randomized controlled trial (RCT) design [28]. In children, evidence promoting *H. pylori* eradication in ITP patients exists, but the sole influence of *H. pylori* in pediatric ITP is put into question [29,30]. Starting from various hypotheses that sustain the benefit of *H. pylori* treatment in improving platelet numbers in patients with ITP, this comprehensive review aims to establish the influence of *H. pylori* infection and eradication upon platelet counts and recovery in pediatric ITP.

2. Materials and Methods

We searched the Pubmed, Scopus and Web of Science databases for all articles indexed through the 25 May 2023, which assessed the relationship between *H. pylori* and thrombocytopenia in children. The search terms used were "Helicobacter" OR "*Helicobacter pylori*" AND "thrombocytopenia" AND "child". We only aimed to include population-based studies (including prospective cohort and observational studies, retrospective observational studies, longitudinal studies and RCTs) conducted on child populations or studies enrolling both adults and children which conducted a separate analysis on the impact of *H. pylori* infection and/or its eradication on thrombocytopenia in pediatric populations. Exclusion criteria consisted of non-English language literature data, meta-analyses, review articles, case reports/series, editorials, letters to editor, as well as experimental, animal studies and adult population-based studies. Reference lists of the selected articles were also screened for compliance with the inclusion and exclusion criteria, to the review's objectives and for database indexing.

The article selection process firstly consisted of exclusion of duplicates and triplicates, a task which was performed by authors SM and KAM. Each of the three authors of the article examined the title and abstracts of the identified reports in order to exclude irrelevant articles for the reviewer's objectives. SM and KAM accessed the full-length text of the elected manuscripts and checked for compliance to the aforementioned inclusion criteria. Eventual disagreements between authors had been thoroughly debated and discussed by all authors. The inclusion of each individual record belonging to this review was established upon mutual agreement.

The following information were extracted from articles belonging to the final selection pool: author name, year of publication, type of the study, target population, study group division and main findings of the article related to *H. pylori* prevalence among children with ITP, the impact of its presence on platelet count and the effect of its eradication upon platelet recovery rates.

3. Results

The initial research resulted in a total of 191 records. After exclusion of 59 duplicate and triplicate articles, 15 non-English language articles and 39 articles which were not in line with the reviewer's objectives, a number of 78 relevant articles were screened. Review articles, meta-analyses, case reports/series, editorials, letters to editor (not reporting results of original studies) were excluded, together with studies conducted on adults. This systematic selection resulted in 21 admissible articles. The article selection process has been detailed in Figure 1, being performed in accordance with the PRISMA 2020 statement [31].

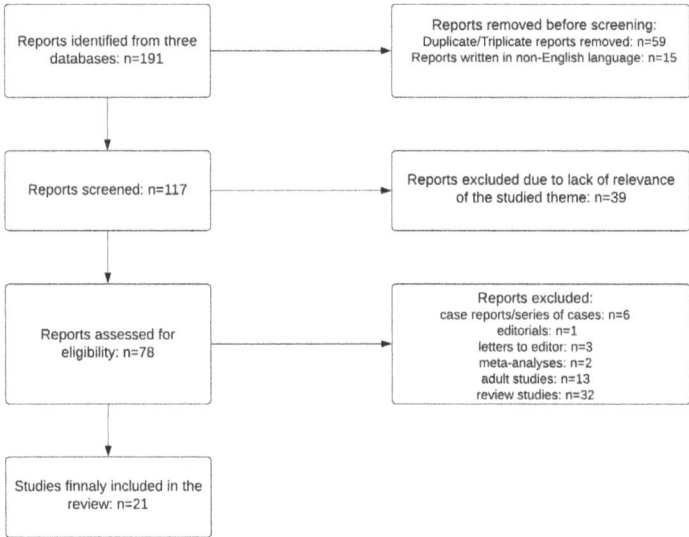

Figure 1. PRISMA flowchart with the eligible studies.

A summary of the main findings of the pediatric studies which complied to our election criteria has been provided through Table 1.

Table 1. Characteristics of pediatric studies which assessed the impact of *H. pylori* infection and eradication upon the course of platelet counts in patients with ITP.

Reference (Author, Year)	Type of Study	Study Group Division	*H. pylori* Detection Method	Main Outcome
Russo et al., 2011 [29]	Prospective, case–control multicentric study	244 children with chronic ITP who were screened for *H. pylori* infection: • 50 children positive for *H. pylori* (37 children receiving eradication therapy) • 194 children negative for *H. pylori*	Stool antigen testing in most cases Urea breath test conducted in 2 cases	Significantly higher platelet response rates among patients who underwent successful eradication in comparison with spontaneous remission rates among *H. pylori* negative patients
Brito et al., 2015 [32]	RCT	85 children with chronic ITP: 63 patients negative for *H. pylori* 22 patients positive for *H. pylori*: • 11 children randomized in the treatment group • 11 children randomized in the control group	Stool antigen test + urea breath test	Significantly higher complete platelet response rates among children who received specific *H. pylori* eradication therapy
Ferrara et al., 2009 [33]	Retrospective observational study	24 children with chronic ITP: • 8 children positive for *H. pylori* • 16 children negative for *H. pylori*	Stool antigen test	Significant increase in platelet counts after eradication therapy among *H. pylori* infected children; no significantly difference in platelet numbers during the follow-up period among the uninfected patients
Baxendell et al., 2019 [34]	Cross-sectional study	1038 school children: • 343 children infected with *H. pylori* • 695 children negative for *H. pylori*	Stool antigen test + *H. pylori* antibody test	Significantly lower platelet and MPV values in children infected with *H. pylori* in comparison with uninfected counterparts
Neefjes et al., 2007 [35]	Observational study	47 children: • 3 children infected with *H. pylori* • 44 children negative for *H. pylori*	Stool antigen test	Significant platelet response within the children who benefited from eradication therapy
Maghbool et al., 2009 [36]	Retrospective study	30 children: • 5 children infected with *H. pylori* • 25 children negative for *H. pylori*	Stool antigen test	Platelet response was consistent after 1 year of follow-up in 4 of the *H. pylori* infected patients after eradication
Jaing et al., 2003 [37]	Observational study	22 children: • 9 children infected with *H. pylori* • 13 children negative for *H. pylori*	Stool antigen test	5 patients from the 9 infected with *H. pylori* showed partial or complete remission of platelet counts after 6 months, this response being sustained for a medium period of 16 months
Hayashi et al., 2005 [38]	Observational study	10 children: • 2 children infected with *H. pylori* • 8 children negative for *H. pylori*	Stool antigen test + urea breath test	A sustained platelet response was reported in only one of the *H. pylori* patient during a follow-up period of over an year

Table 1. *Cont.*

Reference (Author, Year)	Type of Study	Study Group Division	H. pylori Detection Method	Main Outcome
Wu et al., 2018 [39]	Case-control study	280 children with chronic ITP	Stool antigen test	H. pylori infection was not identified in any of the children with ITP
Abdollahi et al., 2015 [40]	Case-control study	106 children: • 42 children with ITP • 64 healthy controls	Stool antigen test	Significantly higher prevalence of H. pylori infection among the case group of children with ITP
Rajantie et al., 2003 [41]	Observational study	17 children with chronic ITP	Stool antigen test + urea breath test + H. pylori IgA/IgG antibodies	H. pylori infection was absent in each of the children included in the study
Kim et al., 2016 [42]	Retrospective observational study	200 children with ITP	Stool antigen test	Absence of H. pylori infection among 5 children with chronic ITP whose stool antigen test were examined
Wu et al., 2007 [43]	Case-control study	62 children: • 32 children with ITP • 30 children in the control group	Stool antigen test	No significant differences between the two study groups in terms of H. pylori prevalence rate Similar characteristics and treatment response ratio between H. pylori positive and H. pylori negative subjects from study group
Săsăran et al., 2020 [44]	Prospective, case–control study	151 children: • 31 patients with H. pylori gastritis • 53 patients with non- H. pylori gastritis • 67 healthy controls	Histology based diagnosis	No significant differences in terms of platelet number and MPV values between the three study groups Platelet numbers and MPV values did not vary with different degrees of gastritis
Afifi et al., 2011 [45]	Case-control study	120 children: • 60 patients with H. pylori positive antibodies • 60 controls with H. pylori negative antibodies	H. pylori antibody testing	No significant differences in platelet counts within the two study groups
Bisogno et al., 2008 [46]	Longitudinal study	24 children with ITP: • 8 children infected with H. pylori • 16 children negative for H. pylori	Stool antigen test + urea breath test	No significant differences in platelet counts between the two study groups Improvement of platelet count in 3 patients who underwent eradication therapy, after six months
Loffredo et al., 2007 [47]	Longitudinal study	39 children with ITP: • 8 children infected with H. pylori • 31 children negative for H. pylori	Stool antigen test + urea breath test + H. pylori specific serum IgG antibodies	No improvement in platelet counts in children in whom H. pylori was successfully eradicated No significant differences in platelet counts between infected and uninfected patients during a follow-up period of one year

Table 1. Cont.

Reference (Author, Year)	Type of Study	Study Group Division	H. pylori Detection Method	Main Outcome
Eghbali et al., 2019 [48]	Open label RCT	28 children with ITP and H. pylori infection: • 14 children receiving ITP and H. pylori therapy • 14 children receiving ITP therapy	Stool antigen test	No significant differences between the two study groups in terms of platelet values at the baseline and after six months of follow-up
Morimoto et al., 2014 [49]	Retrospective observational study	49 children with primary ITP (18 children in whom H. pylori infectious status was examined): • 7 children positive for H. pylori infection • 11 children negative for H. pylori infection	Stool antigen test/blood antigen test/urine antibody test	Short-term response to intravenous Ig treatment was not affected of H. pylori infection
Jaing et al., 2006 [50]	Case-control study	91 children: • 63 patients with acute ITP • 28 healthy controls	Stool antigen test	Similar prevalence of H. pylori infection between the two study groups Similar response to steroid treatment among the study group, irrespective of H. pylori infectious status

Treepongkaruna et al., 2009 [51]	Multicenter RCT	55 children with chronic ITP:
		• 16 patients with H. pylori infection who were randomized as follows:
		  ○ 7 children in the treatment group
		  ○ 9 children in the control group
			Stool antigen test	H. pylori eradication did not bring any improvement in platelet count
				CagA antibodies were positive in 12 patients with documented H. Pylori infection, whereas VacA antibodies were positive in 7 patients

Legend: CagA—cytotoxin-associated gene A; H. pylori—Helicobacter pylori; Ig—immunoglobulin; ITP—immune thrombocytopenic purpura; MPV—mean platelet volume; RCT—randomized controlled trial; VacA—vacuolating cytotoxin A.

Although the causative role of *H. pylori* in pediatric ITP has not been sufficiently investigated, some studies sustain a test-and-treat strategy in children diagnosed with this particular condition. Russo et al. enrolled an impressive pediatric cohort of 244 patients diagnosed with chronic ITP and proved that platelet recovery rates were significantly higher in those patients in whom *H. pylori* was successfully eradicated, when compared to spontaneous remission rates encountered in *H. pylori* negative patients [29]. Brito et al. conducted an RCT on 85 children, including 22 children and adolescents with chronic ITP, equally randomized into a treatment group and a control group with similar baseline platelet counts. The authors found no significant difference in complete platelet response rates, defined as platelet values exceeding 150×10^9/L, between treated and untreated children. However, similarly to the study of Russo et al. [29], *H. pylori* eradication yielded a more frequent complete platelet response than in the case of uninfected patients [32]. In accordance with these findings, the study of Ferrara et al. sustains *H. pylori* screening in chronic, childhood and adolescence ITP, after showing a more frequent complete platelet response in patients in whom *H. pylori* was successfully treated. No differences were seen in this study in pre-therapeutic platelet counts in relation to *H. pylori* presence [33]. Another Ethiopian study found a significant reduction in platelet numbers and mean platelet volume in children with positive *H. pylori* stool antigen test or positive *H. pylori* antibodies [34].

The beneficial effects of *H. pylori* eradication in children with ITP are still being investigated. The numerically limited cohorts of other studies greatly influence the interpretation of their results. A Dutch study sustained the favorable therapeutic response brought up by *H. pylori* eradication in chronic ITP, but its conclusion cannot be perceived at a larger scale, as only 3 children out of the entire study cohort were diagnosed with the infection [35]. In similar fashion, a small scale study conducted in Iran found that *H. pylori* eradication might facilitate a sustained therapeutic response in chronic pediatric ITP, but this infection was diagnosed in a very small subset of patients, as well [36]. Jaing et al. reported a sustained rise in platelet counts after 6 months of follow-up in five out of nine children infected with *H. pylori*, but due to the limited number of patients included in the study, it is unclear whether infection eradication, the course of the disease or standard treatment played the major role in therapeutic favorable outcome [37]. Thus, it is hard to interpretate the impact of *H. pylori* eradication in very small subsets of patients with chronic ITP, which characterize most pediatric studies. For example, Hayashi et al. identified *H. pylori* in only two out of ten patients with chronic ITP and reported a sustained response after 1 year of follow up in only one of these [38]. A larger subgroup, of 280 patients under the age of 18 years, was though included in a nationwide study, conducted in Taiwan. Within this study, *H. pylori* was only associated with adult ITP, the infection being absent in each of the children included [39].

Prevalence of *H. pylori* infection varies with age and geographical region among subjects with ITP [52]. In an adult study enrolling Italian and British populations, the incidence of *H. pylori* infection in patients with ITP was reported to be similar to the one of the general, healthy population [53]. However, one study examining spleen specimens from patients undergoing splenectomy for ITP or trauma identified a higher prevalence of *H. pylori* in the first group. Moreover, the presence of *H. pylori* infection was associated with low expression of the FC gamma receptors IIB (FCGRIIB) within splenic macrophages, which is known to play a role in the etiology of ITP [54]. Furthermore, within a case–control study, Abdollahi et al. reported a higher prevalence of *H. pylori* infection among a pediatric group with ITP, when compared to healthy controls. The study did not analyze the therapeutic outcome in the case group, nor the impact of *H. pylori* eradication [40]. On the other hand, a Finnish study conducted on 17 children with ITP failed to confirm the presence of *H. pylori* infection in any of these subjects [41]. Similarly, one study conducted in Japan which analyzed remission rates of chronic ITP in children, during a follow-up period of 20 years, did not identify the presence of *H. pylori* in any of the included subjects [42]. A slightly higher prevalence of *H. pylori* than in general in population was found in a Taiwanese case–control study, but this difference did not reach statistical significance. The relationship between *H. pylori* infection and platelet response was also analyzed, revealing that its presence is slightly discernible in the course of chronic ITP [43].

The sole presence of *H. pylori* infection might not additionally impact platelet counts and clinical picture in pediatric ITP. Similar platelet values between children study groups were reported, divided based on *H. pylori* infectious status. One study compared multiple hematological parameters between children diagnosed with *H. pylori* gastritis, those diagnosed with non-*H. pylori* gastritis and a control group with functional gastro-intestinal symptoms, without microscopic anomalies of the gastric mucosa. Platelet numbers were found to be similar to the ones of healthy subjects in both study groups [44]. Moreover, the study of Afifi et al. also compared various erythrocyte parameters and platelet numbers between pediatric subjects with *H. pylori* infection and healthy controls. Significant lower values of the mean corpuscular volume (MCV) and mean cell hemoglobin (MCH) were found in the *H. pylori* positive group, but platelet counts did not present significant variations among the two study groups [45].

Hence, uncertainty still surrounds the theory of *H. pylori*'s implications in the pathogenesis of ITP, as Bisogno et al. proved within a small-scale study. The number of patients in whom the bacterial infection was not confirmed and presented spontaneous improvements of platelet counts was similar to the one of patients in whom bacterial eradication showed a beneficial, yet unsustainable, therapeutic response [46]. Efforts to eradicate *H. pylori* might not produce the expected positive outcome over platelet numbers. A multicenter randomized controlled trial showed that *H. pylori* eradication does not bring any improvement in platelet counts, after random assignment of 16 children into two balanced groups of patients, one who benefited from eradication therapy and the other one in which anti-infectious treatment was not considered. An important number of subjects from this particular study presented cytotoxin-associated gene A (CagA) and/or vacuolating cytotoxin A (VacA) antibodies [51]. Loffredo et al. also reported no difference in therapeutic outcome from patients without *H. pylori*, after single or multiple courses of eradication lines were applied to children in whom bacteria was positive upon detection of at least two non-invasive tests [47]. Another study confirmed that *H. pylori* eradication does not bring any additional benefit to standard treatment in children with chronic ITP [48]. *H. pylori* infection does not seem to interfere with short term response to intravenous immunoglobulin (IvIg) treatment, assessed after a time-span of 2 weeks, according to Morimoto et al. [49]. Furthermore, a case–control study described no significant differences in number of subjects infected with *H. pylori*, when comparing children diagnosed with ITP and healthy controls. Within the study group, the therapeutic outcome was also assessed in relation to *H. pylori* infectious status and the bacterial pathogen was found to have no impact on platelet count response [50]. Therefore, it is still unclear if *H. pylori* eradication improves therapeutic outcome in pediatric ITP.

4. Discussion

Extra-gastric manifestations of *H. pylori* infection seem to be largely represented by hematological disorders, such as iron deficiency anemia (IDA), megaloblastic anemia (caused by vitamin B12 deficiency) and ITP [55–57]. This review has focused on the impact that *H. pylori* infection poses upon the clinical course and therapeutic efficacy in pediatric ITP, starting from the long-running debate and controversy surrounding the importance of *H. pylori* eradication in patients with ITP. An update to the pediatric literature data has been provided through inclusion of more recent studies conducted on the subject, which met the inclusion and exclusion criteria, but which are still hindered by several limitations. An older review article, published in 2005, initially pointed out that studies analyzing a relationship between *H. pylori* and ITP which were conducted to that point were small-scale, and the enrolled populations were not followed up for longer periods of time [58]. The studies included in this review are also characterized by numeric limitation of target groups. Moreover, only two of those were longitudinally designed, but the follow-up period was limited to 6 months and one year, respectively.

With the availability of new data derived from adult studies which showed utility of *H. pylori* treatment, in cases where the bacterium was encountered, the 2011 guidelines of the American Society of Hematology recommended against routine screening of *H. pylori* infection in patients with ITP, but supported treatment of the bacterial infection in those patients in whom non-invasive or invasive diagnostic tests delivered positive results [6]. Afterwards, the 2019 guidelines of the American Society of Hematology maintained the same position, recommending against routine testing for *H. pylori*, which was meant to be limited to those subjects with clinical, suggestive symptoms [59]. On the other hand, the 2010 Consensus Guidelines of the Associazione Italiana di Ematologia e Oncologia Pediatrica (AIEOP) recommended the conductance of *H. pylori* stool antigen tests in children with ITP, in order to search for an underlying infectious cause which can be combated [60]. As listed in Table 1, in most of the studies included in this review, the identification of *H. pylori* infection was subject to stool antigen testing as well. However, a handful of these studies assessed the presence of the infection only in a subset of patients. Moreover, only a third of the studies included in this review evaluated platelet outcome after eradication therapy was instituted, with the other studies only assessing response to standard ITP treatment in relation to the presence/absence of *H. pylori* infection. Still, the presence of *H. pylori* in subjects with ITP might prompt the physician towards recommending a therapeutic scheme. One treatment strategy protocol developed based on an adult study conducted in a referral center from Northern Brazil also proposes a screening of *H. pylori* and its subsequent treatment, if diagnostic test results are positive [61].

The success of *H. pylori* eradication in patients with ITP varies greatly among different studies. Eradication rates lower than 1% or 5% have been reported, or even exceeding 60% in research conducted in Italy and Japan [27,62,63]. Stasi et al. found among an adult cohort diagnosed with ITP a similar prevalence of *H. pylori* infection to the one found in general population. Furthermore, the authors described a beneficial effect of *H. pylori* eradication only in those mild to moderate cases of ITP, with recent onset [53]. A French study also reported a similar seroprevalence of *H. pylori* infection between a study group of adults with ITP and controls, whereas a Columbian study identified a compellingly higher prevalence of the same bacteria within an ITP cohort, when compared to healthy subjects [64,65]. Still, *H. pylori* seems to be encountered more rarely in children than in adults suffering from ITP [52]. Kuwana et al. have reviewed the heterogeneity of *H. pylori* therapeutic response rates in subjects with ITP, reporting higher eradication failure rates in the United States and non-Italian European countries. Furthermore, the authors claimed that the very low incidence of *H. pylori* infection reported within pediatric studies questions the utility of the specific eradication treatment among these patients, as opposed to adult counterparts [66]. As a matter of fact, from the reports included in this review, one study conducted in Taiwan and another one enrolling a Finish pediatric population failed to identify *H. pylori* in any of the enrolled subjects [39,41].

Secondary ITP forms are accompanied by a more pronounced thrombocytopenia, splenomegaly, hepatomegaly and lower hemoglobin counts, according to an adult study [67]. In children in particular, search for a secondary cause of ITP and treatment of possible causative agents could represent an important therapeutic aid which can lead to avoidance of standard treatment and its widely known side effects, which are more extensive at this particular age group [68]. One study conducted on a numerous cohort of pediatric ITP patients, identified that the two most frequent causes of secondary ITP cases are recent immunizations and viral infections, followed by autoimmune disorders and immunodeficiency [16]. Within this study, post-immunization and post-viral infections ITPs showed the best remission rates [16]. Although *H. pylori* infection is usually acquired during childhood, physicians are less familiar with its extra-gastric, hematological manifestations. Hence, screening of this bacterium is not routinely performed in children with ITP and is reported as a rare practice among adult studies as well [69,70]. One meta-analysis of six randomized trials sustained the importance of *H. pylori* eradication in adults with ITP, but failed to identify a therapeutic benefit in children diagnosed with the same condition, in whom the infection was successfully treated [71]. One systematic review study drew this same conclusion, in light of the frequent limitations of pediatric studies addressing a potential association between *H. pylori* and ITP, such as the lack of controls, the small sample sizes, the low prevalence of *H. pylori* infection among the studied subjects and the short period of follow-ups. Furthermore, the same review concluded that the poor statistical power of pediatric studies hinders the establishment of benefits to *H. pylori* eradication in children, in both gastric and extra-gastric manifestations [72]. Another meta-analysis of 7 Middle-Eastern, adult studies, highlighted the same advantages of *H. pylori* screening and treatment in ITP, but was hindered by several limitations, which the authors acknowledged. Among these, the small population samples, the heterogeneity of the *H. pylori* detection methods used and of the complete versus partial platelet response criteria were the ones that stood out [73]. Although a correlation between *H. pylori* eradication and platelet count increase in children seems obvious, another meta-analysis of miscellaneous studies points out their limitations related to the design, and the need for further evidence delivered by RCTs [74]. Unicentric studies, even those performed on significantly larger cohorts, identified *H. pylori* only in small subsets of patients with ITP and found very low platelet recovery rates in case of successful infection eradication [75]. Hence, due to the bias-prone studies conducted in both pediatric and adult populations, the utility of a test and treat strategy for *H. pylori* is still in question. Moreover, as shown in Table 1, most of the studies included in this review, which assessed the effect of *H. pylori* eradication, showed no significant improvement in platelet counts.

As the persistence of chronic gastric inflammation might be responsible for mild thrombocytosis, controversial results were reported by Matsukawa et al., who claimed through their study that *H. pylori* eradication leads to a decrease in platelet numbers in adults with gastritis and gastric ulcer, as opposed to non-eradicated patients [76]. However, one study, which assessed the impact of chronic gastric inflammation upon platelet numbers and mean platelet volume (MPV), found no significant differences between two study groups of subjects, divided depending on *H. pylori* infectious status. Furthermore, MPV did not correlate with severity of chronic gastric inflammation [77]. Two pediatric studies also confirmed these findings, describing lack of significant differences in MPV values between non-*H. pylori* gastritis and *H. pylori* gastritis subjects, eradicated and non-eradicated patients, and lack of correlations between this parameters and different degree of gastritis severity [44,78]. Mean platelet volume has been for a long time regarded as a marker of platelet activation, which might increase with enhanced thromobocytopoiesis in inflammation and infections [79]. Therefore, it is yet unclear whether concurring *H. pylori* infection and chronic gastritis influence platelet parameters in both adults and children.

In various adult cohorts, the eradication of *H. pylori* has been followed by a sustained, favorable platelet response after follow-up periods of one year [80]. However, platelet response rates seem to be higher in patients with milder thrombocytopenia and countries with higher prevalence of *H. pylori* infection [81]. One previous systematic review of studies performed on pediatric populations concluded that platelet response rates in pediatric populations are expected to be similar to the ones found so far in adults and that *H. pylori* eradication should constitute a first-line treatment approach in children with ITP as well [82]. There is still a discrepancy between the results reported by cohort studies, such as those included in the review, and individual case reports which sustain the need for *H. pylori* infection eradication in pediatric ITP. The case of a 12-year-old male patient who presented recovery of platelet counts after *H. pylori* eradication distinguishes among others, due to a reported higher efficacy of the bacterial eradication when compared to corticosteroid treatment [83]. In another case report on an 11-year-old, a sustained platelet response was reported only after *H. pylori* re-eradication, in spite of previous therapy with IvIg and cepharantine, administered as a substitute of corticosteroids [84]. The report of a female of 13 years of age with *H. pylori* induced atrophic gastritis also details the remission of the associated conditions, namely IDA and ITP, with infection eradication [85]. A temporary increase in platelet numbers was also reported in relation to omeprazole monotherapy [84], which had previously been described to eventually lead to *H. pylori* eradication and to remission of ITP, when administered for a period of approximately 1 year and a half in an elderly woman [86]. Ikeda et al. describe a peculiar case of neonatal thrombocytopenia related to maternal ITP, diagnosed during pregnancy. The neonate benefited from IvIg treatment, but in the mother's case, ITP was found to be related to *H. pylori* and infection eradication led to recovery of platelet counts. Moreover, the case brought into attention the neonatal impact of gestational platelet auto-antibodies [87]. Although case reports offer insufficient evidence to sustain *H. pylori* screening and treatment in pediatric ITP, they prove that for certain individuals, this strategy might be helpful in improving platelet numbers.

In spite of the multiple pediatric studies which have thoroughly investigated the impact of *H. pylori* infection and its eradication upon platelet counts, their main limitations remain the small population samples of available studies and the short follow-up periods of the included patients, which have been highlighted through Table 1. Furthermore, there are currently only three RCTs [32,48,51] which randomized children with ITP into two groups, depending on the choice of adding *H. pylori* treatment to conventional therapy. Hence, available pediatric studies with higher statistical power, such as RCTs, are very scarce. Therefore, there are insufficient data available to certify the negative impact of *H. pylori* infection upon platelet count in pediatric populations [88], and the long-term stability of platelet numbers after *H. pylori* eradication is yet uncertain in children.

5. Conclusions

The generally low prevalence of *H. pylori* in children with ITP might suggest that this infection only plays a minor role in the pathogenesis of this condition, at pediatric ages. Controversy still surrounds the utility of *H. pylori* identification and treatment in children with ITP. Several studies reported the benefits of *H. pylori* screening, but evidence is scarcer than in adult populations and it is yet unclear how the treatment of this particular infection influences platelet counts in the long term. The lack of longitudinal design of most of the available pediatric research calls for future studies which should also consistently follow up the enrolled study populations.

Author Contributions: M.O.S. and C.O.M. conceptualized and designed the study and conducted the literature search and drafted the initial manuscript. M.O.S. and C.O.M. reviewed and revised the manuscript. A.M.K. participated in collecting literature data and helped in drafting the manuscript tables. All authors have read and agreed to the published version of the manuscript.

Funding: This research received no external funding.

Institutional Review Board Statement: Not applicable.

Informed Consent Statement: Not applicable.

Conflicts of Interest: The authors declare no conflict of interest.

References

1. Cooper, N.; Bussel, J. The Pathogenesis of Immune Thrombocytopaenic Purpura. *Br. J. Haematol.* **2006**, *133*, 364–374. [CrossRef] [PubMed]
2. Rodeghiero, F.; Stasi, R.; Gernsheimer, T.; Michel, M.; Provan, D.; Arnold, D.M.; Bussel, J.B.; Cines, D.B.; Chong, B.H.; Cooper, N.; et al. Standardization of Terminology, Definitions and Outcome Criteria in Immune Thrombocytopenic Purpura of Adults and Children: Report from an International Working Group. *Blood* **2009**, *113*, 2386–2393. [CrossRef] [PubMed]
3. Cines, D.B.; Bussel, J.B.; Liebman, H.A.; Luning Prak, E.T. The ITP Syndrome: Pathogenic and Clinical Diversity. *Blood* **2009**, *113*, 6511–6521. [CrossRef] [PubMed]
4. McMillan, R.; Wang, L.; Tomer, A.; Nichol, J.; Pistillo, J. Suppression of in Vitro Megakaryocyte Production by Antiplatelet Autoantibodies from Adult Patients with Chronic ITP. *Blood* **2004**, *103*, 1364–1369. [CrossRef] [PubMed]
5. Arnold, D.M. Bleeding Complications in Immune Thrombocytopenia. *Hematol. Am. Soc. Hematol. Educ. Program.* **2015**, *2015*, 237–242. [CrossRef]

6. Neunert, C.; Lim, W.; Crowther, M.; Cohen, A.; Solberg, L.; Crowther, M.A. American Society of Hematology The American Society of Hematology 2011 Evidence-Based Practice Guideline for Immune Thrombocytopenia. *Blood* **2011**, *117*, 4190–4207. [CrossRef]
7. Provan, D.; Arnold, D.M.; Bussel, J.B.; Chong, B.H.; Cooper, N.; Gernsheimer, T.; Ghanima, W.; Godeau, B.; González-López, T.J.; Grainger, J.; et al. Updated International Consensus Report on the Investigation and Management of Primary Immune Thrombocytopenia. *Blood Adv.* **2019**, *3*, 3780–3817. [CrossRef]
8. Moulis, G.; Palmaro, A.; Montastruc, J.-L.; Godeau, B.; Lapeyre-Mestre, M.; Sailler, L. Epidemiology of Incident Immune Thrombocytopenia: A Nationwide Population-Based Study in France. *Blood* **2014**, *124*, 3308–3315. [CrossRef]
9. Segal, J.B.; Powe, N.R. Prevalence of Immune Thrombocytopenia: Analyses of Administrative Data. *J. Thromb. Haemost.* **2006**, *4*, 2377–2383. [CrossRef]
10. Franchini, M.; Vescovi, P.P.; Garofano, M.; Veneri, D. *Helicobacter pylori*-Associated Idiopathic Thrombocytopenic Purpura: A Narrative Review. *Semin. Thromb. Hemost.* **2012**, *38*, 463–468. [CrossRef]
11. Psaila, B.; Bussel, J.B. Immune Thrombocytopenic Purpura. *Hematol. Oncol. Clin. N. Am.* **2007**, *21*, 743–759. [CrossRef] [PubMed]
12. Hedman, A.; Henter, J.I.; Hedlund, I.; Elinder, G. Prevalence and Treatment of Chronic Idiopathic Thrombocytopenic Purpura of Childhood in Sweden. *Acta Paediatr.* **1997**, *86*, 226–227. [CrossRef] [PubMed]
13. Matzdorff, A.; Meyer, O.; Ostermann, H.; Kiefel, V.; Eberl, W.; Kühne, T.; Pabinger, I.; Rummel, M. Immune Thrombocytopenia—Current Diagnostics and Therapy: Recommendations of a Joint Working Group of DGHO, ÖGHO, SGH, GPOH, and DGTI. *Oncol. Res. Treat.* **2018**, *41* (Suppl. S5), 1–30. [CrossRef] [PubMed]
14. Rosu, V.E.; Roșu, S.T.; Ivanov, A.V.; Starcea, I.M.; Streanga, V.; Miron, I.C.; Mocanu, A.; Lupu, A.; Lupu, V.V.; Gavrilovici, C. Predictor Factors for Chronicity in Immune Thrombocytopenic Purpura in Children. *Children* **2023**, *10*, 911. [CrossRef] [PubMed]
15. Palau, J.; Sancho, E.; Herrera, M.; Sánchez, S.; Mingot, M.E.; Upegui, R.I.; Rodríguez Salazar, M.J.; de la Cruz, F.; Fernández, M.C.; González López, T.J.; et al. Characteristics and Management of Primary and Other Immune Thrombocytopenias: Spanish Registry Study. *Hematology* **2017**, *22*, 484–492. [CrossRef]
16. Berrueco, R.; Sebastián, E.; Solsona, M.; González de Pablo, J.; Ruiz-Llobet, A.; Mesegué, M.; Gálvez, E.; Sevilla, J. Secondary Immune Thrombocytopenia in Children: Characteristics and Outcome of a Large Cohort from Two Spanish Centres. *Acta Paediatr.* **2021**, *110*, 1952–1958. [CrossRef]
17. Sadia, H.; Abro, S.; Ali, M.; Uddin, K.; Agboola, A.A.; Bano, S.; Anigbo, C.L.; Singh, R. Immune Thrombocytopenia Induced by *Helicobacter pylori* Infection: A Case Report and Literature Review. *Cureus* **2022**, *14*, e27809. [CrossRef]
18. Vanegas, Y.A.M.; Vishnu, P. Management of *Helicobacter pylori* in Patients with Immune Thrombocytopenia. *Hamostaseologie* **2019**, *39*, 279–283. [CrossRef]
19. Stasi, R.; Provan, D. *Helicobacter pylori* and Chronic ITP. *Hematol. Am. Soc. Hematol. Educ. Program.* **2008**, *2008*, 206–211. [CrossRef]
20. Takahashi, T.; Yujiri, T.; Shinohara, K.; Inoue, Y.; Sato, Y.; Fujii, Y.; Okubo, M.; Zaitsu, Y.; Ariyoshi, K.; Nakamura, Y.; et al. Molecular Mimicry by *Helicobacter pylori* CagA Protein May Be Involved in the Pathogenesis of H. Pylori-Associated Chronic Idiopathic Thrombocytopenic Purpura. *Br. J. Haematol.* **2004**, *124*, 91–96. [CrossRef]
21. Emilia, G.; Luppi, M.; Zucchini, P.; Morselli, M.; Potenza, L.; Forghieri, F.; Volzone, F.; Jovic, G.; Leonardi, G.; Donelli, A.; et al. *Helicobacter pylori* Infection and Chronic Immune Thrombocytopenic Purpura: Long-Term Results of Bacterium Eradication and Association with Bacterium Virulence Profiles. *Blood* **2007**, *110*, 3833–3841. [CrossRef] [PubMed]
22. Cines, D.B. ITP: Time to "Bug Off"? *Blood* **2007**, *110*, 3818–3819. [CrossRef]
23. Asahi, A.; Nishimoto, T.; Okazaki, Y.; Suzuki, H.; Masaoka, T.; Kawakami, Y.; Ikeda, Y.; Kuwana, M. *Helicobacter pylori* Eradication Shifts Monocyte Fcgamma Receptor Balance toward Inhibitory FcgammaRIIB in Immune Thrombocytopenic Purpura Patients. *J. Clin. Investig.* **2008**, *118*, 2939–2949. [CrossRef]
24. Veneri, D.; De Matteis, G.; Solero, P.; Federici, F.; Zanuso, C.; Guizzardi, E.; Arena, S.; Gaio, M.; Pontiero, P.; Ricetti, M.M.; et al. Analysis of B- and T-Cell Clonality and HLA Class II Alleles in Patients with Idiopathic Thrombocytopenic Purpura: Correlation with *Helicobacter pylori* Infection and Response to Eradication Treatment. *Platelets* **2005**, *16*, 307–311. [CrossRef] [PubMed]
25. Liu, C.; Cheng, L.; Ji, L.; Li, F.; Zhan, Y.; Wu, B.; Ke, Y.; Chen, P.; Hua, F.; Yuan, L.; et al. Intestinal Microbiota Dysbiosis Play a Role in Pathogenesis of Patients with Primary Immune Thrombocytopenia. *Thromb. Res.* **2020**, *190*, 11–19. [CrossRef]
26. Cines, D.B.; Liebman, H.; Stasi, R. Pathobiology of Secondary Immune Thrombocytopenia. *Semin. Hematol.* **2009**, *46*, S2–S14. [CrossRef]
27. Gasbarrini, A.; Franceschi, F.; Tartaglione, R.; Landolfi, R.; Pola, P.; Gasbarrini, G. Regression of Autoimmune Thrombocytopenia after Eradication of *Helicobacter pylori*. *Lancet* **1998**, *352*, 878. [CrossRef]
28. Han, B.; Kim, H.J.; Yhim, H.-Y.; Oh, D.; Bae, S.H.; Shin, H.-J.; Lee, W.-S.; Kwon, J.; Lee, J.-O.; Kim, H.J.; et al. Sequential Eradication of *Helicobacter pylori* as a Treatment for Immune Thrombocytopenia in Patients with Moderate Thrombocytopenia: A Multicenter Prospective Randomized Phase 3 Study. *Ann. Hematol.* **2022**, *101*, 1435–1445. [CrossRef]
29. Russo, G.; Miraglia, V.; Branciforte, F.; Matarese, S.M.R.; Zecca, M.; Bisogno, G.; Parodi, E.; Amendola, G.; Giordano, P.; Jankovic, M.; et al. Effect of Eradication of *Helicobacter pylori* in Children with Chronic Immune Thrombocytopenia: A Prospective, Controlled, Multicenter Study. *Pediatr. Blood Cancer* **2011**, *56*, 273–278. [CrossRef]
30. Yetgin, S.; Demir, H.; Arslan, D.; Unal, S.; Koçak, N. Autoimmune Thrombocytopenic Purpura and *Helicobacter pylori* Infection Effectivity during Childhood. *Am. J. Hematol.* **2005**, *78*, 318. [CrossRef]

31. Page, M.J.; McKenzie, J.E.; Bossuyt, P.M.; Boutron, I.; Hoffmann, T.C.; Mulrow, C.D.; Shamseer, L.; Tetzlaff, J.M.; Akl, E.A.; Brennan, S.E.; et al. The PRISMA 2020 Statement: An Updated Guideline for Reporting Systematic Reviews. *BMJ* 2021, *372*, n71. [CrossRef] [PubMed]
32. Brito, H.S.H.; Braga, J.A.P.; Loggetto, S.R.; Machado, R.S.; Granato, C.F.H.; Kawakami, E. *Helicobacter pylori* Infection & Immune Thrombocytopenic Purpura in Children and Adolescents: A Randomized Controlled Trial. *Platelets* 2015, *26*, 336–341. [CrossRef] [PubMed]
33. Ferrara, M.; Capozzi, L.; Russo, R. Effect of *Helicobacter pylori* Eradication on Platelet Count in Children with Chronic Idiopathic Thrombocytopenic Purpura. *Hematology* 2009, *14*, 282–285. [CrossRef] [PubMed]
34. Baxendell, K.; Walelign, S.; Tesfaye, M.; Wordofa, M.; Abera, D.; Mesfin, A.; Wolde, M.; Desta, K.; Tsegaye, A.; Taye, B. Association between Infection with *Helicobacter pylori* and Platelet Indices among School-Aged Children in Central Ethiopia: A Cross-Sectional Study. *BMJ Open* 2019, *9*, e027748. [CrossRef] [PubMed]
35. Neefjes, V.M.E.; Heijboer, H.; Tamminga, R.Y.J.H. Pylori Infection in Childhood Chronic Immune Thrombocytopenic Purpura. *Haematologica* 2007, *92*, 576. [CrossRef]
36. Maghbool, M.; Maghbool, M.; Shahriari, M.; Karimi, M. Does *Helicobacter pylori* Play a Role in the Pathogenesis of Childhood Chronic Idiopathic Thrombocytopenic Purpura? *Pediatr. Rep.* 2009, *1*, e2. [CrossRef]
37. Jaing, T.H.; Yang, C.P.; Hung, I.J.; Chiu, C.H.; Chang, K.W. Efficacy of *Helicobacter pylori* Eradication on Platelet Recovery in Children with Chronic Idiopathic Thrombocytopenic Purpura. *Acta Paediatr.* 2003, *92*, 1153–1157. [CrossRef]
38. Hayashi, H.; Okuda, M.; Aoyagi, N.; Yoshiyama, M.; Miyashiro, E.; Kounami, S.; Yoshikawa, N. *Helicobacter pylori* Infection in Children with Chronic Idiopathic Thrombocytopenic Purpura. *Pediatr. Int.* 2005, *47*, 292–295. [CrossRef]
39. Wu, S.-R.; Kuo, H.-C.; Huang, W.-C.; Huang, Y.-F.; Chiou, Y.-H.; Chang, Y.-H.; Nong, B.-R. Incidence, Clinical Characteristics, and Associated Diseases in Patients with Immune Thrombocytopenia: A Nationwide Population-Based Study in Taiwan. *Thromb. Res.* 2018, *164*, 90–95. [CrossRef]
40. Abdollahi, A.; Shoar, S.; Ghasemi, S.; Zohreh, O.-Y. Is *Helicobacter pylori* Infection a Risk Factor for Idiopathic Thrombocytopenic Purpura in Children? *Ann. Afr. Med.* 2015, *14*, 177–181. [CrossRef]
41. Rajantie, J.; Klemola, T. *Helicobacter pylori* and Idiopathic Thrombocytopenic Purpura in Children. *Blood* 2003, *101*, 1660. [CrossRef] [PubMed]
42. Kim, C.Y.; Lee, E.H.; Yoon, H.S. High Remission Rate of Chronic Immune Thrombocytopenia in Children: Result of 20-Year Follow-Up. *Yonsei Med. J.* 2016, *57*, 127–131. [CrossRef] [PubMed]
43. Wu, K.-S.; Hsiao, C.-C.; Yu, H.-R.; Huang, E.-Y.; Mai, W.-L.; Sheen, J.-M. *Helicobacter pylori* Infection and Childhood Idiopathic Thrombocytopenic Purpura. *Acta Paediatr. Taiwan.* 2007, *48*, 263–266.
44. Săsăran, M.O.; Meliț, L.E.; Mocan, S.; Ghiga, D.V.; Dobru, E.D. Pediatric Gastritis and Its Impact on Hematologic Parameters. *Medicine* 2020, *99*, e21985. [CrossRef]
45. Afifi, R.A.-R.; Ali, D.K.; Shaheen, I.A.-M. A Localized Case-Control Study of Extra-Gastric Manifestations of *Helicobacter pylori* Infection in Children. *Indian J. Pediatr.* 2011, *78*, 418–422. [CrossRef] [PubMed]
46. Bisogno, G.; Errigo, G.; Rossetti, F.; Sainati, L.; Pusiol, A.; Da Dalt, L.; Colleselli, P.; Grotto, P.; Carli, M. The Role of *Helicobacter pylori* in Children with Chronic Idiopathic Thrombocytopenic Purpura. *J. Pediatr. Hematol. Oncol.* 2008, *30*, 53–57. [CrossRef]
47. Loffredo, G.; Marzano, M.G.; Migliorati, R.; Miele, E.; Menna, F.; Poggi, V.; Staiano, A. The Relationship between Immune Thrombocytopenic Purpura and *Helicobacter pylori* Infection in Children: Where Is the Truth? *Eur. J. Pediatr.* 2007, *166*, 1067–1068. [CrossRef]
48. Eghbali, A.; Siavashan, V.R.; Bagheri, B.; Afzal, R.R. Impact of *Helicobacter pylori* Eradication in Children with Acute Immune Thrombocytopenia: A Randomized Controlled Study. *Arch. Pediatr. Infect. Dis.* 2019, *7*, e90522. [CrossRef]
49. Morimoto, Y.; Yoshida, N.; Kawashima, N.; Matsumoto, K.; Kato, K. Identification of Predictive Factors for Response to Intravenous Immunoglobulin Treatment in Children with Immune Thrombocytopenia. *Int. J. Hematol.* 2014, *99*, 597–602. [CrossRef]
50. Jaing, T.-H.; Tsay, P.-K.; Hung, I.-J.; Chiu, C.-H.; Yang, C.-P.; Huang, I.-A. The Role of *Helicobacter pylori* Infection in Children with Acute Immune Thrombocytopenic Purpura. *Pediatr. Blood Cancer* 2006, *47*, 215–217. [CrossRef]
51. Treepongkaruna, S.; Sirachainan, N.; Kanjanapongkul, S.; Winaichatsak, A.; Sirithorn, S.; Sumritsopak, R.; Chuansumrit, A. Absence of Platelet Recovery Following *Helicobacter pylori* Eradication in Childhood Chronic Idiopathic Thrombocytopenic Purpura: A Multi-Center Randomized Controlled Trial. *Pediatr. Blood Cancer* 2009, *53*, 72–77. [CrossRef] [PubMed]
52. Kuwana, M. *Helicobacter pylori*-Associated Immune Thrombocytopenia: Clinical Features and Pathogenic Mechanisms. *World J. Gastroenterol.* 2014, *20*, 714–723. [CrossRef] [PubMed]
53. Stasi, R.; Rossi, Z.; Stipa, E.; Amadori, S.; Newland, A.C.; Provan, D. *Helicobacter pylori* Eradication in the Management of Patients with Idiopathic Thrombocytopenic Purpura. *Am. J. Med.* 2005, *118*, 414–419. [CrossRef] [PubMed]
54. Wu, Z.; Zhou, J.; Prsoon, P.; Wei, X.; Liu, X.; Peng, B. Low Expression of FCGRIIB in Macrophages of Immune Thrombocytopenia-Affected Individuals. *Int. J. Hematol.* 2012, *96*, 588–593. [CrossRef]
55. Santambrogio, E.; Orsucci, L. *Helicobacter pylori* and Hematological Disorders. *Minerva Gastroenterol. Dietol.* 2019, *65*, 204–213. [CrossRef]
56. Mărginean, C.D.; Mărginean, C.O.; Meliț, L.E. *Helicobacter pylori*-Related Extraintestinal Manifestations—Myth or Reality. *Children* 2022, *9*, 1352. [CrossRef]

57. Sherman, P.M.; Lin, F.Y.H. Extradigestive Manifestation of *Helicobacter pylori* Infection in Children and Adolescents. *Can. J. Gastroenterol.* **2005**, *19*, 421–424. [CrossRef]
58. Fujimura, K. *Helicobacter pylori* Infection and Idiopathic Thrombocytopenic Purpura. *Int. J. Hematol.* **2005**, *81*, 113–118. [CrossRef]
59. Sahi, P.K.; Chandra, J. Immune Thrombocytopenia: American Society of Hematology Guidelines, 2019. *Indian Pediatr* **2020**, *57*, 854–856. [CrossRef]
60. De Mattia, D.; Del Vecchio, G.C.; Russo, G.; De Santis, A.; Ramenghi, U.; Notarangelo, L.; Jankovic, M.; Molinari, A.C.; Zecca, M.; Nobili, B.; et al. Management of Chronic Childhood Immune Thrombocytopenic Purpura: AIEOP Consensus Guidelines. *Acta Haematol.* **2010**, *123*, 96–109. [CrossRef]
61. Ribeiro, R.d.A.; de Galiza Neto, G.C.; Furtado, A.d.S.; Ribeiro, L.L.P.A.; Kubrusly, M.S.; Kubrusly, E.S. Proposal of Treatment Algorithm for Immune Thromocytopenia in Adult Patients of a Hematology Service at a Referral Center in Northeastern Brazil. *Hematol. Transfus. Cell Ther.* **2019**, *41*, 253–261. [CrossRef] [PubMed]
62. Liebman, H.A.; Stasi, R. Secondary Immune Thrombocytopenic Purpura. *Curr. Opin. Hematol.* **2007**, *14*, 557–573. [CrossRef] [PubMed]
63. Michel, M.; Cooper, N.; Jean, C.; Frissora, C.; Bussel, J.B. Does Helicobater Pylori Initiate or Perpetuate Immune Thrombocytopenic Purpura? *Blood* **2004**, *103*, 890–896. [CrossRef] [PubMed]
64. Michel, M.; Khellaf, M.; Desforges, L.; Lee, K.; Schaeffer, A.; Godeau, B.; Bierling, P. Autoimmune Thrombocytopenic Purpura and *Helicobacter pylori* Infection. *Arch. Intern. Med.* **2002**, *162*, 1033–1036. [CrossRef] [PubMed]
65. Campuzano-Maya, G. Proof of an Association between *Helicobacter pylori* and Idiopathic Thrombocytopenic Purpura in Latin America. *Helicobacter* **2007**, *12*, 265–273. [CrossRef]
66. Kuwana, M.; Ikeda, Y. *Helicobacter pylori* and Immune Thrombocytopenic Purpura: Unsolved Questions and Controversies. *Int. J. Hematol.* **2006**, *84*, 309–315. [CrossRef]
67. Cirasino, L.; Robino, A.M.; Cattaneo, M.; Pioltelli, P.E.; Pogliani, E.M.; Morra, E.; Colombo, P.; Palmieri, G.A. Reviewed Diagnosis of Primary and Secondary Immune Thrombocytopenic Purpura in 79 Adult Patients Hospitalized in 2000–2002. *Blood Coagul. Fibrinolysis* **2011**, *22*, 1–6. [CrossRef]
68. Cooper, N. A Review of the Management of Childhood Immune Thrombocytopenia: How Can We Provide an Evidence-Based Approach? *Br. J. Haematol.* **2014**, *165*, 756–767. [CrossRef]
69. Pacifico, L.; Osborn, J.F.; Tromba, V.; Romaggioli, S.; Bascetta, S.; Chiesa, C. *Helicobacter pylori* Infection and Extragastric Disorders in Children: A Critical Update. *World J. Gastroenterol.* **2014**, *20*, 1379–1401. [CrossRef]
70. Hamzah, R.; Yusof, N.; Tumian, N.R.; Abdul Aziz, S.; Mohammad Basri, N.S.; Leong, T.S.; Ho, K.W.; Selvaratnam, V.; Tan, S.M.; Muhamad Jamil, S.A. Clinical Epidemiology, Treatment Outcome and Mortality Rate of Newly Diagnosed Immune Thrombocytopenia in Adult Multicentre Study in Malaysia. *J. Blood Med.* **2022**, *13*, 337–349. [CrossRef]
71. Kim, B.J.; Kim, H.S.; Jang, H.J.; Kim, J.H. *Helicobacter pylori* Eradication in Idiopathic Thrombocytopenic Purpura: A Meta-Analysis of Randomized Trials. *Gastroenterol. Res. Pract.* **2018**, *2018*, 6090878. [CrossRef] [PubMed]
72. Sierra, M.S.; Hastings, E.V.; Goodman, K.J. What Do We Know about Benefits of H. Pylori Treatment in Childhood? *Gut Microbes* **2013**, *4*, 549–567. [CrossRef] [PubMed]
73. Pezeshki, S.M.S.; Saki, N.; Ghandali, M.V.; Ekrami, A.; Avarvand, A.Y. Effect of *Helicobacter pylori* Eradication on Patients with ITP: A Meta-Analysis of Studies Conducted in the Middle East. *Blood Res.* **2021**, *56*, 38–43. [CrossRef] [PubMed]
74. Franchini, M.; Cruciani, M.; Mengoli, C.; Pizzolo, G.; Veneri, D. Effect of *Helicobacter pylori* Eradication on Platelet Count in Idiopathic Thrombocytopenic Purpura: A Systematic Review and Meta-Analysis. *J. Antimicrob. Chemother.* **2007**, *60*, 237–246. [CrossRef] [PubMed]
75. Estrada-Gómez, R.A.; Parra-Ortega, I.; Martínez-Barreda, C.; Ruiz-Argüelles, G.J. *Helicobacter pylori* Infection and Thrombocytopenia: A Single-Institution Experience in Mexico. *Rev. Investig. Clin.* **2007**, *59*, 112–115.
76. Matsukawa, Y.; Kato, K.; Hatta, Y.; Iwamoto, M.; Mizuno, S.; Kurihara, R.; Arakawa, Y.; Kurosaka, H.; Hayashi, I.; Sawada, S. *Helicobacter pylori* Eradication Reduces Platelet Count in Patients without Idiopathic Thrombocytopenic Purpura. *Platelets* **2007**, *18*, 52–55. [CrossRef]
77. Akar, T. Can Mean Platelet Volume IndIcate HelIcobacter posItIvIty and severIty of gastrIc InflammatIon? An orIgInal Study and revIew of the lIterature. *Acta Clin. Croat.* **2019**, *58*, 576–582. [CrossRef]
78. Sahin, Y.; Gubur, O.; Tekingunduz, E. Relationship between the Severity of *Helicobacter pylori* Infection and Neutrophil and Lymphocyte Ratio and Mean Platelet Volume in Children. *Arch. Argent. Pediatr.* **2020**, *118*, e241–e245. [CrossRef]
79. Aktas, G.; Sit, M.; Tekce, H.; Alcelik, A.; Savli, H.; Simsek, T.; Ozmen, E.; Isci, A.Z.; Apuhan, T. Mean Platelet Volume in Nasal Polyps. *West Indian Med. J.* **2013**, *62*, 515–518. [CrossRef]
80. Lee, A.; Hong, J.; Chung, H.; Koh, Y.; Cho, S.-J.; Byun, J.M.; Kim, S.G.; Kim, I. *Helicobacter pylori* Eradication Affects Platelet Count Recovery in Immune Thrombocytopenia. *Sci. Rep.* **2020**, *10*, 9370. [CrossRef]
81. Stasi, R.; Sarpatwari, A.; Segal, J.B.; Osborn, J.; Evangelista, M.L.; Cooper, N.; Provan, D.; Newland, A.; Amadori, S.; Bussel, J.B. Effects of Eradication of *Helicobacter pylori* Infection in Patients with Immune Thrombocytopenic Purpura: A Systematic Review. *Blood* **2009**, *113*, 1231–1240. [CrossRef] [PubMed]
82. Ikuse, T.; Toda, M.; Kashiwagi, K.; Maruyama, K.; Nagata, M.; Tokushima, K.; Ito, N.; Tokita, K.; Kyodo, R.; Hosoi, K.; et al. Efficacy of *Helicobacter pylori* Eradication Therapy on Platelet Recovery in Pediatric Immune Thrombocytopenic Purpura-Case Series and a Systematic Review. *Microorganisms* **2020**, *8*, 1457. [CrossRef] [PubMed]

83. Kurekci, A.E.; Atay, A.A.; Sarici, S.U.; Ozcan, O. Complete Platelet Recovery after Treatment of *Helicobacter pylori* Infection in a Child with Chronic Immune Thrombocytopenic Purpura: A Case Report. *Pediatr. Hematol. Oncol.* **2004**, *21*, 593–596. [CrossRef]
84. Takechi, T.; Unemoto, J.; Ishihara, M.; Hosokawa, T.; Zushi, N.; Shiraishi, T.; Ogura, H.; Wakiguchi, H. Idiopathic Thrombocytopenic Purpura Associated with *Helicobacter pylori* Infection. *Pediatr. Int.* **2006**, *48*, 76–78. [CrossRef]
85. Todo, K.; Ohmae, T.; Osamura, T.; Imamura, T.; Imashuku, S. Severe *Helicobacter pylori* Gastritis-Related Thrombocytopenia and Iron Deficiency Anemia in an Adolescent Female. *Ann. Hematol.* **2016**, *95*, 835–836. [CrossRef]
86. Kumagai, T.; Sekigawa, K.; Hashimoto, N.; Shirato, R. Remission of Idiopathic Thrombocytopenic Purpura by Eradicating *Helicobacter pylori* after Omeprazole Monotherapy. *Int. J. Hematol.* **2001**, *74*, 237–238. [CrossRef]
87. Ikeda, N.; Shoji, H.; Ikuse, T.; Ohkawa, N.; Kashiwagi, K.; Saito, Y.; Shimizu, T. A Case of Neonatal Thrombocytopenia Due to Maternal *Helicobacter pylori*-Associated Immune Thrombocytopenia. *Helicobacter* **2023**, *28*, e12976. [CrossRef]
88. Kühne, T.; Michaels, L.A. *Helicobacter pylori* in Children with Chronic Idiopathic Thrombocytopenic Purpura: Are the Obstacles in the Way Typical in Pediatric Hematology? *J. Pediatr. Hematol. Oncol.* **2008**, *30*, 2–3. [CrossRef]

Disclaimer/Publisher's Note: The statements, opinions and data contained in all publications are solely those of the individual author(s) and contributor(s) and not of MDPI and/or the editor(s). MDPI and/or the editor(s) disclaim responsibility for any injury to people or property resulting from any ideas, methods, instructions or products referred to in the content.

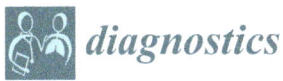

Article

Helicobacter pylori Infection in Children: A Possible Reason for Headache?

Ancuta Lupu [1], Cristina Gavrilovici [1], Vasile Valeriu Lupu [1,*], Anca Lavinia Cianga [1,*], Andrei Tudor Cernomaz [2], Iuliana Magdalena Starcea [1,*], Cristina Maria Mihai [3,*], Elena Tarca [4], Adriana Mocanu [1] and Silvia Fotea [5]

1. Pediatrics, "Grigore T. Popa" University of Medicine and Pharmacy, 700115 Iasi, Romania
2. III-rd Medical Department, "Grigore T. Popa" University of Medicine and Pharmacy, 700115 Iasi, Romania
3. Pediatrics, Faculty of General Medicine, Ovidius University, 900470 Constanta, Romania
4. Department of Surgery II—Pediatric Surgery, "Grigore T. Popa" University of Medicine and Pharmacy, 700115 Iasi, Romania
5. Medical Department, Faculty of Medicine and Pharmacy, "Dunarea de Jos" University of Galati, 800008 Galati, Romania
* Correspondence: valeriulupu@yahoo.com (V.V.L.); ancalaviniacianga@gmail.com (A.L.C.); magdabirm@yahoo.com (I.M.S.); cristina2603@yahoo.com (C.M.M.)

Abstract: (1) Background: The correlation between infection with *Helicobacter pylori* (*H. pylori*) and headache has been argued and explored for a long time, but a clear association between the simultaneous presence of the two in children has not been established yet. In this study, we aimed to explore this relationship in children from the Northeast region of Romania. (2) Methods: A retrospective study exploring the correlation between children having *H. pylori* infection and headache or migraine was conducted on a batch of 1757 children, hospitalized over 3 years in a pediatric gastroenterology department in Northeast Romania. (3) Results: A total of 130 children of both sexes had headache. From 130 children, 54 children (41.5%) also presented *H. pylori* infection. A significant association between headache and *H. pylori* infection ($\chi 2$; $p < 0.01$) was noticed. (4) Conclusions: More studies are needed on this relationship, and we emphasize the importance of further analyses, as they present great clinical importance for both prompt diagnosis and treatment.

Keywords: headache; *Helicobacter pylori*; children; migraine

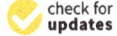

1. Introduction

Headache represents a common complaint among the pediatric population, which, as well as in adults, is frequently underdiagnosed, although it affects the quality of life. The prevalence of migraine, one of the most common types of primary headache, is estimated at approximately 9% among the pediatric population, and a perpetual increase in its incidence has been registered over the last three decades. Among the indicative factors of an increased incidence of headache, Anttila et al. mention sleep deprivation, an increase in the use of information technology, and soft drink consumption [1]. In children, migraine and tension-type headache usually occur simultaneously with a mixed symptomatology [2]. They are usually considered to be self-limited conditions, but they can persist from childhood to adulthood, affecting the quality of life [3]. Being a burdensome condition, headache plays an important role in mental and physical health, and in children, it can impair school performance or lead to social isolation [4,5]. Thus, headache can interfere negatively with the entire education path in childhood and adolescence [6]. In children, headache can present through neurobehavioral symptoms such as agitation, sleep disturbances, irritability, and trouble concentrating [7]. Various factors such as sleep disorders, genetics, environmental factors such as humidity, light, or noise, severe trauma, and menstruation have been indicated as risk factors and possible triggers of migraine

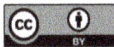

headaches [8]. The literature suggests that there may be a significant connection between *Helicobacter pylori* (*H. pylori*) infection and headaches. However, though this association has been explored in adults, there is still a significant gap in data regarding this issue in the pediatric population [9].

H. pylori is a gram-negative, microaerophilic, spiral bacterium with increased motility as a result of the presence of multiple unipolar flagella [10]. It generates urease and colonizes the mucus layer adjacent to the gastric mucosa, usually being responsible for gastrointestinal impairments such as chronic active gastroenteritis, infection, gastric and duodenal ulcer, and, more rarely, stomach cancer [11]. The bacterium possesses adaptive characteristics that allows the body's survival in an acidic environment. It produces urease that consequently converts urea into bicarbonate and ammonium and leads to the neutralization of the gastric acid [12]. However, numerous studies claim that infection with *H. pylori* may be the result of various extra-digestive conditions such as neurological, cardiovascular, metabolic, hematologic, ocular, or dermatological ones.

Along with various extra-digestive impairments, the relationship between the infection with *H. pylori* and neurological manifestations such as mild cognitive impairment, migraine, or Alzheimer's disease have been extensively studied, but there are no clear results concerning the pathophysiology of the process [13]. However, it was shown that the systemic effects of the infection with *H. pylori* are the result of the modulation of the gut–brain axis (GBA), which consists of a two-way signaling pathway between the gastro-intestinal tract (GIT) and the brain, and which plays a pivotal role in infections and additional clinical outcomes [14–16].

Among the stated hypotheses, *H. pylori* infection may trigger a host immune response to the presence of bacteria and a consequent release of vasoactive substances [17]. The pathological process encompasses immunological events such as migration of lymphocytic, monocytic, and neutrophilic invasion into the gastric mucosa and submucosa, along with the release of chemokines or pro-inflammatory cytokines such as IL-6, IL-1β, TNF-α, or IL-8 at the site of infection [18,19]. Moreover, *H. pylori* infection disturbs the balance in the microbiota, influences the host–pathogen interaction, and plays an important role in the modulation of the gastric microenvironment, thus causing changes in homeostasis [20,21].

H. pylori type I cagA-positive strains are also thought to have the ability to induce a significant release of proinflammatory substances by the gastric mucosa, leading consequently to systemic vasospasms [22]. As described in the literature, for patients with *H. pylori* infection who complain of headache, bacteria eradication might improve the symptoms or reduce the migraine-related disability level [19].

There exist multiple pharmaceutical treatment plans for managing both digestive and extra-digestive infections and diseases caused by *H. pylori*. Timely and precise identification of *H. pylori* plays a critical role in the effective treatment and eradication of the bacterium. Due to *H. pylori*'s specific localization in the gastric mucus layer, pharmacotherapy must be effective in penetrating this layer to prevent *H. pylori* colonization. As such, the medication used must be able to penetrate the gastric mucosal layer [23].

The data on children in Romania regarding *H. pylori* infection reveals a declining trend that might be the result of improving socio-economic conditions [24]. However, Yuan et al. highlighted in their review that despite advances in medical science, *H. pylori* infection continues to exhibit a high incidence rate among children worldwide, emphasizing the significance of this infection [25].

Although the data regarding the link between *H. pylori* infection and headache have been explored for many years, and the results of this association are controversial, we present the results we obtained on a pediatric population in Northeast Romania.

2. Materials and Methods

We performed a retrospective study on 1757 children, hospitalized over 3 years in a pediatric gastroenterology department in "St. Maria" Emergency Hospital for Children in Iasi, Romania, complaining of symptoms suggestive of gastric or duodenal ulcer. Thus, according to Jones et al.'s recommendations from 2017 [26], all the 1757 patients underwent superior digestive endoscopy. With a treatment that was likely to be offered, biopsies and cultures were taken for the examined patients. The diagnostic of infection with *H. pylori* was established by having *H. pylori*-positive gastritis on histopathology examination, along with positive cultures. For these patients, we focused on the association between the *Helicobacter pylori* infection and the presence of headache/migraine. Out of the 1757 patients of both sexes, we selected based on the anamnestic findings those who complained of migraine or headache at admission. To assess the importance of headache, the Migraine Disability Assessment Test (MIDAS) along with the Visual Analogue Scale (VAS) were utilized.

We excluded children who previously received eradication treatment of *H. pylori*, those who previously had treatment with acetaminophen or antibiotics, children with evidence of bleeding of the gastro-intestinal tract at endoscopy, those who complained of headache or migraine during previous hospitalizations or had a medical past history of headache/migraine, patients with gastrointestinal disorders known to be associated with headache such as inflammatory bowel syndrome, celiac disease, or functional abdominal pain, and patients with a history of drug use, including H2 blockers, antibiotics, or proton pump inhibitors, within 4 weeks [27–29].

Based on the available information in the literature, migraine was defined as the presence of severe and recurrent headache attacks, along with neurological and autonomic symptoms. The diagnostic criteria for pediatric migraine were realized according to the second edition of the International Classification of Headache Disorders (ICHD-2) [30].

All patients enrolled underwent upper gastrointestinal endoscopic examination with intravenous sedation, and video pediatric gastroduodenoscopes from Pentax and Olympus were used. For children under 10 years old, the procedure was performed under general anesthesia. Biopsies were collected from the antrum and gastric corpus during endoscopy for rapid urease testing and histological and bacteriological examination [27–29].

Informed consent was taken from all caregivers, and the study was approved by the "St. Mary" Emergency Hospital for Children Ethics Committee's (no.31490/29.10.2021).

Data were extracted from the hospital database, patient observation charts, endoscopy results, and discharge papers. IBM SPSS 17.0 platform, GraphPad Prism, and Microsoft Excel were used to analyze the data.

3. Results

From the 1757 patients, 542 had infection with *H. pylori*. We reported the structure of the study group in Table 1.

Table 1. Study group presenting or not presenting *H. pylori* infection.

Infection with *H. pylori*		%
absent	1215	69.2
present	542	30.8
Headache		
absent	1627	92.6
present	130	7.4
Sex		
female	1210	68.9
male	547	31.1
Area of living		
urban	643	36.6
rural	1114	63.4

The main symptoms that led to admission to the pediatric gastroenterology clinic and that later resulted in the diagnosis of gastritis were represented in order of frequency by: abdominal pain in 1664 cases (94.7%), nausea in 668 cases (38.0%), vomiting in 468 cases (27.2%), inappetence in 243 cases (13.8%), heartburn in 144 cases (8.2%), headache in 130 cases (7.4%), vertigo in 87 cases (5.0%), constipation in 57 cases (3.2%), abdominal flatulence in 56 cases (6.2%), asthenia in 26 cases (1.5%), and early satiety in 17 cases (1.0%).

Among the non-specific symptoms, we found a strongly significant association between headache and infection with *H. pylori* (χ^2; $p < 0.01$) (Table 2). Of the 130 children who had headaches, 54 children (41.5%) were also diagnosed with infection with *H. pylori*.

Table 2. Estimated parameters in testing the association between *H. pylori* infection and headache.

	Headache (+)	Headache (−)
HP (+)	54	488
HP (−)	76	1139
	p value = 0.006	

HP—Helicobacter pylori.

Important differences between sex-stratified subgroups regarding *H. pylori* infection and headache were also noticed. Our evaluation showed that the prevalence of headache was almost five times higher in girls, out of the total number of 130 cases (83.1% females vs. 16.9% males). (Table 3).

Table 3. Differences between sex-stratified subgroups.

	HP (+)	HP (−)	Headache (+)	Headache (−)
Sex				
male	145	402	22	525
female	397	813	108	1102
		$p = 0.0002$ chi-squared		

HP—Helicobacter pylori.

Moreover, regarding the area of living, we noticed a higher number of children from rural areas—104 children (80%), compared to 26 children (20%) from urban areas—among all cases with headache.

Subsequently, we evaluated the environmental distribution of *H. pylori* (+) and (−) patients. The distribution of children with *H. pylori* (+) according to the area of living revealed a frequency of 75.3% in rural environments compared to 24.7% in urban areas (Figure 1).

In addition, the exploration of the age distribution of all the patients from the initial batch showed a mean value of 13.19 years (SD = +3.501) (Figure 2).

Considering the population analyzed, which is represented by hospital-referred pediatric patients with clinical pictures suggestive of gastritis, there seems to be a significant difference in the odds of having chronic headache complaints between the *H. pylori* positive and negative subgroups: odds ratio = 1.658 (95% confidence interval [CI]: 1.15–2.38)—as indicated by a post-hoc binary logistic regression model including the presence of headache as the dependent variable and *H. pylori* infection status, gender, and living conditions as covariates. The computed power was 77% (given the sample size of 1757 and an effect size of 0.065), and the goodness of fit of the model was deemed low. More data would be useful, but given the retrospective nature of our analysis, no viable solution to enlarge the data pool was identified.

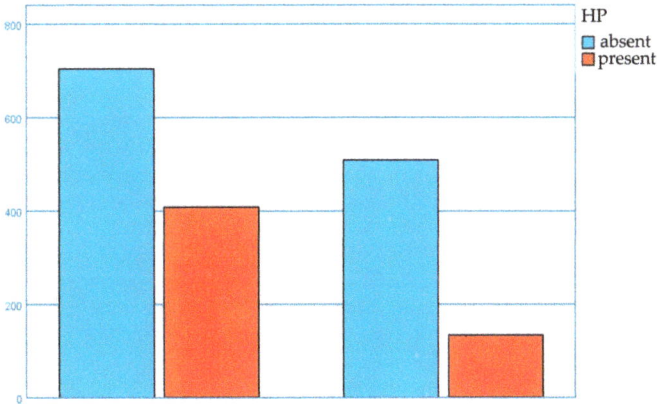

Left bars= rural area; Right bars= urban area.

Figure 1. Environmental distribution of patients with or without infection with *H. pylori*.

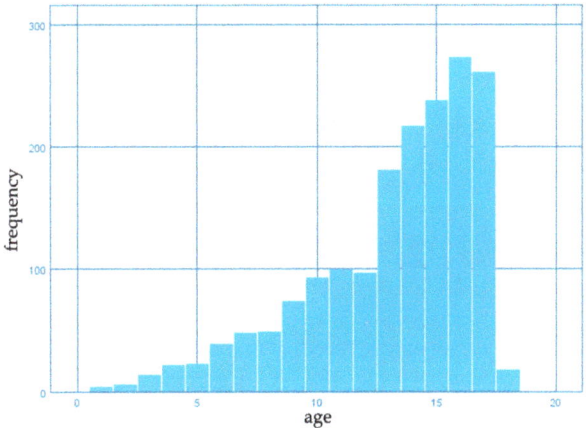

Figure 2. Age distribution of patients with or without infection with *H. pylori*.

4. Discussion

Migraine is a common condition consisting of primary headaches with a prevalence of 15% in Western societies [31]. Secondary headache is frequently reported by patients with various gastrointestinal disorders such as gastroesophageal reflux disease, inflammatory bowel syndrome, constipation, functional abdominal pain, or *H. pylori* infection, but the potential causal link remains unclear [32,33]. However, in recent years, research has focused on the implication of *H. pylori* activity in the pathogenesis of migraine, as this microorganism was identified as a cause for multiple extra digestive manifestations [22]. It has been hypothesized that the recurrence of headaches following *H. pylori* infection may be due to the systemic vasospastic effects of proinflammatory substances that are released by the infected gastric mucosa [34]. Other authors indicate the production of platelet-activating factor in *H. pylori* infections and claim that the migraine attacks may be the result of the high level of serotonin released from platelets [35]. Eradication of *H. pylori* infection resulted in a significant reduction in the intensity, frequency, and duration of migraine attacks [36,37]. However, the studies conducted on the correlation between *H. pylori* infection and headache have provided mixed and controversial results.

Kikui et al. showed in their study that in comparison to non-migraine individuals of similar characteristics, migraine sufferers exhibit a higher prevalence of gastrointestinal comorbidities—specifically, increased odds of irritable bowel syndrome (adjusted odds ratio (95% CI: 3.8 (2.7 to 5.4)), heartburn (3.6 (95% CI 2.8 to 4.7)), gastroesophageal reflux disease (3.5 (2.5, 4.8)), ulcers (3.1 (95% CI 2.0 to 4.8)), frequent diarrhea (3.1 (95% CI 2.3 to 4.1)), and chronic constipation (2.5 (95% CI 1.9 to 3.3)) [38].

Our study found a strongly significant association between headache and infection with *H. pylori* ($\chi2$; $p < 0.01$). Out of the 130 children who complained of headaches, 54 of them (41.5%) also had concomitant *H. pylori* infection. Thereby, a high prevalence of infection with *H. pylori* in patients with headache/migraine is indicated. These results are in agreement with the findings of Cavestro et al., who conducted an impressive cross-sectional study on the relationship between *H. pylori* infection and headache and found a significant association between these two entities ($p = 0.009$) [39]. Moreover, in their case-control study, Yiannopoulou et al. presumed the same association and found that *H. pylori* infection prevalence was significantly higher in 49 patients with headache than in 51 control subjects ($p = 0.016$) [40]. In their study on 70 patients, Hosseinzadeh et al. also showed that the prevalence of migraine was significantly correlated with the IgG and IgM titer against *H. pylori* ($p \leq 0.048$ and $p \leq 0.03$, respectively) [41].

In addition, the eradication treatment for *H. pylori* infection proved a beneficial effect on the patients suffering from migraine compared to controls in a study conducted by Tunca et al. [36]. Comparable results were obtained in 2012 by Faraji et al., who showed that their patients with migraine who received *H. pylori* eradication treatment presented a lower headache-related disability level than those in the placebo batch. The mechanisms involved could be linked to oxidative stress and nitric oxide imbalance secondary to acute inflammation caused by *H. pylori* infection [42]. The same improvement was obtained by Karkelis et al., who evaluated a number of 65 children suffering from headache and migraine and discovered that 17 of them had concomitant *H. pylori* infection. After completing the anti-Helicobacter infection therapy, a complete resolution of migraine symptoms was noticed for all the patients in the study [43].

All these studies agree with the results reported by Gasbarrini et al. in 1997 and 1998, who described both an association between *H. pylori* infection and headache, as well as a significant alleviation of the intensity of headache along with the eradication of *H. pylori* infection [44,45]. In their case-control study, Hassan et al. obtained a similar result with a significant prevalence of infection with *H. pylori* in 77 migraine patients ($p < 0.001$, OR = 3.439), but at the same time, they obtained no correlation between *H. pylori* infection and migraine attacks, migraine disability assessment test, or the visual analogue scale. In addition, *H. pylori* infection did not represent a trigger for the migraine attacks or a risk factor for an increased frequency of headache episodes [46].

Su et al. also described in their meta-analysis of five case-control studies that *H. pylori* infection was positive in approximately 45% of patients with migraine compared to a prevalence rate of 33% among healthy controls (OR = 1.92, 95%CI: 1.05–3.51, $p = 0.001$). Moreover, the infection rate of *H. pylori* was higher in Asian patients with migraine, but the same could not be established for European ones (OR = 3.48 and 1.19, respectively) [47].

In contradiction with the results above, Lee et al. found a higher frequency of *H. pylori* infection in patients with migraines or headaches than in the control groups, but no statistical significance was obtained ($p = 0.51$) [48]. In Iran, a study was conducted on 84 patients that revealed a significant correlation between the severity of headache and the IgG antibody. However, there was no statistically significant difference observed in levels of IgG in migraine versus control subjects. On the other hand, they observed a statistical significance in the IgM antibody titer against *H. pylori* among the patients with migraine compared to those in the control batches ($p = 0.004$) [49]. The role of interleukin-10 was also speculated, on one hand because its elevation was associated with both migraine and *H. pylori* infection (cagA-positive strains, in particular), and on the other hand, due to the fact that sumatriptan (5-HT1D receptor agonist) decreases the levels of this cytokine during a migraine attack [50,51].

In another study conducted on 31 children complaining of migraine and abdominal pain, an impressive high prevalence of esophagitis (41.9%), antral gastritis (38.7%), duodenitis (87.1%), and corpus gastritis (51.6%) was found. However, only seven patients out of the total had simultaneous *H. pylori* infection, and no association between migraine and *H. pylori* infection could be made [52]. In the same manner, Ciancarelli et al. evaluated 30 subjects suffering from migraine and found that for only 16.7% of them, the infection with *H. pylori* was confirmed, leading to the absence of a certain association between infection with *H. pylori* and migraine [53].

Interestingly, a retrospective study from Turkey performed on 526 subjects with migraine described that the infection with *H. pylori*, as a chronic infection, can be more aggressive and may represent one of the risk factors of the apparition and development of matter lesions in these patients. Here, Ocal et al. found that white matter lesions (WMLs) were present in 178 (33.8%) *H. pylori*-positive subjects ($p < 0.05$), and more than that, there was a 2.5-fold higher incidence of WMLs on the brain MRIs of migraine patients with *H. pylori* infection [54]. In an impressive cross-sectional study from 2021 that covered 489,753 participants, Welander et al. found a significant association between migraine and *H. pylori* infection when entered separately, but with other gastro-intestinal conditions added to the same adjusted model, the statistical significance could not be validated (OR = 1.34, $p = 0.024$) [55].

Having a multifactorial susceptibility with hormonal, genetic, and environmental factors each playing different, but important roles, headache affects over 17% of females and only 5–8% of males [56]. In our study, we also found that out of the 130 patients who complained of headache, 108 were females (83.1%), and only 22 were males (16.9%). Hormati et al. also described in their research on 341 patients the presence of a higher prevalence of migraine among females ($p = 0.003$) [57]. Akbari et al. described in their research performed on 305 patients with dyspepsia that the prevalence of migraine was significantly higher in female patients compared to male patients (48.9% vs. 35.5%, respectively, $p < 0.010$) [58]. This idea may be explained by the fact that girls are, firstly, usually more aware of their symptoms; secondly, they are prone to encounter more headache episodes along with the debut of menstrual cycles; and thirdly, females may present a more important bacterial load.

Regarding the area of living, the results of our study describe an increased incidence of headache/migraine among the pediatric population living in the rural area (80%) than those from the urban one (20%). These results are similar to the environmental distribution among the *H. pylori*-positive patients in our study, where 75.3% came from rural environments, whereas 24.7% lived in urban areas. These facts are consistent with Martin et al., who found that along with females and white people, the individuals residing in rural areas were more likely to suffer from headache than their respective comparison batches [59]. This hypothesis may be explained by the lack of specialist care in rural regions, thus leading to a lower adherence to headache or migraine management and treatment.

Knowing that *H. pylori* may lead to a low luminal pH by decreasing the bicarbonate secretion and increasing the acid secretion, this microorganism is recognized for its capacity to weaken the mucosa in the areas of gastric metaplasia and to make the mucosa more vulnerable to acid secretion. With many findings that associated the presence of *H. pylori* infection with migraine, Hormati et al. even postulated that a low value of the gastric pH can represent a trigger for headache, whereas the treatment with proton pump inhibitor (PPI) drugs may contribute to a significant improvement in both the severity and frequency of migraine attacks [57]. Another hypothesis raised by Lileikyte et al. involves the role of *H. pylori* in the development of vestibular migraine through irritation of the respiratory mucosa by the gastric acid, with subsequent inflammation or direct local infection caused by the presence of *H. pylori*, but these interesting affirmations need further explorations [60].

Further, individuals who suffer from migraines may have an increased risk of developing vitamin B12 deficiency due to the use of non-steroidal anti-inflammatory drugs for acute symptom relief and an increased incidence of active *H. pylori* infection [61]. In their article, Urits et al. describe that many individuals with migraines also experience gastro-intestinal damage, and *H. pylori* infection further impairs vitamin B12 absorption by destroying gastric parietal cells and reducing the availability of intrinsic factors [62].

Recently developed antimigraine drugs, such as anti-calcitonin gene-related peptide antibodies (CGRP) and monoclonal antibodies, offer a promising breakthrough in the treatment of migraine. The antimigraine mechanism of action of these drugs is similar to that of a kynurenic acid analogue, which can eliminate nitroglycerin-induced hyperalgesia by increasing CGRP expression. The kynurenine pathway, which is involved in the metabolism of L-tryptophan, is known to be altered in functional gastrointestinal diseases that are associated with migraines. In consequence, targeting this pathway may be an effective approach for treating both migraine and functional gastrointestinal diseases [63].

The present study showed a significant association between the infection with *H. pylori* and headache, but this relationship needs further studies. Although findings about the correlations between *H. pylori* and headache pathogenesis have been accumulating, the existing data do not completely amount to an unequivocal conclusion. However, there are certain effects of *H. pylori* infection, such as a decrease in food sensitivity, a lack of changes in plasma levels of thiobarbituric acid-reactive substances, and nitric oxide metabolites in infected patients compared to control subjects, and there is a similar prevalence of infection with *H. pylori* in patients with migraines compared to healthy subjects. These effects could be interpreted as valid arguments against *H. pylori* being considered a risk factor for migraines [36,47,53].

The need for establishing a definite association between headache and the *H. pylori* infection remains of great importance. Furthermore, our study has its limitations, such as a lack of paraclinical investigations consequent to the irregularity of the funding availability, the impossibility of performing real-time PCR for testing the antimicrobial susceptibility in *H. pylori* infection, along with the inability to conduct a long-term follow-up of the children due to their refractoriness.

5. Conclusions

Currently, there is sufficient evidence that correlates the increased frequency of migraine or headache with various gastro-intestinal disorders, compared to the general pediatric population. However, no clear association between *H. pylori* infection and headache was established to present. The gut–brain axis needs further exploration, as it is indicated in playing an important role between the *H. pylori* infection—migraine relationship.

It is important to note that further investigations should be carried out to evaluate the effectiveness of *H. pylori* eradication on the severity of headaches, the long-term clinical implications of this potential relationship, the assessment of multiple strains of *H. pylori* in children with headache, and the ethnicity of the participants under study. Furthermore, the variation in *H. pylori* in different regions should also be considered as a significant factor in future evaluations. We are certain that a better understanding of this association between headache and gastrointestinal disorders in children is of great clinical importance for both prompt diagnosis and treatment.

Author Contributions: C.G., A.T.C., E.T., I.M.S., C.M.M. and A.M. contributed equally with A.L. to this article. Conceptualization, A.L., A.L.C. and V.V.L.; methodology, C.M.M. and C.G.; software, A.T.C. and I.M.S.; formal analysis, A.T.C., E.T. and A.M.; investigation, A.L., A.L.C. and V.V.L.; data curation, A.T.C.; writing—original draft preparation, A.L., A.T.C., A.L.C. and E.T.; writing—review and editing, C.G., I.M.S., C.M.M., V.V.L., A.M. and S.F.; visualization, A.M. and I.M.S.; supervision, C.M.M. and C.G.; project administration, S.F. All authors have read and agreed to the published version of the manuscript.

Funding: This research received no external funding.

Institutional Review Board Statement: The study was conducted in accordance with the Declaration of Helsinki and approved by the Ethics Committee of the "St. Maria" Emergency Hospital for Children, Iasi, Romania (31490/29.10.2021).

Informed Consent Statement: Informed consent was obtained from all subjects involved in the study.

Data Availability Statement: The data presented in this study are available on request from the corresponding author.

Acknowledgments: We thank the Endoscopy Department and the colleagues for their involvement in managing these patients.

Conflicts of Interest: The authors declare no conflict of interest.

References

1. Anttila, P.; Metsähonkala, L.; Sillanpää, M. Long-term Trends in the Incidence of Headache in Finnish Schoolchildren. *Pediatrics* **2006**, *117*, e1197–e1201. [CrossRef]
2. Blankenburg, M.; Schroth, M.; Braun, S. Chronic headache in children and adolescents. *Klin. Padiatr.* **2019**, *231*, 14–20.
3. Teleanu, R.I.; Vladacenco, O.; Teleanu, D.M.; Epure, D.A. Treatment of Pediatric Migraine: A Review. *Maedica* **2016**, *11*, 136–143.
4. Bigal, M.E.; Lipton, R.B. The epidemiology, burden, and comorbidities of migraine. *Neurol. Clin.* **2009**, *27*, 321–334. [CrossRef]
5. Wöber-Bingöl, Ç. Epidemiology of Migraine and Headache in Children and Adolescents. *Curr. Pain Headache Rep.* **2013**, *17*, 341. [CrossRef]
6. Nieswand, V.; Richter, M.; Gossrau, G. Epidemiology of Headache in Children and Adolescents—Another Type of Pandemia. *Curr. Pain Headache Rep.* **2020**, *24*, 62. [CrossRef]
7. Gazerani, P. Migraine and Mood in Children. *Behav. Sci.* **2021**, *11*, 52. [CrossRef]
8. Deleu, D.; Hanssens, Y.; Worthing, E.A. Symptomatic and prophylactic treatment of migraine: A critical reappraisal. *Clin. Neuropharmacol.* **1998**, *21*, 267–279.
9. Le Gal, J.; Michel, J.F.; Rinaldi, V.E.; Spiri, D.; Moretti, R.; Bettati, D.; Romanello, S.; Berlese, P.; Lualdi, R.; Boizeau, P.; et al. Association between functional gastrointestinal disorders and migraine in children and adolescents: A case-control study. *Lancet Gastroenterol. Hepatol.* **2016**, *1*, 114–121. [CrossRef]
10. Wang, Y.-H.; Lv, Z.-F.; Zhong, Y.; Liu, D.-S.; Chen, S.-P.; Xie, Y. The internalization of Helicobacter pylori plays a role in the failure of H. pylori eradication. *Helicobacter* **2016**, *22*, e12324. [CrossRef]
11. Pinessi, L.; Savi, L.; Pellicano, R.; Rainero, I.; Valfre, W.; Gentile, S.; Cossotto, D.; Rizzetto, M.; Ponzetto, A. Chronic Helicobacter Pylori Infection and Migraine: A Case-Control Study. *Headache* **2000**, *40*, 836–839. [CrossRef]
12. Figueiredo, C.; Machado, J.C.; Yamaoka, Y. Pathogenesis of Helicobacter pylori Infection. *Helicobacter* **2005**, *10*, 14–20. [CrossRef]
13. Pellicano, R.; Ianiro, G.; Fagoonee, S.; Settanni, C.R.; Gasbarrini, A. Review: Extragastric diseases and Helicobacter pylori. *Helicobacter* **2020**, *25*, e12741. [CrossRef]
14. Kountouras, J.; Zavos, C.; Polyzos, S.A.; Deretzi, G. The gut-brain axis: Interactions between Helicobacter pylori and enteric and central nervous systems. *Ann. Gastroenterol.* **2015**, *28*, 506.
15. Budzyński, J. Brain-gut axis in the pathogenesis of Helicobacter pylori infection. *World J. Gastroenterol.* **2014**, *20*, 5212–5225. [CrossRef]
16. Baj, J.; Forma, A.; Flieger, W.; Morawska, I.; Michalski, A.; Buszewicz, G.; Sitarz, E.; Portincasa, P.; Garruti, G.; Flieger, M.; et al. Helicobacter pylori Infection and Extragastric Diseases—A Focus on the Central Nervous System. *Cells* **2021**, *10*, 2191. [CrossRef]
17. Savi, L.; Ribaldone, D.; Fagoonee, S.; Pellicano, R. Is Helicobacter pylori the infectious trigger for headache?: A review. *Infect. Disord.—Drug Targets* **2014**, *13*, 313–317. [CrossRef]
18. Tsai, H.-F.; Hsu, P.-N. Interplay between Helicobacter pylori and immune cells in immune pathogenesis of gastric inflammation and mucosal pathology. *Cell. Mol. Immunol.* **2010**, *7*, 255–259. [CrossRef]
19. Arzani, M.; Jahromi, S.R.; Ghorbani, Z.; Vahabizad, F.; Martelletti, P.; Ghaemi, A.; Sacco, S.; Togha, M.; On behalf of the School of Advanced Studies of the European Headache Federation (EHF-SAS). Gut-brain Axis and migraine headache: A comprehensive review. *J. Headache Pain* **2020**, *21*, 15. [CrossRef]
20. Mayer, E.A.; Tillisch, K.; Bradesi, S. Review article: Modulation of the brain–gut axis as a therapeutic approach in gastrointestinal disease. *Aliment. Pharmacol. Ther.* **2006**, *24*, 919–933. [CrossRef]
21. Sticlaru, L.; Stăniceanu, F.; Cioplea, M.; Nichita, L.; Bastian, A.; Micu, G.; Popp, C. Dangerous Liaison: Helicobacter pylori, Ganglionitis, and Myenteric Gastric Neurons: A Histopathological Study. *Anal. Cell. Pathol.* **2019**, *2019*, 3085181. [CrossRef] [PubMed]
22. Gasbarrini, A.; Gabrielli, M.; Fiore, G.; Candelli, M.; Bartolozzi, F.; De Luca, A.; Cremonini, F.; Franceschi, F.; Di Campli, C.; Armuzzi, A.; et al. Association Between Helicobacter Pylori Cytotoxic Type I Caga-Positive Strains and Migraine with Aura. *Cephalalgia* **2000**, *20*, 561–565. [CrossRef] [PubMed]
23. Ranjbar, R.; Behzadi, P.; Farshad, S. Advances in diagnosis and treatment of Helicobacter pylori infection. *Acta Microbiol. et Immunol. Hung.* **2017**, *64*, 273–292. [CrossRef]
24. Corojan, A.L.; Dumitrașcu, D.; Ciobanca, P.; Leucuta, D. Prevalence of Helicobacter pylori infection among dyspeptic patients in Northwestern Romania: A decreasing epidemiological trend in the last 30 years. *Exp. Ther. Med.* **2020**, *20*, 3488–3492. [CrossRef]

25. Yuan, C.; Adeloye, D.; Luk, T.T.; Huang, L.; He, Y.; Xu, Y.; Ye, X.; Yi, Q.; Song, P.; Rudan, I.; et al. The global prevalence of and factors associated with Helicobacter pylori infection in children: A systematic review and meta-analysis. *Lancet Child Adolesc. Health* **2022**, *6*, 185–194. [CrossRef]
26. Jones, N.L.; Koletzko, S.; Goodman, K.; Bontems, P.; Cadranel, S.; Casswall, T.; Czinn, S.; Gold, B.D.; Guarner, J.; Elitsur, Y.; et al. Joint ESPGHAN/NASPGHAN Guidelines for the Management of Helicobacter pylori in Children and Adolescents (Update 2016). *J. Pediatr. Gastroenterol. Nutr.* **2017**, *64*, 991–1003. [CrossRef] [PubMed]
27. Lupu, A.; Miron, I.C.; Cianga, A.L.; Cernomaz, A.T.; Lupu, V.V.; Munteanu, D.; Ghica, D.C.; Fotea, S. The Relationship between Anemia and Helicobacter Pylori Infection in Children. *Children* **2022**, *9*, 1324. [CrossRef]
28. Lupu, A.; Miron, I.C.; Cianga, A.L.; Cernomaz, A.T.; Lupu, V.V.; Gavrilovici, C.; Stârcea, I.M.; Tarca, E.; Ghica, D.C.; Fotea, S. The Prevalence of Liver Cytolysis in Children with Helicobacter pylori Infection. *Children* **2022**, *9*, 1498. [CrossRef] [PubMed]
29. Lupu, A.; Miron, I.C.; Cernomaz, A.T.; Gavrilovici, C.; Lupu, V.V.; Starcea, I.M.; Cianga, A.L.; Stana, B.; Tarca, E.; Fotea, S. Epidemiological Characteristics of Helicobacter pylori Infection in Children in Northeast Romania. *Diagnostics* **2023**, *13*, 408. [CrossRef] [PubMed]
30. Olesen, J. The international classification of headache disorders, 2nd edn (ICDH-II). *J. Neurol. Neurosurg. Psychiatry* **2004**, *75*, 808–811. [CrossRef] [PubMed]
31. Stewart, W.F.; Lipton, R.B.; Celentano, D.D.; Reed, M.L. Prevalence of migraine headache in the United States. Relation to age, income, race, and other sociodemographic factors. *JAMA* **1992**, *267*, 64–69. [CrossRef] [PubMed]
32. Holtmann, G.; Goebell, H.; Holtmann, M.; Talley, N.J. Dyspepsia in healthy blood donors: Pattern of symptoms and association with Helicobacter pylori. *Dig. Dis. Sci.* **1994**, *39*, 1090–1098. [CrossRef] [PubMed]
33. Imanieh, M.H.; Dehghani, S.M.; Haghighat, M.; Irani, M.; Yousefi, M. Migraine headache and acid peptic diseases in children. *Iran. Red Crescent Med. J.* **2009**, *11*, 181–183.
34. Pacifico, L.; Anania, C.; Osborn, J.F.; Ferraro, F.; Chiesa, C. Consequences of Helicobacter pylori infection in children. *World J. Gastroenterol.* **2010**, *16*, 5181–5194. [CrossRef]
35. Panconesi, A.; Sicuteri, R. Headache induced by serotonergic agonists—A key to the interpretation of migraine pathogenesis? *Cephalalgia* **1997**, *17*, 3–14. [CrossRef]
36. Tunca, A.; Turkay, C.; Tekin, O.; Kargili, A.; Erbayrak, M. Is Helicobacter pylori infection a risk factor for migraine? A case-control study. *Acta Neurol. Belg.* **2004**, *104*, 161–164.
37. Bradbeer, L.; Thakkar, S.; Liu, A.; Nanan, R. Childhood headache and *H. pylori*: A possible association. *Aust. Fam. Physician* **2013**, *42*, 134–136. [PubMed]
38. Kikui, S.; Chen, Y.; Ikeda, K.; Hasebe, M.; Asao, K.; Takeshima, T. Comorbidities in patients with migraine in Japan: A cross-sectional study using data from National Health and Wellness Survey. *BMJ Open* **2022**, *12*, e065787. [CrossRef]
39. Cavestro, C.; Prandi, G.; Manildo, M.; Martini, S.; Genovesi, C.; Premoli, A.; Fraire, F.; Neri, L.; Mandrino, S.; Ferrero, M.; et al. A cross-sectional study on the association between Helicobacter pylori infection and headache. *Neurol. Sci.* **2022**, *43*, 6031–6038. [CrossRef]
40. Yiannopoulou, K.G.; Efthymiou, A.; Karydakis, K.; Arhimandritis, A.; Bovaretos, N.; Tzivras, M. Helicobacter pylori infection as an environmental risk factor for migraine without aura. *J. Headache Pain* **2007**, *8*, 329–333. [CrossRef]
41. Hosseinzadeh, M.; Khosravi, A.; Saki, K.; Ranjbar, R. Evaluation of Helicobacter pylori infection in patients with common migraine headache. *Arch. Med. Sci.* **2011**, *5*, 844–849. [CrossRef] [PubMed]
42. Faraji, F.; Zarinfar, N.; Zanjani, A.T.; Morteza, A. The effect of Helicobacter pylori eradication on migraine: A randomized, double blind, controlled trial. *Pain Physician* **2012**, *15*, 495–498. [PubMed]
43. Karkelis, S.; Papadaki-Papandreou, O.; Lykogeorgou, M.; Papandreou, T.; Lianou, L.; Panayotou, I.; Roma, E.; Chrousos, G. 667 Helicobacter Pylori Infection and Headache in Children and Adolescents. *Pediatr. Res.* **2010**, *68*, 340. [CrossRef]
44. Gasbarrini, A.; De Luca, A.; Fiore, G.; Gambrielli, M.; Franceschi, F.; Ojetti, V.; Torre, E.S.; Gasbarrini, G.; Pola, P.; Giacovazzo, M. Beneficial effects of Helicobacter pylori eradication on migraine. *Hepato-Gastroenterology* **1998**, *45*, 765–770. [PubMed]
45. Gasbarrini, A.; De Luca, A.; Fiore, G.; Franceschi, F.; Ojetti, V.; Torre, E.S.; Di Campli, C.; Candelli, M.; Pola, M.S.R.; Tondi, P.; et al. Primary Headache and Helicobacter Pylori. *Int. J. Angiol.* **1998**, *7*, 310–312. [CrossRef] [PubMed]
46. Hassan, A.; Mehany, D.; Eldin, H.G.; Abdelghaffar, M.; Abdelbaky, H.A.; Kamal, Y.S.; Hussein, M. Helicobacter pylori infection in migraine headache: A true association or an innocent bystander? *Int. J. Neurosci.* **2022**, 1–6. [CrossRef] [PubMed]
47. Su, J.; Zhou, X.Y.; Zhang, G.X. Association between helicobacter pylori infection and migraine: A meta-analysis. *World J. Gastroenterol.* **2014**, *20*, 14965–14972. [CrossRef] [PubMed]
48. Lee, S.H.; Lee, J.J.; Kwon, Y.; Kim, J.H.; Sohn, J.H. Clinical Implications of Associations between Headache and Gastrointestinal Disorders: A Study Using the Hallym Smart Clinical Data Warehouse. *Front. Neurol.* **2017**, *8*, 526. [CrossRef]
49. Ansari, B.; Basiri, K.; Meamar, R.; Chitsaz, A.; Nematollahi, S. Association of Helicobacter pylori antibodies and severity of migraine attack. *Iran. J. Neurol.* **2015**, *14*, 125–129.
50. Kang, J.W.; Shin, Y.I. The role of interleukin 10 in the associations between migraine and Helicobacter pylori infection. *Pain Physician* **2013**, *16*, E450. [CrossRef]
51. Munno, I.; Marinaro, M.; Bassi, A.; Cassiano, M.; Causarano, V.; Centonze, V. Immunological aspects in migraine: Increase of IL-10 plasma levels during attack. *Headache* **2001**, *41*, 764–767. [CrossRef]

52. Mavromichalis, I.; Zaramboukas, T.; Giala, M.M. Migraine of gastrointestinal origin. *Eur. J. Pediatr.* **1995**, *154*, 406–410. [CrossRef] [PubMed]
53. Ciancarelli, I.; Di Massimo, C.; Ciancarelli, M.G.T.; De Matteis, G.; Marini, C.; Carolei, A. Helicobacter Pylori Infection and Migraine. *Cephalalgia* **2002**, *22*, 222–225. [CrossRef] [PubMed]
54. Öcal, S.; Öcal, R.; Suna, N. Relationship between Helicobacter pylori infection and white matter lesions in patients with migraine. *BMC Neurol.* **2022**, *22*, 187. [CrossRef]
55. Welander, N.Z.; Olivo, G.; Pisanu, C.; Rukh, G.; Schiöth, H.B.; Mwinyi, J. Migraine and gastrointestinal disorders in middle and old age: A UK Biobank study. *Brain Behav.* **2021**, *11*, e2291. [CrossRef]
56. Cámara-Lemarroy, C.R.; Rodriguez-Gutierrez, R.; Monreal-Robles, R.; Marfil-Rivera, A. Gastrointestinal disorders associated with migraine: A comprehensive review. *World J. Gastroenterol.* **2016**, *22*, 8149–8160. [CrossRef] [PubMed]
57. Hormati, A.; Akbari, N.; Sharifipour, E.; Hejazi, S.A.; Jafari, F.; Alemi, F.; Mohammadbeigi, A. Migraine and gastric disorders: Are they associated? *J. Res. Med. Sci.* **2019**, *24*, 60. [CrossRef] [PubMed]
58. Akbari, N.; Hormati, A.; Sharifipour, E.; Hejazi, S.A.; Jafari, F.; Mousavi-Aghdas, S.A.; Golzari, S.E. Migraine, dyspepsia, and Helicobacter pylori: Zeroing in on the culprit. *Iran. J. Neurol.* **2019**, *18*, 19–24. [CrossRef]
59. Martin, B.C.; Dorfman, J.H.; McMillan, J.A.; McMillan, C.A. Prevalence of migraine headache and association with sex, age, race, and rural/urban residence: A population-based study of Georgia Medicaid recipients. *Clin. Ther.* **1994**, *16*, 855–872.
60. Lileikytė, V.; Brasas, K.; Vaitkus, A.; Žvirblienė, A. Is vestibular migraine really a separate form of migraine? *Med. Hypotheses* **2022**, *165*, 110880. [CrossRef]
61. Martami, F.; Ghorbani, Z.; Abolhasani, M.; Togha, M.; Meysamie, A.; Sharifi, A.; Jahromi, S.R. Comorbidity of gastrointestinal disorders, migraine, and tension-type headache: A cross-sectional study in Iran. *Neurol. Sci.* **2017**, *39*, 63–70. [CrossRef] [PubMed]
62. Urits, I.; Yilmaz, M.; Bahrun, E.; Merley, C.; Scoon, L.; Lassiter, G.; An, D.; Orhurhu, V.; Kaye, A.D.; Viswanath, O. Utilization of B12 for the treatment of chronic migraine. *Best Pract. Res. Clin. Anaesthesiol.* **2020**, *34*, 479–491. [CrossRef] [PubMed]
63. Fila, M.; Chojnacki, J.; Pawlowska, E.; Szczepanska, J.; Chojnacki, C.; Blasiak, J. Kynurenine Pathway of Tryptophan Metabolism in Migraine and Functional Gastrointestinal Disorders. *Int. J. Mol. Sci.* **2021**, *22*, 10134. [CrossRef] [PubMed]

Disclaimer/Publisher's Note: The statements, opinions and data contained in all publications are solely those of the individual author(s) and contributor(s) and not of MDPI and/or the editor(s). MDPI and/or the editor(s) disclaim responsibility for any injury to people or property resulting from any ideas, methods, instructions or products referred to in the content.

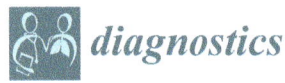

Article

Is There a Potential Link between Gastroesophageal Reflux Disease and Recurrent Respiratory Tract Infections in Children?

Vasile Valeriu Lupu [1], Gabriela Stefanescu [2], Ana Maria Laura Buga [1,*], Lorenza Forna [1], Elena Tarca [3,*], Iuliana Magdalena Starcea [1,*], Cristina Maria Mihai [4], Laura Florescu [5], Andrei Tudor Cernomaz [6], Adriana Mocanu [1], Viorel Tarca [7], Aye Aung Thet [8] and Ancuta Lupu [1]

1 Pediatrics, "Grigore T. Popa" University of Medicine and Pharmacy, 700115 Iasi, Romania
2 Gastroenterology, "Grigore T. Popa" University of Medicine and Pharmacy, 700115 Iasi, Romania
3 Department of Surgery II—Pediatric Surgery, "Grigore T. Popa" University of Medicine and Pharmacy, 700115 Iasi, Romania
4 Pediatrics, Faculty of General Medicine, Ovidius University, 900470 Constanta, Romania; cristina2603@yahoo.com
5 Mother and Child Medicine Department, "Grigore T. Popa" University of Medicine and Pharmacy, 700115 Iasi, Romania
6 3rd Medical Department, "Grigore T. Popa" University of Medicine and Pharmacy, 700115 Iasi, Romania
7 Department of Preventive Medicine and Interdisciplinarity, "Grigore T. Popa" University of Medicine and Pharmacy, 700115 Iasi, Romania; viorel.tarca@umfiasi.ro
8 Faculty of General Medicine, "Grigore T. Popa" University of Medicine and Pharmacy, 700115 Iasi, Romania
* Correspondence: anamaria_bnz@yahoo.com (A.M.L.B.); elena.tuluc@umfiasi.ro (E.T.); magdabirm@yahoo.com (I.M.S.)

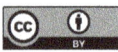

Citation: Lupu, V.V.; Stefanescu, G.; Buga, A.M.L.; Forna, L.; Tarca, E.; Starcea, I.M.; Mihai, C.M.; Florescu, L.; Cernomaz, A.T.; Mocanu, A.; et al. Is There a Potential Link between Gastroesophageal Reflux Disease and Recurrent Respiratory Tract Infections in Children? Diagnostics 2023, 13, 2310. https://doi.org/10.3390/diagnostics13132310

Academic Editor: Padukudru Anand Mahesh

Received: 2 June 2023
Revised: 28 June 2023
Accepted: 4 July 2023
Published: 7 July 2023

Copyright: © 2023 by the authors. Licensee MDPI, Basel, Switzerland. This article is an open access article distributed under the terms and conditions of the Creative Commons Attribution (CC BY) license (https://creativecommons.org/licenses/by/4.0/).

Abstract: Background: The implications of gastroesophageal reflux disease in respiratory tract infections have been investigated over time. The aim of our study was to evaluate the relationship between these two pathologic entities and the outcome after proper antireflux treatment. Methods: A group of 53 children with recurrent respiratory tract infections admitted in the gastroenterology clinic of a children's hospital in North-East Romania was investigated for gastroesophageal reflux disease through 24 h pH-metry. Those with a Boix-Ochoa score higher than 11.99 received proton pump inhibitor treatment and were reevaluated after 2 months. Results: A total of 41 children were found with a positive Boix-Ochoa score. After 2 months of antireflux therapy, eight patients still had a positive Boix-Ochoa score. Conclusions: Recurrent respiratory tract infections with symptoms resistant to treatment should be considered a reason to investigate for gastroesophageal reflux, because the symptoms may be due to micro- or macro-aspiration of the gastric refluxate or to an esophageal-bronchial reflex mediated through the vagal nerve.

Keywords: recurrent respiratory tract infections; gastroesophageal reflux disease; children; Boix-Ochoa score; pH-metry

1. Introduction

Gastroesophageal reflux becomes a disease when the physiologic retrograde passage of gastric content due to transient lower esophageal sphincter relaxation crosses a biologic threshold and determines disturbing symptoms and complications [1].

In children, unlike adults, there are some particular elements that intervene in the pathogenesis of GERD. These elements are characteristic for a certain age range. First of all, in infants younger than six months, reflux episodes are due to the physiological immaturity of the lower esophageal sphincter, the type of exclusively liquid feeding and the extended periods of time that the newborn and infants spend in a horizontal position. To all this are added elements related to the anatomical dynamic of the esophagus and stomach, by which we refer to the lower volumetric capacity of the esophagus and its shorter intraabdominal portion, as well as the relationship between the volume of food that a child at this age consumes relative to his body mass [2,3]. Beyond this age, the mechanisms through which GERD occurs tend to resemble those of adults.

The connection through which GERD can interfere with the functioning of the respiratory tract has its origins in embryonic life. Several events that take place during this stage of human evolution—the organ formation phase—represent the basis for the links between the digestive tract and the pathology of the respiratory tract. Due to the cross between the respiratory and digestive tracts in the pharynx, there are both anatomical and neural connections among these two pathways. Therefore, there are a series of reflexes at this level intended to protect the airways from the penetration of reflux liquid: the pharyngeal swallow reflex, the esophago-upper esophageal sphincter contractile reflex and the esophago-glottal closure reflex. Also, the fact that on the laryngeal surface of the epiglottis there are "taste buds" similar to those present on the tongue, determines the closure of glottis when water and hydrochloric acid reach its surface, to keep away substances that should not enter the respiratory tract [4]. Respiratory symptoms such as cough, hoarseness and odynophagia can sometimes be the only signs of gastroesophageal reflux, many patients (especially pediatric ones) are lacking in typical reflux signs or symptoms [5].

Epidemiological data regarding pediatric gastroesophageal reflux disease (GERD) is limited; it is estimated that 1.8% to 8.2% of all children have GERD, with an incidence that decreases until the age of 1 and then rises again to a maximum at the age of 16 [6].

Manifestations that can occur due to GERD can be grouped into two large categories: esophageal and extraesophageal syndromes. The esophageal symptoms refer to those pathological entities related to the esophagus or the anatomical region where it is located, and the extraesophageal syndromes include mainly pathology of the respiratory tract as follows: reflux cough syndrome, reflux laryngitis syndrome, reflux asthma syndrome, reflux dental erosion syndrome, pharyngitis, sinusitis, idiopathic pulmonary fibrosis and recurrent otitis media [7].

Studies have already established a clear link between the esophageal syndromes listed above, but with regard to the other extraesophageal pathological entities—the recurrent respiratory tract infections—data from literature suggest that GER could be in fact one of the multiple factors that contribute to their occurrence and not a single etiological factor [8]. On the same note, when GERD does not manifest itself with the typically known symptoms of regurgitation or heartburn, it may be not suspected as a leading cause for respiratory disorder, and hence the treatment result may be unsatisfactory and the disease could be mistakenly considered refractory to treatment [9].

The correlation between gastroesophageal reflux and pulmonary pathology was first noted by Mendelson in 1887, who reported symptoms similar to those seen in asthmatic patients [5]. Since then, numerous studies have elucidated and strengthened the evidence provided that supports the link between a series of respiratory pathologies and the presence of gastroesophageal reflux. For example, asthma refractory to treatment was a challenge for clinicians until research revealed that in several studies more than a half of patients with asthma tested through continuous pH-metry presented with GERD [10,11]. Considering these new findings, the suspicion was raised that wheezing, although a symptom commonly seen in asthmatic patients, could also be linked to GERD, an extra-respiratory pathology that acts as a trigger factor [12,13]. Last but not least, the negative effects of acid reflux which can extend even to the level of the oral cavity should not be ignored. Caries is a public health issue, with GERD being a contributing factor to dental erosion, for patients of all ages as data in literature suggests [14–16].

The aim of the study presented in this paper was to determine the relationship between recurrent respiratory tract infections and GERD in pediatric patients aged 6 months to 162 months and to evaluate patients' response after antireflux treatment.

2. Materials and Methods

The study took place in the gastroenterology clinic of a regional emergency hospital for children in North-East Romania that serves pediatric patients from seven surrounding counties. It is a retrospective study that involved 234 patients admitted to the clinic in a 5-year interval out of which we focused on those with recurrent respiratory tract infections. Informed consent was signed by all the patients' caregivers at admission and approval from the hospital's ethics committee was obtained.

Patients were diagnosed with GERD after being monitored for 24 h through continuous esophageal pH-metry and the diagnosis of respiratory pathology was established following anamnesis, objective clinical examination, laboratory tests and imaging explorations. Cases were selected for the study after they met the inclusion criteria listed in Table 1 and patients were excluded based on the criteria presented in the same table.

Table 1. Inclusion and exclusion criteria for the study.

Inclusion Criteria	Exclusion Criteria
Regurgitation/vomiting unrelated to other pathology	Treatment with proton pump inhibitors over the last 3 months
Poor weight gain/ weight loss in infants and small children	Treatment with aspirin or other non-steroidal anti-inflammatory drugs
Protracted crying in infants	Treatment for *H. pylori* infection
Chronic cough that did not improve under treatment	Foreign body aspiration
Cough that occurred at night time	Systemic diseases that caused esophageal lesions
Diagnosis of recurrent upper respiratory tract infection (sinusitis, pharyngitis, laryngitis, rhinitis, tonsillitis, acute otitis media)	Known diagnosis of bronchopulmonary dysplasia, primary ciliary dyskinesia, cystic fibrosis, sleep apnea, asthma
Diagnosis of recurrent lower respiratory tract infection (pneumonia, bronchiolitis)	Gastrointestinal blood loss identified at endoscopic examination
	Surgery for esophageal or gastric pathology
	Known food allergy
	Cardiac abnormalities

The pH measurement procedure involves a series of steps. First, the patient must stop the ingestion of both liquids and solids for a minimum of 6 h (if the patient is older than 12 months) or 3 h (if the patient is 12 months or less) prior to investigation. Use of medication known to modify the gastric secretion must also be stopped before the procedure within a certain timeframe specific to each drug (6 h for antacid drugs, 48 h for prokinetic drugs, 3 days for H2 receptor inhibitors and 7 days for proton pump inhibitors). The second step implies calibrating the device; this is done by performing two measurements in fluids with different pH levels of 1 and 7. After calibrating the device, the measurement can begin. In order to insert the electrode, the patient is seated in left lateral decubitus (for infants and small children) or in seated position (for children over the age of six). Then the lubricated electrode is inserted through one nostril until it reaches 5 cm above the lower esophageal sphincter. Next, the patient's caregiver or the patient itself, depending on age, is advised to register symptoms and changes in body position (supine or standing) and to press the device's button when these occur.

In order to monitor the esophageal pH, the Medtronic Digitrapper® pH 100 SN 37660 with Zinetics 24 and ComforTEc by Sandhill multiuse catheters was used. The measurements were recorded using Polygram.Net™ pH software (version 4.21). Physiological and pathological reflux episodes were differentiated by the pH values above, respectively, below 4. The Boix-Ochoa score was used to establish that the reflux episodes were pathological, cases scoring a value higher than 11.99 were included in the statistics [17–19].

To consider whether patients had recurrent respiratory tract infections, we used as a guide the next three criteria for defining recurrent respiratory tract infections: a minimum of 6 respiratory infections over the last 12 months; a minimum 1 episode of upper respiratory tract infection per month between September and April; a minimum 3 episodes of lower respiratory tract infection over the last 12 months [20]. In order to be included in the study, the patients had to check at least 1 of the 3 criteria mentioned above.

After being diagnosed with GERD, all patients received a two-month treatment course with PPIs (esomeprazole 1 mg/kg/day for children aged 1 month to 1 year, 20 mg/day for children with a weight below 55 kg, and 40 mg/day for those weighing over 55 kg) during which they came for the monthly check-up.

Data was processed using IBM SPSS Statistics 20 and correlation analysis was performed with Pearson parametric correlation. The correlation coefficients were established for a 95% confidence interval.

3. Results

After establishing the diagnosis of GERD and history of recurrent respiratory tract infection and applying the inclusion and exclusion criteria, we found that of all 234 children, 53 (22.64%) patients had recurrent respiratory tract infections and 41 (77.36%) were associated with GERD ($p = 0.0470$, 95% confidence interval) (Figure 1).

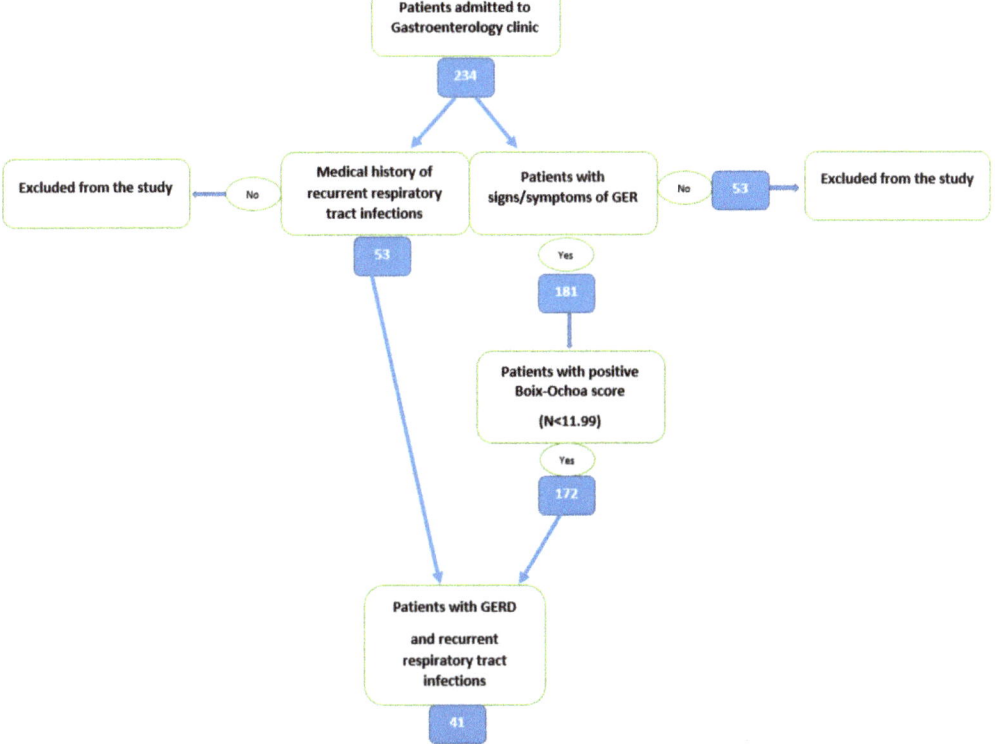

Figure 1. Flowchart of the selection process.

Furthermore, we analyzed the number of cases that associated GERD and infectious respiratory pathology depending on the respiratory tract portion involved. We observed that 66% of all cases with respiratory tract infections were located above the larynx. Of these 35 cases, 27 (77.14%) were associated with GERD. A similar pattern was seen in children with lower respiratory tract infections and GERD, even if they were fewer in number (18 cases), the proportion was preserved, 77.7% were associated GERD (see Table 2). Data on gender distribution and place of living are presented in Tables 3 and 4. We observed that there was a higher number of male patients with respiratory tract infections than female patients (39 vs. 14, with a p value of 0.038) and the same pattern was seen in patients that associated GERD and respiratory pathology (31 vs. 10, with a p value of 0.045). The mean age for children with respiratory tract infections was 42.45 months (with a p value of 0.032), and for those with associated GERD the mean age was almost the same; 41.73 months (with a p value of 0.040).

Table 2. Distribution of cases regarding respiratory tract infection and GERD presence.

		Gastroesophageal Reflux		Total
		Negative	Positive	
Recurrent respiratory tract infections	Upper tract	8	27	35
	Lower tract	4	14	18
Total		12	41	53

Table 3. Data on Gender Distribution and Place of living among patients.

Cases	Gender		Place of Living	
	Male	Female	Urban	Rural
With recurrent respiratory tract infections	39	14	40	13
With recurrent respiratory tract infections and GERD	31	10	24	17

Table 4. Gender distribution according to the type of cases included in the study.

	Gender		Total
	Male (% of Total)	Female (% of Total)	
Cases with RURTI * without GERD	5 (9.43)	3 (5.66)	8 (15.09)
Cases with RURTI and GERD	20 (37.73)	7 (13.20)	27 (50.94)
Cases with RLRTI ** without GERD	3 (5.66)	1 (1.88)	4 (7.54)
Cases with RLRTI and GERD	10 (18.86)	4 (7.54)	14 (26.41)
Total	39 (73.58)	14 (26.41)	53 (100)

* RURTI = recurrent upper respiratory tract infections. ** RLRTI = recurrent lower respiratory tract infections.

All 41 patients with GERD were counseled regarding postural and feeding changes based on each individual's age and treatment with a proton pump inhibitor—omeprazole or esomeprazole—in appropriate dose was initiated (1 mg/kg/day for children between 1 month to 1 year, 20 mg/day for children with a weight below 55 kg and 40 mg/day for those weighing over 55 kg). After 8 weeks of therapy, from a total of 41 patients, 8 (19.51%) screened positive for GERD, with a positive Boix-Ochoa score greater than 11.99, while the other 33 tested negative for GERD after control pH-metry.

4. Discussion

Our study aimed to evaluate the relationship between GERD and recurrent episodes of respiratory infections in pediatric patients. Although we had a small number of cases, only 53 children identified with recurrent respiratory infections (a number that did not allow us to extract many statistical data) and we found that 41 of them (77.35%) were also associated with GERD. From these 41 cases, 27 had a history of recurrent ear-nose-throat infections, while 14 had recurrent lower respiratory tract infections; regarding gender distribution, we observed that these two pathologies were more prevalent among males (31 out of 41 cases). After the 2 months of treatment with PPIs, 33 patients had a Boix-Ochoa score lower than 11.99. At evaluation one month after the end of the treatment, the respiratory symptoms (cough, sneezing, hoarseness, sore throat, rhinorrhea) had improved.

There are two main proposed mechanisms through which acidic reflux determines respiratory symptoms. The first would be an indirect one in which receptors in the esophageal wall that are sensitive to acidic pH are stimulated; this mechanism is suspected of being mediated by the vagal nerve. By stimulating the vagal fibers present in the respiratory tract, a series of inflammation-promoting substances are released, such as tachykinins, neurokinins, P substance and TNF alpha [21]. These pro-inflammatory mediators would then set off an inflammatory reaction and bronchoconstriction. Another hypothesis related to the nervous stimulation would be that the esophagus and airways have numerous transient receptor potential channels that are activated by reflux, thus leading to inflammation and increased bronchial reaction. The second proposed mechanism would be that of the direct action of acidic gastric content on airways and lung when being aspired; if micro-aspiration occurs then the usual manifestations are chronic cough and if there is macro-aspiration then repeated episodes of chemical pneumonitis or aspiration-related bacterial pneumonia appear [22].

There is always a possibility that GERD may manifest only through respiratory symptoms such as chronic cough or wheezing; this form of disease for which typical symptoms are regurgitation and/or vomiting is called "silent reflux". This type of gastroesophageal reflux disease suggests that the degree of severity of reflux is not necessarily correlated with the appearance of respiratory symptoms, as can be demonstrated by studies on groups of children diagnosed with GERD through continuous monitoring with pH-metry. Therefore, whether the refluxed liquid is located in the proximal or distal esophagus, acid reflux plays a role in the occurrence of respiratory disorders; not necessarily through the intensity of the reflux, but through the exposure of the respiratory tissue to both the acidic environment and nonacid components provided by the refluxed liquid [23–25].

A study published in 2022 evaluated the type of symptoms found in 243 eligible patients with GERD, aged 14 to 88, who had pulmonary micro-aspiration diagnosed through reflux micro-aspiration scintigraphy technique, a procedure that can detect even silent micro-aspiration. The results evidenced that the most frequent symptoms were regurgitation, cough and heartburn, while the most encountered combinations were heartburn and regurgitation followed closely by cough and throat clearing. There were also patients that associated three symptoms; heartburn with regurgitation and throat clearing being present in most cases, followed by cough, regurgitation and throat clearing. These findings suggest that cough that appears in a patient with regurgitation or heartburn should guide us to investigate a possible reflux with subsequent micro-aspiration in order to prevent pulmonary damage and further bacterial infection [26].

Results from a study conducted on 65 children aged up to 12 years old with gastroesophageal reflux concluded that different respiratory manifestations in various proportions were present. In descending order of prevalence, the presence of recurrent bronchopneumonia was seen in 79.1% of cases with GERD, cough was positive in 58.3%, and the same percent was seen in patients that had nasal obstruction; 45.8% had rhinosinusitis, 61.6% had tonsillitis, 16.7% presented with asthma, and pharyngitis occurred in 12.5% of cases [27].

Also, a study conducted by a research group in New Delhi, India, on 312 pediatric patients aged 4 months to 11 years, aimed to determine the correlation between recurrent lower respiratory tract infections and silent gastroesophageal reflux using gastroesophageal scintigraphy to diagnose reflux. The results showed that more than a quarter of patients enrolled (34.6%) presented with GERD, highlighting that silent GER has an important prevalence rate, even in children older than 18 months where GER becomes pathologic [28].

Evidence exists for gastroesophageal reflux acting as an etiological factor for otitis media as gastric pepsin was identified in the middle ear fluid. This event determines mucosal inflammation through proteolytic action of pepsin over the eustachian tube cells. Also, a pH lower than 4, as happens in pathologic gastroesophageal reflux, determines ciliostasis which prevents effective clearance, thus favoring the proliferation of pathogens. A study about the clinical implications of the presence of pepsin in middle ear fluid of children with otitis media concluded that 31% of children under the age of 1 had pepsin detected in their ear, this group being definitely larger than other age groups included in the study, suggesting that pepsin from gastroesophageal reflux is a co-factor in the pathogenesis of otitis [29].

A study conducted in Egypt by a research group that aimed to identify the risk factors for recurrent otitis media with effusion (OME) among a group of 2003 children, found that, from 310 patients diagnosed with OME, 66 were associated with gastroesophageal reflux. From the 66 cases with OME and GER, 41 were recorded in children under the age of 6. Gastroesophageal reflux was the fifth risk factor as the number of cases (66) from a list of ten evaluated in the study, close to presence of nasal polyps (68), sinusitis (72) and adenoid hypertrophy (73) or allergic rhinitis (73). Thus, the study highlighted the fact that GER is an important risk factor in the repeated occurrence of otitis media with effusion [30].

In another study on pediatric patients aged 5 to 12 years old, which aimed to establish the relationship between OME and GERD, the results showed that 58% of the cases enrolled associated GERD and OME, suggesting that GERD may have an important role in the etiology of otitis media with effusion [31].

Regarding rhinosinusal pathology, in several studies GERD was found to have a high prevalence especially in cases of chronic rhinosinusitis refractory to treatment. After testing positive for presence of acid reflux in nasal cavity and then giving antireflux therapy, results showed that chronic rhinosinusitis improved, with better results in children than in adults [32].

Moving on to the next anatomical site where frequent respiratory infections in children are located, the tonsils, research data showed that, in addition to the already established mechanism by which tonsillitis occurs, gastroesophageal reflux would also play a role in its etiopathogenesis. It has been demonstrated that tonsil hypertrophy occurs when lymphocytes are stimulated due to bacterial infection but then the hypothesis of reflux mediated tonsillitis emerged. Considering this aspect, an in vitro study using human tonsillar tissue showed that when exposed to pepsin activity, the cells expressed higher levels of IL-2 and IFN-gamma, these being cytokines involved in CD4 lymphocyte proliferation that further led to tonsil hypertrophy. A particular aspect found in this study was that the phenomenon mentioned above, where pepsin acts as an antigen was observed only in pediatric patients and not in adults with tonsillitis [33].

In addition to pepsin, which acts as a trigger for the inflammatory process in the tonsils, other substances from the refluxed fluid can also play a role in the various forms of respiratory tract damage, these being hydrochloric acid, bile and trypsin. Hydrochloric acid exhibits its effects on carbonic anhydrase III, (CA III), E-cadherin and laryngeal H+/K+-ATPase, leading to several processes that ensure the negative impact of reflux over the laryngopharyngeal tissue. Thus, when CA III is missing, the bicarbonate secretion is imbalanced, leading to a pH dysregulation. Next, the reduced expression of E-cadherin, leads to the loss of cell junctions that result in an alteration of the local cell barrier with increased intercellular permeability and further deterioration of cells from the pharyngeal and nasal mucosa. Last but not least, the H+/K+-ATPase, which is found both in the stomach and larynx, as studies have shown, has been found to have a higher rate of expression in neoplastic pharyngeal cells. Bile also plays a role in the occurrence of laryngeal cancer, but this phenomenon is not the purpose of our research. Last but not least, trypsin has been shown to increase pulmonary injury and to contribute to the dentine erosion process [34].

We must mention that even a respiratory infection can be the cause of GERD aggravation, with further pulmonary aspiration and recurrent pulmonary infection. This affirmation is supported by a recent study published in 2022 that presented the role of pertussis in the exacerbation of GERD events in a group of 208 patients aged 16 to 85 years. For inclusion in the study, their profile included GERD exacerbation episodes refractory to treatment and a positive diagnosis of pertussis, resulting in 103 post-pertussis patients and 105 non-pertussis patients. They were further evaluated for presence of laryngopharyngeal reflux and aspiration by SPECT/CT. The results showed that the recent pertussis infection group had higher rates of reflux. The mechanism involved in this case is represented by a change in the thoraco-abdominal pressures due to chronic cough, this leading to GERD, hiatus hernia development and pulmonary micro-aspiration episodes [35].

In relation to the presence of recurrent pneumonia and GERD, a study published in 2021 on the risk factors of recurrent pneumonia encountered in a group of 763 patients with pneumonia, from which 87 had more than 2 episodes in a single year, found that the presence of gastroesophageal reflux was one of the factors that predisposed to repeated episodes of respiratory disease [36]. The mechanism by which this occurs is as discussed above.

Another infectious pathological entity that has a preferred pulmonary location is tuberculosis. In order to explore the impact of GERD on the risk of tuberculosis, a nationwide cohort study was conducted in Taiwan exploring patients diagnosed with GERD over a period of nine years. The results of the study showed that the presence of GERD represented an independent risk factor for pulmonary tuberculosis [37]. Considering that at global level and in our country in particular, the prevalence of tuberculosis is still high, even among children, we consider that this aspect is one that we must take into account when we are in front of a child with GERD, to whom other factors with known role in determining tuberculosis are added.

Considering diagnosis methods in GERD manifesting with respiratory symptoms, a study conducted on 515 adults with GERD diagnosed through pH-metry and who were also investigated by upper digestive endoscopy, concluded that patients who presented esophageal lesions detected by endoscopy were associated more frequently with episodes of respiratory manifestations, including infectious ones that affected their quality of life [38]. Even though it implied adult patients, the study emphasizes the important role of upper digestive endoscopy in the diagnostic algorithm of GERD and also encourages its use in pediatric reflux cases that associate important respiratory symptoms or recurrent episodes of airway infections in order to determine the degree to which reflux is involved in their occurrence, in the same manner observed in the mentioned study carried out in adults.

Regarding the treatment options in GERD, recent guidelines recommend that before initiating drug treatment, changes in lifestyle and diet must be implemented, especially in the case of infants and young children, the ages at which most presentations to the doctor due to the suspicion of GERD are registered. Therefore, initially it is recommended to use thickened or extensively hydrolyzed milk formulas for a period of 2 to 4 weeks (where there is the case to rule out a possible cow's milk proteins allergy). In parallel with these dietary changes, it is indicated that meals should be small and frequent, the child should be kept in a vertical position for at least 30 min after each meal, the last meal of the day should be eaten 2 h before bedtime, the position during sleep should be 30 degrees from the horizontal, infants should be placed on their left side during sleep (and during the day for those that do not sit on their own yet) [1,39].

If these general and dietary measures fail, anti-secretory treatment can be initiated. The mechanisms by which the antireflux medications act in treating GERD are that of inhibiting gastric acid secretion and of reducing inflammation through their action on neutrophils, where they inhibit the production of reactive oxygen species [40].

A study presenting the GERD implication in respiratory events (recurrent pneumonia, bronchial asthma, chronic cough, chronic nasal obstruction, recurrent acute middle ear infection, recurrent tonsillitis) performed on a group of 45 children aged 3 months to 12 years, showed that antireflux treatment combined with antiallergic or surgical treatment resulted in the improvement of respiratory pathology in various degrees, suggesting that antireflux therapy has an important role in the management scheme, but does not help if used alone; other treatment methods being necessary depending on the pathology [41].

In 2022, a narrative review revised studies in which the efficacy of proton pump inhibitors and histamine H2 receptor antagonists as treatment options for pediatric GERD was tested. There were studies that evaluated only children under the age of 1 year, studies that exclusively enrolled pediatric patients aged 1 year and older and studies that included children of all ages. While the results showed that PPIs are the treatment of choice in pediatric GERD for patients aged 1 year and up, it did not find them useful in treating children under the age of 1 year that presented with unspecific symptoms such as crying, irritability, or apnea, particularly when they had no proven esophagitis or complications due to gastroesophageal reflux. Also, it concluded that there is no strong evidence in treating with PPIs asthma symptoms in children with GERD as they might actually be caused by the quantity of refluxed fluid and not by its quality, i.e., by its pH [42].

Our study showed that proper treatment with PPIs for two months lead to the resolution of GERD which was diagnosed through a Boix-Ochoa score lower than 11.99 after pH-metry. These results advocate for the effective detection and treatment of GERD in order to remove it from the equation as a risk factor for recurrent respiratory tract infections. Our results regarding the efficient use of PPIs are supported by those in the specialized literature [43,44].

Maybe the pH is not a direct trigger factor for respiratory symptoms in children compared to adults, due to the short time of exposure to the effects of acid on the respiratory tract, but reflux episodes definitely play a role in the occurrence of respiratory manifestations, not only of asthmatic ones but also of infectious ones.

Last but not least, one must bear in mind that although for the practitioner the diagnosis of GERD or silent reflux is frequently encountered in current practice and he knows that in most cases the symptoms improve as the child reaches the age of 1 year, for parents this diagnosis or the uncertainty of its confirmation is a cause of anxiety and depression, especially for young mothers who are usually the main caregivers for children particularly those under the age of 2, in which reflux symptoms (both esophageal and extraesophageal ones) are a frequent cause of hospitalization [45]. Parental mental health is an important aspect as it always influences a child's mental and physical development.

Our study had certain limitations. First, the included lot was small and did not allow us to obtain statistically relevant data, according to a value of $p = 0.0470$. Second, pH-metry measurement is an invasive procedure, therefore it is more difficult to perform in pediatric patients, especially small ones. Also, the technique is performed exclusively in hospital, which does not respect the child's regular schedule, pattern of meals, or daily routine. But, despite these impediments, we consider that our study contributes one more step to the attempt to establish to what extent GERD contributes as a trigger for respiratory tract infections or causes the occurrence of repeated episodes by creating an irritating and at the same time favorable environment for microbial agents.

5. Conclusions

Gastroesophageal reflux and respiratory infections are two of the most frequent reasons for pediatric patients to be consulted by a doctor. When respiratory symptoms do not improve under appropriate treatment, persist or infections are frequent, even in the absence of typical symptoms of reflux, the clinician should consider its presence as a source of the unfavorable evolution.

Although in our study the results did not register statistical significance, according to a value of $p = 0.0470$, the fact that approximately a quarter of the children examined in the study had repeated episodes of respiratory infections, and of these more than three-quarters also had associated GERD, shows that reflux is an important factor that contributes to airway inflammation and creates a favorable environment for repeated infectious episodes.

Author Contributions: Conceptualization, V.V.L. and A.L.; methodology, E.T. and C.M.M.; software, A.T.C. and I.M.S.; validation, G.S., E.T., L.F. (Laura Florescu) and C.M.M.; formal analysis, A.M., A.A.T., V.T. and A.T.C.; investigation, V.V.L. and A.L.; data curation, A.M.L.B.; writing—original draft preparation, A.M.L.B., V.V.L., L.F. (Lorenza Forna), A.A.T. and A.L.; writing—review and editing, G.S., I.M.S., A.T.C., E.T., C.M.M., L.F. (Laura Florescu), V.T. and A.M.; visualization, A.M.L.B., V.T. and L.F. (Lorenza Forna); supervision, G.S.; project administration, V.V.L. G.S., A.M.L.B., L.F. (Laura Florescu), E.T., I.M.S., C.M.M., L.F. (Lorenza Forna), A.T.C., A.M., V.T., A.A.T. and A.L contributed equally with V.V.L. to this article. All authors have read and agreed to the published version of the manuscript.

Funding: This research received no external funding.

Institutional Review Board Statement: The study was conducted according to the guidelines of the Declaration of Helsinki. The research was approved by the Ethics Committee of "Saint Mary" Emergency Children's Hospital.

Informed Consent Statement: Informed consent was obtained from all subjects involved in the study.

Data Availability Statement: Data available on request from the corresponding author.

Conflicts of Interest: The authors declare no conflict of interest.

References

1. Rosen, R.; Vandenplas, Y.; Singendonk, M.; Cabana, M.; DiLorenzo, C.; Gottrand, F.; Gupta, S.; Langendam, M.; Staiano, A.; Thapar, N.; et al. Pediatric Gastroesophageal Reflux Clinical Practice Guidelines: Joint Recommendations of the North American Society for Pediatric Gastroenterology, Hepatology, and Nutrition and the European Society for Pediatric Gastroenterology, Hepatology, and Nutrition. *J. Pediatr. Gastroenterol. Nutr.* **2018**, *66*, 516–554. [CrossRef]
2. Pados, B.F.; Davitt, E.S. Pathophysiology of Gastroesophageal Reflux Disease in Infants and Nonpharmacologic Strategies for Symptom Management. *Nurs. Women's Health* **2020**, *24*, 101–114. [CrossRef]
3. Jones, A.B. Gastroesophageal reflux in infants and children. When to reassure and when to go further. *Can. Fam. Physician* **2001**, *47*, 2045–2050, 2053. [PubMed]
4. Orenstein, S.R. Update on gastroesophageal reflux and respiratory disease in children. *Can. J. Gastroenterol.* **2000**, *14*, 131–135. [CrossRef] [PubMed]
5. Karbasi, A.; Ardestani, M.E.; Ghanei, M.; Harandi, A.A. The association between reflux esophagitis and airway hyper-reactivity in patients with gastro-esophageal reflux. *J. Res. Med. Sci.* **2013**, *18*, 473–476. [PubMed]
6. Mousa, H.; Hassan, M. Gastroesophageal Reflux Disease. *Pediatr. Clin. N. Am.* **2017**, *64*, 487–505. [CrossRef]
7. Vakil, N.; van Zanten, S.V.; Kahrilas, P.; Dent, J.; Jones, R.; Global Consensus Group. The Montreal definition and classification of gastroesophageal reflux disease: A global evidence-based consensus. *Am. J. Gastroenterol.* **2006**, *101*, 1900–1943. [CrossRef]
8. Katzka, D.A.; Pandolfino, J.E.; Kahrilas, P.J. Phenotypes of Gastroesophageal Reflux Disease: Where Rome, Lyon, and Montreal Meet. *Clin. Gastroenterol. Hepatol.* **2020**, *18*, 767–776. [CrossRef]
9. Young, M.A.; Reynolds, J.C. Respiratory complications of gastrointestinal diseases. *Gastroenterol. Clin. N. Am.* **1998**, *27*, 721–746. [CrossRef]
10. Kaplan, A.; Szefler, S.J.; Halpin, D.M.G. Impact of comorbid conditions on asthmatic adults and children. *NPJ Prim. Care Respir. Med.* **2020**, *30*, 36. [CrossRef]
11. Lupu, V.V.; Miron, I.; Tarca, E.; Trandafir, L.M.; Anton-Paduraru, D.T.; Moisa, S.M.; Starcea, M.; Cernomaz, A.; Miron, L.; Lupu, A. Gastroesophageal Reflux in Children with Asthma. *Children* **2022**, *9*, 336. [CrossRef]
12. Patra, S.; Singh, V.; Chandra, J.; Kumar, P.; Tripathi, M. Gastro-esophageal reflux in early childhood wheezers. *Pediatr. Pulmonol.* **2011**, *46*, 272–277. [CrossRef]
13. Lupu, V.V.; Miron, I.C.; Lupu, A.; Moscalu, M.; Mitrofan, E.C.; Munteanu, D.; Luca, A.C. The relationship between gastroesophageal reflux disease and recurrent wheezing in children. *Medicine* **2021**, *100*, e27660. [CrossRef]
14. Chakraborty, A.; Anjankar, A.P. Association of Gastroesophageal Reflux Disease with Dental Erosion. *Cureus* **2022**, *14*, e30381. [CrossRef]
15. Ignat, A.; Burlea, M.; Lupu, V.V.; Paduraru, G. Oral manifestations of gastroesophageal reflux disease in children. *Rom. J. Oral Rehabil.* **2017**, *9*, 40–43.

16. Borysenko, A.; Timokhina, T.; Kononova, O. Combined caries and gastroesophageal reflux disease. *Georgian Med. News* **2021**, *319*, 22–27.
17. Lupu, V.V.; Burlea, M.; Nistor, N.; Streanga, V.; Starcea, M.I.; Paduraru, G.; Ghica, D.C.; Mitrofan, E.C.; Moscalu, M.; Ignat, A. Correlation between esophageal pH-metry and esophagitis in gastroesophageal reflux disease in children. *Medicine* **2018**, *97*, e12042. [CrossRef] [PubMed]
18. Butt, I.; Kasmin, F. *Esophageal pH Monitoring*; StatPearls Publishing: Treasure Island, FL, USA, 2023.
19. Lupu, V.V.; Miron, I.; Buga, A.M.L.; Gavrilovici, C.; Tarca, E.; Adam Raileanu, A.; Starcea, I.M.; Cernomaz, A.T.; Mocanu, A.; Lupu, A. Iron Deficiency Anemia in Pediatric Gastroesophageal Reflux Disease. *Diagnostics* **2023**, *13*, 63. [CrossRef]
20. Jesenak, M.; Ciljakova, M.; Rennerova, Z.; Babusikova, E.; Banovci, P. Recurrent Respiratory Infections in Children—Definition, Diagnostic Approach, Treatment and Prevention. In *Bronchitis*; IntechOpen: London, UK, 2011. [CrossRef]
21. Harding, S.M.; Allen, J.E.; Blumin, J.H.; Warner, E.A.; Pellegrini, C.A.; Chan, W.W. Respiratory manifestations of gastroesophageal reflux disease. *Ann. N. Y. Acad. Sci.* **2013**, *1300*, 43–52. [CrossRef] [PubMed]
22. Griffiths, T.L.; Nassar, M.; Soubani, A.O. Pulmonary manifestations of gastroesophageal reflux disease. *Expert Rev. Respir. Med.* **2020**, *14*, 767–775. [CrossRef]
23. Gorenstein, A.; Levine, A.; Boaz, M.; Mandelberg, A.; Serour, F. Severity of acid gastroesophageal reflux assessed by pH metry: Is it associated with respiratory disease? *Pediatr. Pulmonol.* **2003**, *36*, 330–334. [CrossRef]
24. Jiang, M.Z.; Wang, T.L.; Yu, J.D.; Zhou, X.L.; Ou, B.Y. Role of proximal gastric acid reflux in causation of respiratory symptoms in children with gastroesophageal reflux. *Indian Pediatr.* **2007**, *44*, 575–579. [PubMed]
25. Ramaiah, R.N.; Stevenson, M.; McCallion, W.A. Hypopharyngeal and distal esophageal pH monitoring in children with gastroesophageal reflux and respiratory symptoms. *J. Pediatr. Surg.* **2005**, *40*, 1557–1561. [CrossRef] [PubMed]
26. Khoma, O.; Park, J.S.; Lee, F.M.; Van der Wall, H.; Falk, G.L. Different clinical symptom patterns in patients with reflux micro-aspiration. *ERJ Open Res.* **2022**, *8*, 00508–02021. [CrossRef] [PubMed]
27. Santos, V.J.; Comes, G.T.; Gonçalves, T.M.; Carvalho, M.D.A.; Weber, S.A. Prevalence of bronchopulmonary and otorhinolaryngologic symptoms in children under investigation for gastroesophageal reflux disease: Retrospective analysis. *Braz. J. Otorhinolaryngol.* **2011**, *77*, 328–333. [CrossRef] [PubMed]
28. Thomas, E.J.; Kumar, R.; Dasan, J.B.; Bal, C.; Kabra, S.K.; Malhotra, A. Prevalence of silent gastroesophageal reflux in association with recurrent lower respiratory tract infections. *Clin. Nucl. Med.* **2003**, *28*, 476–479. [CrossRef]
29. He, Z.; O'Reilly, R.C.; Mehta, D. Gastric pepsin in middle ear fluid of children with otitis media: Clinical implications. *Curr. Allergy Asthma Rep.* **2008**, *8*, 513–518. [CrossRef]
30. Saad, K.; Abdelmoghny, A.; Abdel-Raheem, Y.F.; Gad, E.F.; Elhoufey, A. Prevalence and associated risk factors of recurrent otitis media with effusion in children in Upper Egypt. *World J. Otorhinolaryngol.-Head Neck Surg.* **2020**, *7*, 280–284. [CrossRef]
31. Elbeltagy, R.; Abdelhafeez, M. Outcome of Gastroesophageal Reflux Therapy in Children with Persistent Otitis Media with Effusion. *Int. Arch. Otorhinolaryngol.* **2021**, *26*, e058–e062. [CrossRef]
32. Katle, E.J.; Hatlebakk, J.G.; Steinsvåg, S. Gastroesophageal reflux and rhinosinusitis. *Curr. Allergy Asthma Rep.* **2013**, *13*, 218–223. [CrossRef]
33. Kim, J.H.; Jang, S.J.; Yun, J.W.; Jung, M.H.; Woo, S.H. Effects of pepsin and pepstatin on reflux tonsil hypertrophy in vitro. *PLoS ONE* **2018**, *13*, e0207090. [CrossRef] [PubMed]
34. Li, Y.; Xu, G.; Zhou, B.; Tang, Y.; Liu, X.; Wu, Y.; Wang, Y.; Kong, J.; Xu, T.; He, C.; et al. Effects of acids, pepsin, bile acids, and trypsin on laryngopharyngeal reflux diseases: Physiopathology and therapeutic targets. *Eur. Arch. Oto-Rhino-Laryngol.* **2022**, *279*, 2743–2752. [CrossRef] [PubMed]
35. Burton, L.; Weerasinghe, D.P.; Joffe, D.; Saunders, J.; Falk, G.L.; Van der Wall, H. A putative link between pertussis and new onset of gastroesophageal reflux an observational study. *Multidiscip. Respir. Med.* **2022**, *17*, 832. [CrossRef]
36. Abdel Baseer, K.A.; Sakhr, H. Clinical profile and risk factors of recurrent pneumonia in children at Qena governorate, Egypt. *Int. J. Clin. Pract.* **2021**, *75*, e13695. [CrossRef]
37. Fan, W.C.; Ou, S.M.; Feng, J.Y.; Hu, Y.W.; Yeh, C.M.; Su, V.Y.; Hu, L.Y.; Chien, S.H.; Su, W.J.; Chen, T.J.; et al. Increased risk of pulmonary tuberculosis in patients with gastroesophageal reflux disease. *Int. J. Tuberc. Lung Dis.* **2016**, *20*, 265–270. [CrossRef] [PubMed]
38. Maher, M.M.; Darwish, A.A. Study of respiratory disorders in endoscopically negative and positive gastroesophageal reflux disease. *Saudi J. Gastroenterol.* **2010**, *16*, 84–89. [CrossRef] [PubMed]
39. Papachrisanthou, M.M.; Davis, R.L. Clinical Practice Guidelines for the Management of Gastroesophageal Reflux and Gastroesophageal Reflux Disease: 1 Year to 18 Years of Age. *J. Pediatr. Health Care* **2016**, *30*, 289–294. [CrossRef]
40. Hait, E.J.; McDonald, D.R. Impact of Gastroesophageal Reflux Disease on Mucosal Immunity and Atopic Disorders. *Clin. Rev. Allergy Immunol.* **2019**, *57*, 213–225. [CrossRef]
41. Megale, S.R.; Scanavini, A.B.; Andrade, E.C.; Fernandes, M.I.; Anselmo-Lima, W.T. Gastroesophageal reflux disease: Its importance in ear, nose, and throat practice. *Int. J. Pediatr. Otorhinolaryngol.* **2006**, *70*, 81–88. [CrossRef]
42. Cuzzolin, L.; Locci, C.; Chicconi, E.; Antonucci, R. Clinical use of gastric antisecretory drugs in pediatric patients with gastroesophageal reflux disease: A narrative review. *Transl. Pediatr.* **2023**, *12*, 260–270. [CrossRef]
43. Ummarino, D.; Miele, E.; Masi, P.; Tramontano, A.; Staiano, A.; Vandenplas, Y. Impact of antisecretory treatment on respiratory symptoms of gastroesophageal reflux disease in children. *Dis. Esophagus* **2012**, *25*, 671–677. [CrossRef] [PubMed]

44. Lin, H.C.; Xirasagar, S.; Chung, S.D.; Huang, C.C.; Tsai, M.C.; Chen, C.H. Fewer acute respiratory infection episodes among patients receiving treatment for gastroesophageal reflux disease. *PLoS ONE* **2017**, *12*, e0172436. [CrossRef] [PubMed]
45. Aizlewood, E.G.; Jones, F.W.; Whatmough, R.M. Paediatric gastroesophageal reflux disease and parental mental health: Prevalence and predictors. *Clin. Child Psychol. Psychiatry* **2023**, *28*, 1024–1037. [CrossRef] [PubMed]

Disclaimer/Publisher's Note: The statements, opinions and data contained in all publications are solely those of the individual author(s) and contributor(s) and not of MDPI and/or the editor(s). MDPI and/or the editor(s) disclaim responsibility for any injury to people or property resulting from any ideas, methods, instructions or products referred to in the content.

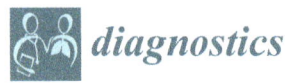

Article

Iron Deficiency Anemia in Pediatric Gastroesophageal Reflux Disease

Vasile Valeriu Lupu [1], Ingrith Miron [1], Ana Maria Laura Buga [1,*], Cristina Gavrilovici [1], Elena Tarca [2,*], Anca Adam Raileanu [1], Iuliana Magdalena Starcea [1], Andrei Tudor Cernomaz [3,*], Adriana Mocanu [1] and Ancuta Lupu [1]

1. Pediatrics Department, "Grigore T. Popa" University of Medicine and Pharmacy, 700115 Iasi, Romania
2. Department of Surgery II—Pediatric Surgery, "Grigore T. Popa" University of Medicine and Pharmacy, 700115 Iasi, Romania
3. 3rd Medical Department, "Grigore T. Popa" University of Medicine and Pharmacy, 700115 Iasi, Romania
* Correspondence: anamaria_bnz@yahoo.com (A.M.L.B.); elena.tuluc@umfiasi.ro (E.T.); a_cernomaz@yahoo.com (A.T.C.)

Abstract: (1) Background: Gastroesophageal reflux disease (GERD) can cause several complications as a result of the acidic pH over various cellular structures, which have been demonstrated and evaluated over time. Anemia can occur due to iron loss from erosions caused by acidic gastric content. In children, anemia has consequences that, in time, can affect their normal development. This study evaluates the presence of anemia as a result of pediatric gastroesophageal reflux disease. (2) Methods: 172 children were diagnosed with gastroesophageal reflux in the gastroenterology department of a regional children's hospital in northeast Romania by esophageal pH-metry and they were evaluated for presence of anemia. (3) Results: 23 patients with GERD from the studied group also had anemia, showing a moderate correlation ($r = -0.35$, $p = 0.025$, 95% confidence interval) and lower levels of serum iron were found in cases with GERD, with statistical significance ($F = 8.46$, $p = 0.012$, 95% confidence interval). (4) Conclusions: The results of our study suggest that there is a relationship between anemia or iron deficiency and gastroesophageal reflux due to reflux esophagitis in children, which needs to be further studied in larger groups to assess the repercussions on children's development.

Keywords: gastroesophageal reflux; anemia; esophagitis; children

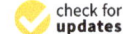

Citation: Lupu, V.V.; Miron, I.; Buga, A.M.L.; Gavrilovici, C.; Tarca, E.; Adam Raileanu, A.; Starcea, I.M.; Cernomaz, A.T.; Mocanu, A.; Lupu, A. Iron Deficiency Anemia in Pediatric Gastroesophageal Reflux Disease. *Diagnostics* **2023**, *13*, 63. https://doi.org/10.3390/diagnostics13010063

Academic Editor: Cristina Oana Marginean

Received: 7 December 2022
Revised: 19 December 2022
Accepted: 23 December 2022
Published: 26 December 2022

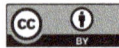

Copyright: © 2022 by the authors. Licensee MDPI, Basel, Switzerland. This article is an open access article distributed under the terms and conditions of the Creative Commons Attribution (CC BY) license (https:// creativecommons.org/licenses/by/ 4.0/).

1. Introduction

Gastroesophageal reflux represents the retrograde movement of gastric content into the esophagus. This phenomenon is physiological and can occur several times a day, for all age groups [1].

According to the Montreal consensus in 2006, when gastroesophageal reflux leads to symptoms that interfere with a person's well-being and/or the occurrence of complications, it is referred to as gastroesophageal reflux disease (GERD). The complications included in the definition of gastroesophageal reflux disease can be grouped into esophageal and extraesophageal syndromes, as presented in Figures 1 and 2 [2].

In pediatric gastroesophageal reflux disease, the symptomatology varies according to age and is non-specific. If for older children and adolescents this is similar to those present in the adult patient, in infants, the manifestations are often general or superimposed on the onset of other diseases (regurgitations, arching, feeding refusal, weight loss or weight stagnation, agitation, irritability, inconsolable crying, etc.) [3].

The diagnosis of GERD is established both clinically, based on symptoms and signs, and paraclinical, by identifying lesions caused by acidic pH through upper digestive endoscopy (esophagitis of various degrees, Barrett's esophagus, or adenocarcinoma) or by determining the presence of low pH in the esophagus by esophageal pH-metry. Continuous esophageal pH-metry was introduced in the 1990s and represented the gold standard for the diagnosis of GERD until the introduction of impedance pH-metry. Technological advances led to the possibility of performing wireless esophageal pH-metry, by means of a capsule that attaches to the esophageal mucosa and detaches after 48 h, as an alternative to classical monitoring, but at the moment, this technique is mainly used in the United States of America [4].

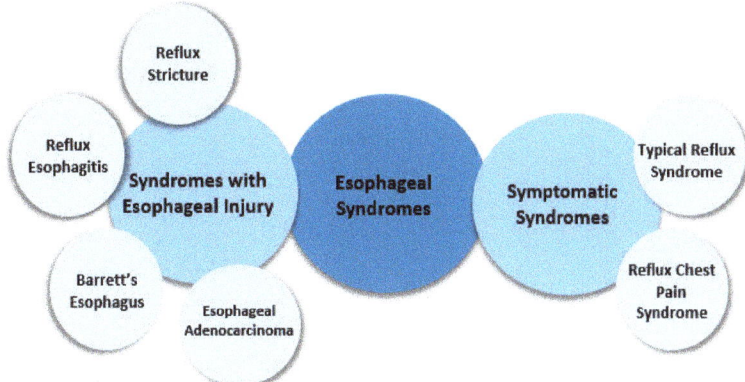

Figure 1. Esophageal syndromes of GERD [2].

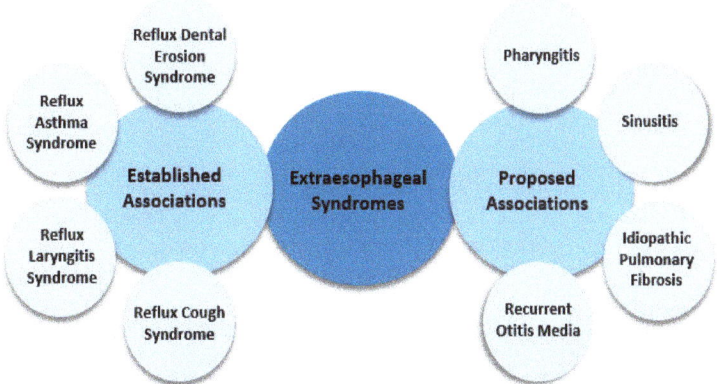

Figure 2. Extraesophageal syndromes of GERD [2].

The prolonged action of acidic pH on the esophageal epithelial cells can lead to various important consequences, from feeding intolerance and malnutrition in infants to respiratory pathology in those predisposed (i.e., children with Down syndrome or neuromuscular diseases) and, in extreme situations, to Barrett's esophagus at older ages. Last, but not least, iron loss from bleedings along the esophagus wall can determine iron deficiency or hypochromic hyposideremic anemia in the long term [5].

Iron deficiency anemia (IDA) is the most frequent types of anemia and for pediatric patients has an incidence between 39% and 48.1% in developing countries and between 5.9% and 20%, depending on age, in developed countries [6]. The main mechanism that leads to iron deficiency anemia is low nutritional sources of iron from diet both in industrialized and developing countries, the prevalence for iron deficiency being four times higher in developing countries as opposed to developed ones. In the long run, anemia has a negative impact on growth, cognitive function, and behavior of children, but also in the case of adults, it produces unwanted effects such as physical and mental asthenia, restless leg syndrome, for pregnant women it can cause premature birth, low birth weight children, or even mortality for both mother and fetus [7]. Beside low dietary intake being the main cause of iron deficiency, there are other sources that ultimately lead to iron deficiency anemia, as summarized in Table 1 [8].

Table 1. Causes of iron deficiency anemia according to age and different pathologies [8].

	Newborn	Low birth weight Perinatal blood loss Low maternal iron stores
Age	Infants, Small Children	Excessive consumption of cow's milk Inadequate dietary intake Intake of foods that disrupt iron absorption
	Adolescents	Growth spurt Menstrual period Von Willebrand disease
Pathologies	Occult Bleeding	Peptic ulcer Meckel's diverticulum Intestinal polyp Hemangioma Inflammatory bowel disease
	Insensible Blood Loss	Celiac disease Chronic diarrhea Pulmonary hemosiderosis Parasitosis

Since in our daily clinical practice we encountered many cases of anemia in which other etiologies were excluded through anamnesis and various paraclinical explorations, and at the same time we also observed the large number of patients with gastroesophageal reflux, we proposed to analyze in this study the relationship between these two pathologies.

2. Materials and Methods

We conducted a retrospective study over a period of 5 years, on 234 patients hospitalized in the gastroenterology department of a regional children's hospital in north–east Romania with suspicion of GERD. The diagnosis of gastroesophageal reflux was established following the results of esophageal pH-metry and that of iron deficiency anemia through the measurement of hemoglobin, hematocrit, mean cellular volume, mean cellular hemoglobin concentration, and serum ferritin.

Informed consent was obtained from all patients' carers, and the "St. Mary" Children Emergency Hospital Ethics Committee's approval was obtained.

Indications for esophageal pH-metry were the presence of GERD symptoms and signs: cough unresponsive to treatment, nocturnal cough, odynophagia, frequent regurgitation or vomiting without other cause, prolonged crying in infants, unsatisfactory weight gain in infants and small children.

The exclusion criteria from the study were: treatment with antacid medication in the last 3 months, treatment with non-steroidal anti-inflammatory drugs or aspirin, treatment for Helicobacter pylori eradication, gastrointestinal bleeding diagnosed through endoscopy, esophageal strictures or esophagitis in the context of systemic diseases, personal history of surgery on the esophagus or stomach [9], and other causes of iron deficiency anemia (excluded through detailed medical history, physical examination).

To determine the pH, the equipment used was Medtronic Digitrapper^R pH 100, SN 37660, the catheters used were Zinetics 24 and ComforTec by Sandhill. Software used for recording the measurements was Polygram.Net^{TM} pH. The values were recorded continuously for 24 h through a probe placed 5 cm above the lower esophageal sphincter;

the difference between the physiological and pathological reflux periods were made by the pH values below 4. The diagnosis of GERD was established according to the obtained values of the Boix-Ochoa score, a value lower than 11.99 being considered normal, according to the literature [9,10].

The diagnosis of anemia was established based on the low values for the age range for hemoglobin and hematocrit (see Table 2). We also quantified mean cellular volume (MCV), mean cellular hemoglobin (MCH), mean cellular hemoglobin concentration (MCHC), and serum iron values and compared them to the normal values (see Tables 3 and 4).

Table 2. Normal hemoglobin and hematocrit values for age groups [11].

Age	Gender	Hemoglobin (g/dL)		Hematocrit (%)	
		IF	SL	IL	SL
6 months up to 2 years		11	13.5	31	42
2–6 years		11	13.7	34	44
6–12 years		11.2	14.5	35	44
12–18 years	Girls	11.4	14.7	36	46
	Boys	12.4	16.4	40	51

IL = inferior limit; SL = superior limit.

Table 3. Erythrocyte parameters values for age groups [11].

Age	MCV (fL)		MCH (pg)		MCHC (g/dL)	
	IL	SL	IL	SL	IL	SL
0–1 years	70.5	94.9	22.9	32.7	32.3	35
1–3 years	72.8	85.2	22.7	29		
3–6 years	77.4	89.9	25.2	29.3		
6–13 years			25.4	30.8		
13–18 years	77.6	95.7	25.9	32.4		

IL = inferior limit; SL = superior limit.

Table 4. Serum iron normal values for age groups [11].

Age	Serum Iron (mcg/dL)	
	IL	SL
0–1 year	20	153
1–5 years	9	151
6–10 years	6	148
11–14 years	19	156
15–18 years	14	156

IL = inferior limit; SL = superior limit.

Software used for data processing was IBM SPSS Statistics 20 and the Pearson parametric correlation was used for correlation analysis. Furthermore, the correlation coefficients were calculated for a confidence interval of 95%.

3. Results

Among the 234 children included in the study, 32 patients had anemia and 172 patients were identified with gastroesophageal reflux disease through a positive Boix-Ochoa score (N < 11.99). From the 32 patients with anemia, 23 were associated with GERD, a higher number than those without GERD ($F = 7.86$, $p = 0.0173$, 95% confidence interval). The statistical data analysis shows a moderate correlation between anemia and GERD ($r = -0.35$,

$p = 0.025$, 95% confidence interval). At least two erythrocyte parameters are significantly affected, namely, MCH and MCV, which translates into interpretating terms indicating a tendency towards deficiency anemia (Tables 5 and 6). The decrease in MCH is obvious and meets the conditions of statistical significance even when statistical correlation tests are applied. This aspect actually confirms that these children have a marked tendency to become anemic during the evolution of the disease and the erythrocyte parameters can be the first detectable changes with indicative value.

Table 5. Statistical indicators for MCV in relation to GERD.

	Median MCV	Mean −95%	Mean +95%	Standard Deviation	Standard Error	Min	Max	Q25	Median	Q75
With GERD	77.02	75.82	78.23	7.66	0.61	56.25	102	74	77.89	82
Without GERD	80.75	78.89	82.62	7.02	0.93	61	92	77	81	86

Table 6. Statistical indicators for MCH in relation to GERD.

	Median MCH	Mean −95%	Mean +95%	Standard Deviation	Standard Error	Min	Max	Q25	Median	Q75
With GERD	25.94	25.5	26.37	2.74	0.22	17.29	33.8	24.8	26.35	27.5
Without GERD	27.2	26.56	27.83	2.38	0.32	19.36	31.1	26.07	27.6	28.5

The serum iron level was investigated in patients who had modified erythrocyte parameters even if the hemoglobin and hematocrit values were normal. We identified lower levels of serum iron in cases with GERD, with statistical significance ($F = 8.46$, $p = 0.012$, 95% confidence interval). We must emphasize the fact that this serum parameter also correlates very well with the imminence of anemia as suggested by the other parameters. The values found in patients with GERD are much lower compared to the control group and compared to the normal inferior limit of sideremia (Table 7), suggesting the fact that the origin of the tendency towards anemia is in fact the iron deficiency achieved both by chronic losses and by affecting the intake.

Table 7. Statistical indicators for serum iron in relation to GERD.

	Median Serum Iron	Mean −95%	Mean +95%	Standard Deviation	Standard Error	Min	Max	Q25	Median	Q75
With GERD	58.93	50.82	67.04	27	4.02	15	131	35	54	77
Without GERD	73.37	51.5	95.24	36.19	10.04	1.78	143	52	66	100

Gender distribution and the area of living for the patients in the studied group are summarized in Table 8.

Table 8. Distribution of cases according to gender and area of living.

	Gender		Area of Living	
	Boys	Girls	Urban	Rural
With GERD	92	80	110	62
With anemia	20	12	21	11
With GERD and anemia	14	9	15	8

4. Discussion

From a pathophysiological point of view, in infants, gastroesophageal reflux is due to the immaturity of the smooth muscle fibers of the lower esophageal sphincter, which allows the passage of the gastric contents back into the esophagus, leading to the destruction of the esophageal epithelial cells through its acidic pH, with inflammation and irritation [12]. Furthermore, there is a lower resting pressure in the lower esophageal sphincter of the infants compared to that of the adult, starting at 3.8 mmHg for premature infants born at 27 weeks of gestation, 12.2 mmHg for the ones born at 35 weeks of gestation, and reaching 18 mmHg for full-term infants versus 19 up to 28 mmHg for an adult [13]. At the same time, the exclusively liquid diet and prolonged periods in a horizontal position also contribute to the occurrence of GERD in infants under the age of 6 months [12]. Also, there are more cases of GER at younger ages due to another series of peculiarities at that stage in life: the esophageal capacity is 5–10 mL, unlike that of an adult that has approximately 180 mL, the intra-abdominal part of the esophagus is shorter than in the adult, which is about 3 cm, and last, but not least, infants ingest a volume of food per kilogram of body five to eight times greater than adults [14]. Usually, physiological reflux begins between the ages of 1 to 6 months and improves progressively until the age of 12 months when it should resolve. If the symptoms start outside this age range or do not disappear around the age of 1, then the occurrence of GERD must be considered [5].

When it comes to pediatric patients, for children older than 8 years and adolescents, the same diagnostic criteria for GERD apply as for adults, since the typical symptoms are similar to theirs (i.e., heartburn, regurgitation). Nevertheless, in infants and small children differentiating between GER and GERD is more difficult, as the symptoms are varied and non-specific, among the most common being regurgitation, prolonged crying episodes, back arching, irritability (in Table 9 more symptoms are listed as well as signs by age groups) [15].

Table 9. GERD signs and symptoms in children by age group [15].

Children Aged 1 to 5 Years	Children Aged 6 to 18 Years
Recurrent vomiting	Heartburn
Weight loss	Epigastric pain
Failure to thrive	Retrosternal pain
Refusal to feed	Nocturnal abdominal/retrosternal pain
Abdominal pain	Dysphagia
Difficulty swallowing	Nausea
Recurrent pneumonia	Nocturnal coughing
Anemia	Hoarseness
Chronic sinusitis or otitis	Sore throat
Dental erosions	Halitosis
Sleep disturbances, fatigue	Wheezing
Behavioral disorders, irritability	Recurrent pneumonia
	Chronic sinusitis or recurrent otitis media
	Laryngitis
	Dental erosions
	Sleep disturbances, irritability, behavioral disorder

Also, in infants, the same constellation of symptoms can be found in cow's milk protein allergy, making the two pathologies difficult to differentiate from a clinical point of view, especially when these symptoms do not correlate with the occurrence of reflux in esophageal pH-metry studies or do not remit after initiation of proton pump inhibitor treatment [16].

Regarding the epidemiological data, a systematic review on GERD in pediatric patients carried out in 2019, which included 25 eligible studies on the prevalence and characteristic symptoms of GERD, concluded that, in children aged 0 to 18 months, symptoms were present in more than one quarter of the cases, with their gradual decrease until disappearance until the age of 1. As for children over 18 months old, the percentage of those symptoms varied between 0 and 38% [17].

As mentioned above, anemia is recognized as one of the signs of GERD in children. The underlying mechanism by which it occurs is through corrosive esophagitis, and anemia might be the only presenting sign of this lesion due to GERD [14].

As stated in the beginning of the article, the effects of iron deficiency anemia in the human body are multiple, affecting several systems. On the short list, we note: in the central nervous system, it leads to mental and motor developmental delay, reduced cognitive function, irritability, and a shorter attention span. In the cardiovascular system, it can determine cardiac hypertrophy; in the immunologic system, it reduces the recovery rate after illnesses and increases the rate of respiratory infections, and decreases myeloperoxidase expression in leukocytes and the small intestine. At different cellular levels, it determines several perturbances such as ineffective erythropoiesis, increased auto hemolysis, decreased red cell survival, and oxidative damage to cell membranes [18].

It is known that there are multiple other causes of iron deficiency anemia, but for several, special attention must be paid. First of all, infants born prematurely have a faster growth rate that decreases the iron supply accumulated during pregnancy, but in premature births they are low already, because they are usually formed in the third trimester. Second of all, menstrual blood losses and, rarely, Von Willebrand disease are another source of IDA in adolescents; third of all, children with neuromotor pathology are an additional group predisposed to IDA due to needing gavage or a predominantly liquid diet that may be deficient in certain nutrients such as iron. Last, but not least, several gastrointestinal tract pathologies such as celiac disease, *Helicobacter pylori* infection, chronic inflammatory bowel disease intolerance to cow's milk proteins, Meckel's diverticulum, hiatal hernia, or parasitosis can lead to the path of insufficient iron absorption [6]. If gastroesophageal reflux adds to these particular situations, then the iron deficiency or IDA aggravates it.

The involvement of pediatric GERD in the pathophysiology of other entities such as asthma [19], recurrent pneumonia, recurrent wheezing [20], dental erosions [21,22], Sandifer syndrome [23], and sleep apnea [24] has been the subject of other adult or pediatric studies over time, but the relationship between iron deficiency anemia and gastroesophageal reflux disease, especially in children, was not the goal of many researchers. A query of PubMed Central electronic databases with the terms ("anaemia"[All Fields] OR "anemia"[MeSH Terms] OR "anemia"[All Fields]) AND ("gastroesophageal reflux"[MeSH Terms] OR ("gastroesophageal"[All Fields] AND "reflux"[All Fields]) OR "gastroesophageal reflux"[All Fields]) AND ("child"[MeSH Terms] OR "child"[All Fields] OR "children"[All Fields]) returned 1987 results, from which only a few, at a quick glance, contained the terms "Gastroesophageal reflux", "anemia" or "iron deficiency" and "children" or "pediatric" united in the title [25–28]. In other articles relevant to the subject of our study, anemia was mentioned in the body of the text, as a sign of GERD or as a red flag for this pathology [1,4,5,29].

We identified studies that searched for causes of iron deficiency anemia unresponsive to treatment, among which GERD was counted as well. A retrospective study from 2006, conducted by a research group in Naples, Italy, found that 10 cases from a total of 238 studied had anemia due to blood losses determined by reflux esophagitis [30]. Another study published in 2007 in Cairo, Egypt determined the prevalence of celiac disease, *Helicobacter pylori,* and gastroesophageal reflux among a small group of 25 patients with iron deficiency anemia unresponsive to iron treatment received for 3 months. The research group concluded that gastroesophageal reflux was positive in 11 of the studied cases, but only 6 of them had gastroesophageal reflux solely, while the other 5 had an associated *H. pylori* infection or a combination of celiac disease and *H. pylori* infection in addition to GERD [25]. Another article published by a research group from the United States of America in 2022 described a series of five cases with iron deficiency anemia as a result of gastroesophageal reflux in children with congenital esophageal atresia or neurologic impairment. The article highlighted that these two conditions are at risk of developing GER and reflux can further lead to columnar metaplasia of the esophagus wall cells. This often leads to anemia even in the absence of gastrointestinal symptoms, suggesting that unexplained iron deficiency anemia in children with neurological disorders or esophageal atresia should be considered a consequence of gastroesophageal reflux and additional investigations would be useful in order to diagnose or rule out GERD [26].

A particular and infrequent form of gastroesophageal reflux disease seen typically in infants is Sandifer syndrome. This pathology associates certain movements and postures (spasmodic dystonia and opisthotonos) in the presence of reflux, it being considered that posturing is a way to alleviate pain caused by acidic reflux. Even though it represents less than 1% of pediatric cases of GERD, it must be taken into consideration as a form of gastrointestinal disorder and not be misinterpreted as a neurological disease in order to receive proper antiacid treatment [31]. Regarding the prevalence of anemia in this form of gastroesophageal reflux, we identified cases in the literature that are associated with anemia also or articles that pointed the presence of anemia as a complication of Sandifer syndrome [23,32,33].

Even if our study shows moderate correlation between GERD and anemia, there are still more patients that have associated anemia and GERD than those that have only anemia (23 versus 9). In addition, the results show an increased rate of iron deficiency among patients with GERD. Therefore, we consider it opportune to develop new studies in this direction, with larger groups, to evaluate the impact that this hematological pathology has on the pediatric population with gastroesophageal reflux disease.

5. Conclusions

Cumulating the hematological changes obtained in our study, we can say that GERD is accompanied by a degree of iron deficiency that opens the way to iron deficiency anemia. Considering the fact that anemia can be one of the signs of gastroesophageal reflux disease, especially among pediatric patients, this complication should not be neglected due to its long-term effects in a child's development and further in adult life. When faced with a case of hypochromic hyposideremic anemia in which other causes have been excluded, the clinician should consider it as a result of a gastroesophageal reflux if the patient presents signs and symptoms suggestive for this gastrointestinal pathology, and also if the anemia does not respond to oral iron therapy. In addition, the small number of studies found in the literature regarding the prevalence of anemia in gastroesophageal reflux disease in children opens the road to further investigation.

Author Contributions: Conceptualization, V.V.L. and A.M.; methodology, E.T.; software, A.T.C. and I.M.S.; validation, I.M., E.T. and C.G.; formal analysis, A.M. and A.T.C.; investigation, V.V.L. and A.L.; data curation, A.M.L.B.; writing—original draft preparation, A.M.L.B., V.V.L., A.A.R. and A.L.; writing—review and editing, I.M., I.M.S., A.T.C., E.T., A.M. and C.G.; visualization, A.M.L.B. and A.A.R.; supervision, I.M. and C.G.; project administration, V.V.L., I.M., C.G., A.A.R., I.M.S. and A.M. contributed equally with V.V.L. to this article. All authors have read and agreed to the published version of the manuscript.

Funding: This research received no external funding.

Institutional Review Board Statement: The study was conducted according to the guidelines of the Declaration of Helsinki. The research was approved by the Ethics Committee of "Saint Mary" Emergency Children's Hospital, Iasi, Romania (16832 from 13.08.2015.).

Informed Consent Statement: Informed consent was obtained from all subjects involved in the study.

Data Availability Statement: The data presented in this study are available on request from the corresponding author. The data are not publicly available due to ethical issues.

Acknowledgments: We would like to thank Mihaela Moscalu for statistics, and the clinic's staff from the "St. Mary" Children's Emergency Hospital for their help.

Conflicts of Interest: The authors declare no conflict of interest.

References

1. Singendonk, M.M.J.; Rosen, R.R.; Tabbers, M.M. Gastroesophageal Reflux Disease (GERD) in Children. In *Encyclopedia of Gastroenterology*, 2nd ed.; Kuipers, E.J., Ed.; Academic Press: Cambridge, MA, USA, 2019; pp. 682–691.
2. Vakil, N.; van Zanten, S.V.; Kahrilas, P.; Dent, J.; Jones, R.; Global Consensus Group. The Montreal definition and classification of gastroesophageal reflux disease: A global evidence-based consensus. *Am. J. Gastroenterol.* **2006**, *101*, 1900–1920.E1. [CrossRef] [PubMed]
3. Rosen, R.; Vandenplas, Y.; Singendonk, M.; Cabana, M.; DiLorenzo, C.; Gottrand, F.; Gupta, S.; Langendam, M.; Staiano, A.; Thapar, N.; et al. Pediatric Gastroesophageal Reflux Clinical Practice Guidelines: Joint Recommendations of the North American Society for Pediatric Gastroenterology, Hepatology, and Nutrition and the European Society for Pediatric Gastroenterology, Hepatology, and Nutrition. *J. Pediatr. Gastroenterol. Nutr.* **2018**, *66*, 516–554. [CrossRef] [PubMed]
4. Gonzalez Ayerbe, J.I.; Hauser, B.; Salvatore, S.; Vandenplas, Y. Diagnosis and Management of Gastroesophageal Reflux Disease in Infants and Children: From Guidelines to Clinical Practice. *Pediatr. Gastroenterol. Hepatol. Nutr.* **2019**, *22*, 107–121. [CrossRef]
5. Bingham, S.M.; Muniyappa, P. Pediatric gastroesophageal reflux disease in primary care: Evaluation and care update. *Curr. Probl. Pediatr. Adolesc. Health Care* **2020**, *50*, 100784. [CrossRef] [PubMed]
6. Moscheo, C.; Licciardello, M.; Samperi, P.; La Spina, M.; Di Cataldo, A.; Russo, G. New Insights into Iron Deficiency Anemia in Children: A Practical Review. *Metabolites* **2022**, *12*, 289. [CrossRef] [PubMed]
7. Piskin, E.; Cianciosi, D.; Gulec, S.; Tomas, M.; Capanoglu, E. Iron Absorption: Factors, Limitations, and Improvement Methods. *ACS Omega* **2022**, *7*, 20441–20456. [CrossRef] [PubMed]
8. Özdemir, N. Iron deficiency anemia from diagnosis to treatment in children. *Turk. Pediatr. Ars.* **2015**, *50*, 11–19. [CrossRef]
9. Lupu, V.V.; Burlea, M.; Nistor, N.; Streanga, V.; Starcea, M.I.; Paduraru, G.; Ghica, D.C.; Mitrofan, E.C.; Moscalu, M.; Ignat, A. Correlation between esophageal pH-metry and esophagitis in gastroesophageal reflux disease in children. *Medicine* **2018**, *97*, e12042. [CrossRef]
10. Pandolfino, J.E.; Vela, M.F. Esophageal-reflux monitoring. *Gastrointest. Endosc.* **2009**, *69*, 917–930. [CrossRef]
11. Wong, E.C.C.; Brugnara, C.; Straseski, J.A.; Kellogg, M.D.; Adeli, K. (Eds.) 2-Hematology tests. In *Pediatric Reference Intervals*, 8th ed.; Academic Press: Cambridge, MA, USA, 2020; pp. 209–266.
12. El-Mahdy, M.A.; Mansoor, F.A.; Jadcherla, S.R. Pharmacological management of gastroesophageal reflux disease in infants: Current opinions. *Curr. Opin. Pharmacol.* **2017**, *37*, 112–117. [CrossRef]
13. Pados, B.F.; Davitt, E.S. Pathophysiology of Gastroesophageal Reflux Disease in Infants and Nonpharmacologic Strategies for Symptom Management. *Nurs. Women's Health* **2020**, *24*, 101–114. [CrossRef] [PubMed]
14. Jones, A.B. Gastroesophageal reflux in infants and children. When to reassure and when to go further. *Can. Fam. Physician* **2001**, *47*, 2045–2050. [PubMed]
15. Papachrisanthou, M.M.; Davis, R.L. Clinical Practice Guidelines for the Management of Gastroesophageal Reflux and Gastroesophageal Reflux Disease: 1 Year to 18 Years of Age. *J. Pediatr. Health Care* **2016**, *30*, 289–294. [CrossRef] [PubMed]
16. Mousa, H.; Hassan, M. Gastroesophageal Reflux Disease. *Pediatr. Clin. N. Am.* **2017**, *64*, 487–505. [CrossRef]
17. Singendonk, M.; Goudswaard, E.; Langendam, M.; van Wijk, M.; van Etten-Jamaludin, F.; Benninga, M.; Tabbers, M. Prevalence of Gastroesophageal Reflux Disease Symptoms in Infants and Children: A Systematic Review. *J. Pediatr. Gastroenterol. Nutr.* **2019**, *68*, 811–817. [CrossRef]
18. Powers, J.M. Chapter 4—Nutritional anemias. In *Lanzkowsky's Manual of Pediatric Hematology and Oncology*, 7th ed.; Fish, J.D., Lipton, J.M., Lanzkowsky, P., Eds.; Academic Press: Cambridge, MA, USA, 2021; pp. 61–80.
19. Lupu, V.V.; Miron, I.; Tarca, E.; Trandafir, L.M.; Anton-Paduraru, D.T.; Moisa, S.M.; Starcea, M.; Cernomaz, A.; Miron, L.; Lupu, A. Gastroesophageal Reflux in Children with Asthma. *Children* **2022**, *9*, 336. [CrossRef]
20. Lupu, V.V.; Miron, I.C.; Lupu, A.; Moscalu, M.; Mitrofan, E.C.; Munteanu, D.; Luca, A.C. The relationship between gastroesophageal reflux disease and recurrent wheezing in children. *Medicine* **2021**, *100*, e27660. [CrossRef]
21. Ellis, A.W.; Kosaraju, A.; Ruff, R.R.; Miller, C.B.; Francis, J.M.; Vandewalle, K.S. Dental erosion as an indicator of gastroesophageal reflux disease. *Gen. Dent.* **2022**, *70*, 46–51.
22. Ignat, A.; Burlea, M.; Lupu, V.V.; Paduraru, G. Oral manifestations of gastroesophageal reflux disease in children. *Rom. J. Oral Rehabil.* **2017**, *9*, 40–43.
23. Shrestha, A.B.; Rijal, P.; Sapkota, U.H.; Pokharel, P.; Shrestha, S. Sandifer Syndrome: A Case Report. *JNMA J. Nepal Med. Assoc.* **2021**, *59*, 1066–1068. [CrossRef]
24. Mahfouz, R.; Barchuk, A.; Obeidat, A.E.; Mansour, M.M.; Hernandez, D.; Darweesh, M.; Aldiabat, M.; Al-Khateeb, M.H.; Yusuf, M.H.; Aljabiri, Y. The Relationship Between Obstructive Sleep Apnea (OSA) and Gastroesophageal Reflux Disease (GERD) in Inpatient Settings: A Nationwide Study. *Cureus* **2022**, *14*, e22810. [CrossRef]
25. Fayed, S.B.; Aref, M.I.; Fathy, H.M.; Abd El Dayem, S.M.; Emara, N.A.; Maklof, A.; Shafik, A. Prevalence of celiac disease, Helicobacter pylori and gastroesophageal reflux in patients with refractory iron deficiency anemia. *J. Trop. Pediatr.* **2008**, *54*, 43–53. [CrossRef] [PubMed]
26. Van Arsdall, M.R.; Nair, S.; Moye, L.M.; Nguyen, T.T.; Saleh, Z.M.; Rhoads, J.M. Columnar Metaplasia of the Esophagus Presenting as Iron Deficiency Anemia in Children with Neurologic Impairment or Congenital Esophageal Atresia. *Am. J. Case Rep.* **2022**, *23*, e937255. [CrossRef]
27. Dietrich, C.G.; Hübner, D.; Heise, J.W. Paraesophageal hernia and iron deficiency anemia: Mechanisms, diagnostics and therapy. *World J. Gastrointest. Surg.* **2021**, *13*, 222–230. [CrossRef] [PubMed]

28. Massolo, F.; Laudizi, L.; Sturloni, N.; Cellini, M.; Cordioli, A.; Laudizi, Z. Anemia ipocromica iposideremica come primo sintomo di reflusso gastroesofageo [Hypochromic hyposideremic anemia as the first symptom of gastroesophageal reflux]. *Pediatr. Med. Chir.* **1989**, *11*, 533–535. (In Italian) [PubMed]
29. Rybak, A.; Pesce, M.; Thapar, N.; Borrelli, O. Gastro-Esophageal Reflux in Children. *Int. J. Mol. Sci.* **2017**, *18*, 1671. [CrossRef]
30. Ferrara, M.; Coppola, L.; Coppola, A.; Capozzi, L. Iron deficiency in childhood and adolescence: Retrospective review. *Hematology* **2006**, *11*, 183–186. [CrossRef]
31. Patil, S.; Tas, V. Sandifer Syndrome. In *StatPearls*; StatPearls [Internet]: Treasure Island, FL, USA, 2022.
32. Cafarotti, A.; Bascietto, C.; Salvatore, R.; Breda, L.; Chiarelli, F.; Piernicola, P. A 6-month-old boy with uncontrollable dystonic posture of the neck. Sandifer syndrome. *Pediatr. Ann.* **2014**, *43*, 17–19. [CrossRef]
33. Moore, D.M.; Rizzolo, D. Sandifer syndrome. *JAAPA Off. J. Am. Acad. Physician Assist.* **2018**, *31*, 18–22. [CrossRef]

Disclaimer/Publisher's Note: The statements, opinions and data contained in all publications are solely those of the individual author(s) and contributor(s) and not of MDPI and/or the editor(s). MDPI and/or the editor(s) disclaim responsibility for any injury to people or property resulting from any ideas, methods, instructions or products referred to in the content.

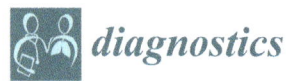

Article

The Usefulness of the Eosinophilic Esophagitis Histology Scoring System in Predicting Response to Proton Pump Inhibitor Monotherapy in Children with Eosinophilic Esophagitis

Jovan Jevtić [1,*], Nina Ristić [2], Vedrana Pavlović [3], Jovana Svorcan [2], Ivan Milovanovich [2], Milica Radusinović [2], Nevena Popovac [2], Ljubica Simić [1], Aleksandar Ćirović [4], Miloš Đuknić [1], Maja Životić [1], Nevena Poljašević [5], Danilo Obradović [1], Jelena Filipović [1] and Radmila Janković [1,*]

[1] Institute of Pathology, Faculty of Medicine, University of Belgrade, 11000 Belgrade, Serbia; ljubica.simic87@gmail.com (L.S.); djuknicmilos996@gmail.com (M.Đ.); majajoker@gmail.com (M.Ž.); drdaniloobradovic@gmail.com (D.O.); vjesticaj@gmail.com (J.F.)

[2] Department of Gastroenterology, Hepatology and GI Endoscopy, University Children's Hospital, 11000 Belgrade, Serbia; nina.ristic13@gmail.com (N.R.); svorcanjovana@yahoo.com (J.S.); imilovanovich@gmail.com (I.M.); milicaradusinovic@hotmail.com (M.R.); nevena.popovac@gmail.com (N.P.)

[3] Institute of Medical Statistics and Informatics, Faculty of Medicine, University of Belgrade, 11000 Belgrade, Serbia; vedrana.pavlovic@med.bg.ac.rs

[4] Institute of Anatomy, Faculty of Medicine, University of Belgrade, 11000 Belgrade, Serbia; aleksandar.cirovic.7@gmail.com

[5] Department of Pathology, University Clinical Center Tuzla, 75000 Tuzla, Bosnia and Herzegovina; nevena.poljasevic@gmail.com

* Correspondence: lordstark90@gmail.com (J.J.); radmila.jankovic@med.bg.ac.rs (R.J.); Tel.: +381-644013120 (J.J.); +381-113643339 (R.J.)

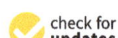

Citation: Jevtić, J.; Ristić, N.; Pavlović, V.; Svorcan, J.; Milovanovich, I.; Radusinović, M.; Popovac, N.; Simić, L.; Ćirović, A.; Đuknić, M.; et al. The Usefulness of the Eosinophilic Esophagitis Histology Scoring System in Predicting Response to Proton Pump Inhibitor Monotherapy in Children with Eosinophilic Esophagitis. *Diagnostics* 2023, 13, 3445. https://doi.org/10.3390/diagnostics13223445

Academic Editor: Cristina Oana Marginean

Received: 7 October 2023
Revised: 8 November 2023
Accepted: 12 November 2023
Published: 15 November 2023

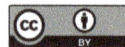

Copyright: © 2023 by the authors. Licensee MDPI, Basel, Switzerland. This article is an open access article distributed under the terms and conditions of the Creative Commons Attribution (CC BY) license (https://creativecommons.org/licenses/by/4.0/).

Abstract: Background: Eosinophilic esophagitis (EoE) is an immune-mediated esophageal disease with rising incidence. While proton pump inhibitors (PPIs) are the first-line treatment, a significant proportion of patients do not respond. This study aimed to determine if the EoE Histology Scoring System (EoEHSS) can predict PPI responsiveness. Methods: A cross-sectional study was conducted on 89 pediatric patients diagnosed with EoE between 2016 and 2022. Patients were categorized into PPI responders (PPIREoE) and non-responders (PPINREoE) based on post-treatment biopsies. EoEHSS values from biopsies of the esophagus (distal, middle, and proximal segments) were compared between the two groups. Results: No significant differences in EoEHSS scores were observed for the distal and proximal esophagus between the groups. However, the middle esophagus showed a significantly higher EoEHSS grade score in the PPINREoE group, indicating a more pronounced disease severity. Specific histological features, particularly eosinophilic abscesses and surface layering of the middle segment of the esophagus, were significantly different between the groups. Conclusions: Performing a biopsy of each esophageal segment, particularly the middle, is crucial for diagnostic precision and predicting PPI responsiveness. The EoEHSS can serve as a valuable tool in predicting therapy response, emphasizing the need for personalized therapeutic approaches in EoE management.

Keywords: eosinophilic esophagitis; pediatrics; EoEHSS; score; EREFS

1. Introduction

Eosinophilic esophagitis (EoE) is an immune-mediated disease characterized by esophageal dysfunction and a peak eosinophil count (PEC) ≥ 15 eosinophils per high-power field (HPF) on histological examination, in the absence of other conditions and diseases that could cause eosinophilia of the esophagus [1]. The incidence of EoE is consistently increasing, in both children and adults. Although it was initially believed that the incidence was rising due to increased awareness and appropriate diagnostic evaluation, recent studies have shown a real increase in the occurrence of EoE [2,3]. EoE is usually not a life-threatening disease, but nevertheless requires timely treatment. Prolonging the time of diagnosis or applying inappropriate therapy can lead to complications [1] such as esophageal stenosis or perforation, the latter of which can prove fatal [4]. Treatment modalities for EoE include proton pump inhibitors (PPIs), topical corticosteroids, and a strict dietary regimen (the elimination of certain foods). Considering that they are safe, inexpensive, and easily applicable, PPIs are the first–line therapy [5]. However, a certain proportion of patients (51%) with EoE does not respond to PPI treatment and they require a different therapeutic approach [6,7]. Given that there is a population of patients who do not respond to PPIs, predicting the response to these drugs would shorten the time to effective treatment.

In 2017, Collins et al. developed the EoE Histology Scoring System (EoEHSS) which has proven to be superior to peak eosinophil count in terms of diagnosis and patient monitoring [8]. This raises the question whether EoEHSS can also be used to predict response to therapy. The objective of our study is to compare EoEHSS values from biopsies of the distal, middle, and proximal segments of the esophagus, as well as clinical parameters, between two patient groups based on their response to PPI therapy, with the aim of predicting therapy response.

2. Materials and Methods

2.1. Study Design and Patient Selection

This cross-sectional study included 89 pediatric patients, aged between 0 and 18 years, who were diagnosed and treated for EoE at a tertiary healthcare center between 2016 and 2022. The diagnosis of EoE was made according to guidelines [1]. Biopsies were taken from all segments of the esophagus (proximal, middle, distal). A minimum of four tissue samples were taken from at least two locations, typically proximally and distally. In cases where all three segments of the esophagus were biopsied, a minimum of six tissue samples were taken. This sampling approach was applied both during the initial diagnosis and in the evaluation of the PPI therapy's effectiveness. After the diagnosis was established, all patients received PPI treatment at a dosage of 1–2 mg/kg per day. Three months after treatment, a follow-up endoscopy with multiple biopsies was performed to evaluate the treatment's effectiveness. Based on their response to the PPI therapy, patients were divided into two groups: responders (PPIREoE) and non-responders (PPINREoE). Responders were defined as those patients who had fewer than 15 eosinophils per HPF within their esophageal biopsies. Analyses for this study were conducted based on data from the initial endoscopy and initial biopsies. We analyzed 151 tissue samples (35 samples of PPIREoE and 116 samples of PPINREoE) from the distal esophageal segment, 64 tissue samples (28 samples of PPIREoE and 36 samples of PPINREoE) from the middle esophageal segment, and 148 samples (32 samples of PPIREoE and 116 samples of PPINREoE) from the proximal esophageal segment. The inclusion criteria for patients into the study were: at least two esophageal biopsies, before and after the administration of therapy. The exclusion criteria were if the patient initially received some other form of therapy other than PPI, if the patient did not undergo a follow up endoscopy with biopsy after treatment, or if the slides were inadequate for analysis because they had faded or for other reasons. This study was conducted with the approval of the Ethics Committee of the Faculty of Medicine, University of Belgrade.

2.2. Demographics, Clinical Characteristics and Endoscopy

The data collected included demographic information, allergy details, laboratory values, comorbidities, and symptoms at the time of the initial endoscopy. Endoscopic data related to EoE were collected using the EREFS score, which is actually an acronym derived from the initial letters of the endoscopic features of EoE (Edema, Rings, Exudates, Furrows, and Strictures) [9].

2.3. Tissue Processing and Preparation of H&E Slides for Scoring

After performing esophageal endoscopic biopsies, the samples were fixed for 24 h in 10% buffered formalin, then rinsed with distilled water, and subsequently dehydrated in increasing concentrations of alcohol (from 70% to pure alcohol). After dehydration in alcohol, the samples were lipophilized in xylene and, following lipophilization, embedded in paraffin blocks. The obtained paraffin blocks were cut with a standard microtome into sections 3–5 µm thick. The sections were further stained with hematoxylin and eosin (H&E).

2.4. Biopsy Scoring

Biopsy scoring was carried out according to the modified validated EoEHSS system developed by Collins et al. [8]. The EoEHSS encompasses more than just eosinophil count; it also considers various histological characteristics of EoE. This scoring system includes eight characteristics: peak eosinophil count (PEC), basal zone hyperplasia (BZH), eosinophilic abscesses (EA), eosinophil surface layering (SL), dilated intercellular spaces (DIS), surface epithelial alterations (SEA), lamina propria fibrosis (LPF), and dyskeratotic epithelial cells (DEC). Due to their presence in a limited number of biopsies, LPF, SEA, and DEC were excluded. Therefore, the scoring was based on PEC, EA, SL, BZH, and DIS (Figure 1). A grade and stage were assigned to each of the aforementioned characteristics [8]. For each histological feature, grade and stage values were determined semi-quantitatively, ranging from 0 to 3 (Tables 1 and 2). If the maximum values for grade and stage for each biopsy feature of a patient were 3, then the maximum possible score for grade and stage would be 15. The final score would be calculated by dividing the given biopsy's grade and stage score by the maximum possible values. Scoring was performed using an Olympus BX43 microscope (Pittsford, NY, USA).

Table 1. Grading within the EoEHSS.

Grade Score	
Peak eosinophil count (PEC)	
0	PEC 0
1	PEC < 15/HPF
2	PEC 15–59/HPF
3	PEC > 60/HPF
Basal zone hyperplasia (BZH)	
0	BZH not present
1	BZH occupies >15% but <33% of the total thickness
2	BZH occupies 33–66% of the total thickness
3	BZH occupies >66% of the total thickness
Eosinophilic abscesses (EA)	
0	EA not present
1	EA consists of 4–9 eosinophils
2	EA consists of 10–20 eosinophils
3	EA consists of >20 eosinophils

Table 1. *Cont.*

Grade	Score
Eosinophil surface layering (SL)	
0	SL not present
1	SL consists of 3–4 eosinophils
2	SL consists of 5–10 eosinophils
3	SL consists of >10 eosinophils
Dilated intercellular spaces (DIS)	
0	DIS not observed at any magnification
1	DIS are observed only at 400× magnification
2	DIS are observed at 200× magnification
3	DIS are observed at 100× magnification or lower

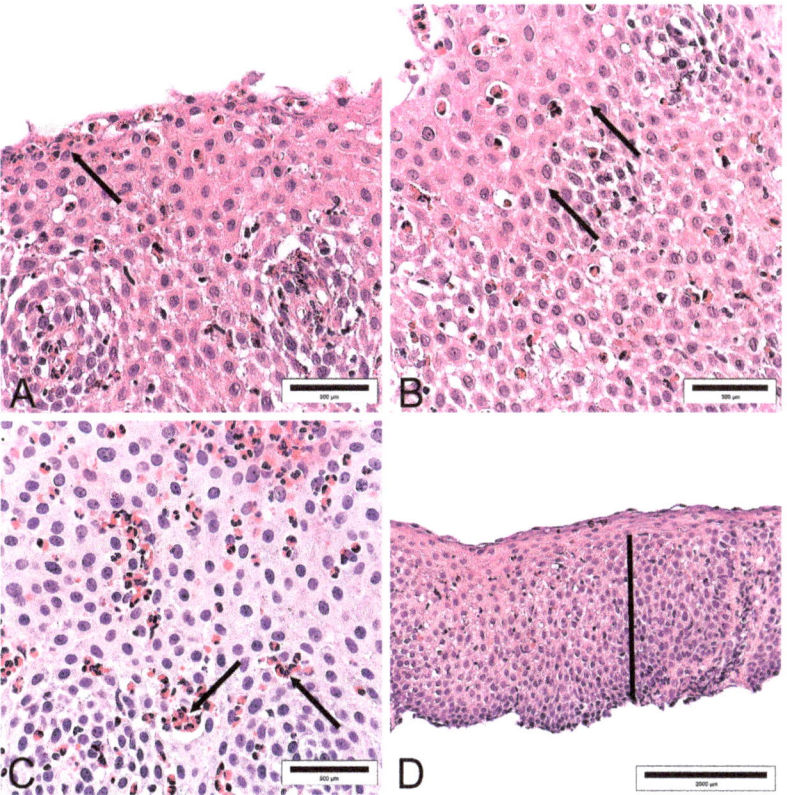

Figure 1. This figure represents a part of the scoring methodology, displaying histological characteristics of EoE that have been scored. ((**A**)—Eosinophil surface layering (arrow), magnification ×100; (**B**)—Dilated intercellular spaces (arrow), magnification ×100; (**C**)—Eosinophilic abscesses (arrow), magnification ×100; (**D**)—Basal zone hyperplasia (The line shows the portion of the esophageal epithelium affected by BZH), magnification ×40; On each image, more than 15 eosinophils per high power field (Eo/HPF) are present).

Table 2. Staging within the EoEHSS.

Stadium	Score
Peak eosinophil count (PEC)	
0	PEC 0–14/HPF
1	PEC $\geq$ 15/HPF in <33% HPFs
2	PEC $\geq$ 15/HPF in 33–66% HPFs
3	PEC $\geq$ 15/HPF in >66% HPFs
Basal zone hyperplasia (BZH)	
0	BZH not present
1	BZH of any grade > 0 occupying < 33% of the biopsy epithelium
2	BZH of any grade > 0 occupying 33–66% of the biopsy epithelium
3	BZH of any grade > 0 occupying > 66% of the biopsy epithelium
Eosinophilic abscesses (EA)	
0	EA not present
1	EA of any grade > 0 occupying < 33% of the biopsy epithelium
2	EA of any grade > 0 occupying 33–66% of the biopsy epithelium
3	EA of any grade > 0 occupying > 66% of the biopsy epithelium
Eosinophil surface layering (SL)	
0	SL not present
1	SL of any grade > 0 occupying < 33% of the biopsy epithelium
2	SL of any grade > 0 occupying 33–66% of the biopsy epithelium
3	SL of any grade > 0 occupying > 66% of the biopsy epithelium
Dilated intercellular spaces (DIS)	
0	DIS not present
1	DIS of any grade > 0 occupying < 33% of the biopsy epithelium
2	DIS of any grade > 0 occupying 33–66% of the biopsy epithelium
3	DIS of any grade > 0 occupying > 66% of the biopsy epithelium

2.5. Statistical Analysis

To characterize the study sample, we used descriptive statistics. For numerical variables, we calculated means, medians, standard deviations, and percentiles. For categorical variables, we determined the numbers and their respective percentages. The Pearson chi-squared test or Fisher's exact test were used to evaluate associations between categorical data. The Student's *t*-test or the Mann-Whitney U test were used for numerical data to evaluate differences between responders and non-responders. Univariate logistic regression analysis was used to establish factors related to overall therapy response. In all analyses, the level of statistical significance was set at $p \leq 0.05$. SPSS version 25 statistical software (Chicago, IL, USA) was used to perform the statistical analysis.

3. Results
3.1. Demographic and Clinical Characteristics

A total of 89 pediatric patients with EoE were included in the study. The average age of study participants was 12.1 ± 3.8 years and more than half were male (78.7%). The youngest patient included was 2 and the eldest was 18 years old. There was no significant age or gender differences between the PPIREoE and PPINREoE groups. Additionally, no differences were observed in terms of allergic factors (Table 3). Regarding symptoms, pain and dyspeptic complaints were more prevalent among PPIREoE, while regurgitation and food impaction were more common among PPINREoE. Vomiting and dysphagia were almost equally represented in both groups. Interestingly, comorbidities were exclusively observed in the non-responder group of patients.

Table 3. Demographic and clinical characteristics of PPINREoE and PPIREoE.

	Total (n = 89)	Response to Therapy		p
		PPINREoE (n = 72)	PPIREoE (n = 17)	
Gender, n (%)				0.284
Male	70 (78.7)	55 (76.4)	15 (88.2)	
Female	19 (21.3)	17 (23.6)	2 (11.8)	
Age, mean ± sd	12.1 ± 3.8	12.3 ± 3.8	11.7 ± 3.5	0.594
Atopy, n (%)	20 (22.5)	17 (23.6)	3 (17.6)	0.596
Food Allergy—SPT, n (%)	12 (13.5)	10 (13.9)	2 (11.8)	0.818
Food Allergy—IGE, n (%)	24 (27.0)	20 (27.8)	4 (23.5)	0.723
Inhalation allergy panel test, n (%)	23 (25.8)	19 (26.4)	4 (23.5)	0.809
Comorbidities, n (%)	17 (19.1)	17 (23.6) *	0 (0.0)	0.026 *
Regurgitation, n (%)	4 (4.5)	4 (5.6)	0 (0)	0.320
Dysphagia, n (%)	31 (34.8)	25 (34.7)	6 (35.3)	0.964
Impaction, n (%)	34 (38.2)	29 (40.3)	5 (29.4)	0.407
Pain, n (%)	21 (23.6)	14 (19.4)	7 (41.2)	0.058
Dyspepsia, n (%)	13 (14.6)	8 (11.1)	5 (29.4)	0.055
Vomiting, n (%)	12 (13.5)	10 (13.9)	2 (11.8)	0.818
EREFS, median (25th–75th percentile)	2 (1–2)	2 (1–2)	2 (0.5–2)	0.291

* Statistically significant. PPINREoE: proton pump inhibitor non-responders; PPIREoE: proton pump inhibitor responders; SPT: skin prick test; EREFS: endoscopic reference score.

3.2. Histological Characteristics

The final EoEHSS grade score for distal segment biopsies was 0.6 (0.5–0.7) for the PPINREoE group and 0.5 (0.4–0.7) for the PPIREoE group, indicating a slight but not statistically significant difference in the overall disease severity score between the two groups. A similar result was observed in biopsies from the proximal segment where the score was 0.6 (0.3–0.7) for the PPINREoE group and 0.4 (0.2–0.6) for the PPIREoE group. When we compared individual components of EoEHSS for grade, no statistically significant difference was observed between PPINREoE and PPIREoE in both distal and proximal segments of the esophagus.

Interestingly, the final EoEHSS grade score for the middle segment was 0.5 (0.5–0.8) for the PPINREoE group, which was significantly higher than the 0.3 (0.3–0.5) observed in the PPIREoE group ($p = 0.037$), indicating a more pronounced severity in the PPIREoE group. Similar results were obtained when comparing individual components of the EoEHSS with respect to grade, revealing a more pronounced disease severity in the PPINREoE group. Specifically, EA and SL demonstrated a statistically significant difference compared with the PPIREoE group ($p = 0.044$ and $p = 0.046$, respectively) (Table 4) (Figure 2).

Table 4. EoEHSS final score and individual components for grade of PPINREoE and PPIREoE.

EoEHSS	Response to Therapy		OR	p
	PPINREoE	PPIREoE		
DG (n = 78)				
PEC	2 (2–3)	2 (2–3)	0.676	0.403
BZH	2 (2–3)	2 (2–3)	0.694	0.296
EA	1 (0–1)	0 (0–1)	0.882	0.734
SL	1 (0–2)	1 (0–1)	0.814	0.495
DIS	3 (2–3)	3 (2–3)	0.755	0.428
Final score	0.6 (0.5–0.7)	0.5 (0.4–0.7)	0.225	0.327
MG (n = 29)				
PEC	3 (2–3)	2 (1–2)	0.392	0.112
BZH	3 (2–3)	1 (1–3)	0.562	0.144
EA	1 (0–1) *	0 (0–0)	0.106	0.044 *
SL	1 (0–2) *	0 (0–0)	0.248	0.046 *
DIS	3 (2–3)	2 (1–3)	0.712	0.305
Final score	0.5 (0.5–0.8) *	0.3 (0.3–0.5)	0.011	0.037 *
PG (n = 76)				
PEC	2 (1–3)	2 (0–3)	0.648	0.154
BZH	3 (2–3)	3 (0–3)	0.669	0.147
EA	0 (0–1)	0 (0–1)	0.852	0.683
SL	0 (0–2)	0 (0–1)	0.914	0.763
DIS	3 (1–3)	3 (0–3)	0.759	0.293
Final score	0.6 (0.3–0.7)	0.4 (0.2–0.6)	0.278	0.253

Data are presented as median (25th–75th percentile). * Statistically significant. EoEHSS: eosinophilic esophagitis histology scoring system; PPINREoE: proton pump inhibitor non-responders; PPIREoE: proton pump inhibitor responders; DG: distal esophagus grade; MG: middle esophagus grade; PG: proximal esophagus grade; PEC: peak eosinophil count; BZH: basal zone hyperplasia; EA: eosinophilic abscesses; SL: eosinophil surface layering; DIS: dilated intercellular spaces.

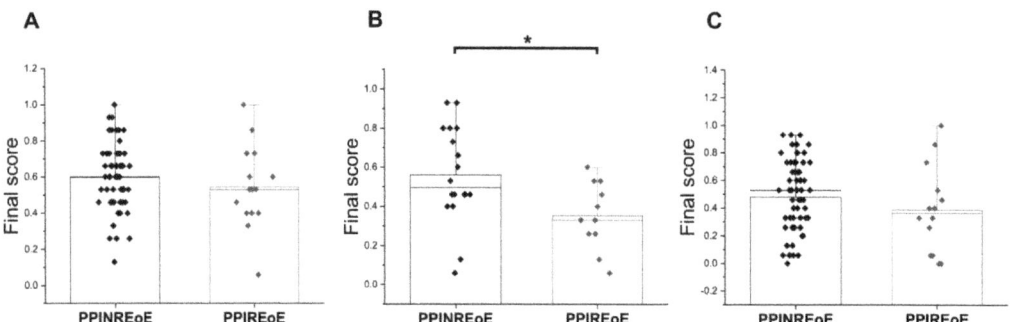

Figure 2. EoEHSS final score for grade of PPINREoE and PPIREoE; (A) EoEHSS final score of the distal esophagus; (B) EoEHSS final score of the middle esophagus; (C) EoEHSS final score of the proximal esophagus. * $p < 0.05$.

None of the EoEHSS stage scores showed a statistically significant difference between PPINREoE and PPIREoE for the proximal, distal, or middle segments of the esophagus. Analysis of the individual EoEHSS parameters for disease stage yielded results consistent with those observed for disease grade. Notably, significant differences between PPINREoE and PPIREoE were identified in the EA values from biopsies of the middle segment and

BZH values from the proximal segment, suggesting a more extensive disease distribution in patients unresponsive to therapy (Table 5) (Figure 3).

Table 5. EoEHSS final score and individual components for stage of PPINREoE and PPIREoE.

EoEHSS	Response to Therapy		OR	p
	PPINREoE	PPIREoE		
DS (n = 78)				
PEC	3 (2–3)	3 (1–3)	0.831	0.512
BZH	3 (3–3)	3 (3–3)	0.730	0.405
EA	1 (0–2)	0 (0–2)	0.890	0.705
SL	1 (0–2)	1 (0–1)	0.713	0.268
DIS	3 (2–3)	3 (2–3)	0.791	0.546
Final score	0.7 (0.5–0.8)	0.6 (0.5–0.8)	0.290	0.339
MS (n = 29)				
PEC	3 (1–3)	1 (0–3)	0.750	0.392
BZH	3 (3–3)	3 (2–3)	0.802	0.570
EA	1 (0–2) *	0 (0–0)	0.126	0.049 *
SL	1 (0–2)	0 (0–0)	0.367	0.077
DIS	3 (2–3)	2 (1–3)	0.784	0.470
Final score	0.5 (0.4–0.8)	0.4 (0.3–0.6)	0.053	0.102
PS (n = 76)				
PEC	2 (1–3)	2 (0–3)	0.738	0.206
BZH	3 (2–3)	3 (0–3)	0.623	0.041 *
EA	0 (0–1)	0 (0–1)	0.769	0.469
SL	0 (0–2)	0 (0–1)	0.852	0.614
DIS	3 (1–3)	3 (0–3)	0.923	0.745
Final score	0.6 (0.3–0.7)	0.4 (0.2–0.6)	0.276	0.212

Data are presented as median (25th–75th percentile). * Statistically significant. EoEHSS: eosinophilic esophagitis histology scoring system; PPINREoE: proton pump inhibitor non-responders; PPIREoE: proton pump inhibitor responders; DS: distal esophagus stadium; MS: middle esophagus stadium; PS: proximal esophagus stadium; PEC: peak eosinophil count; BZH: basal zone hyperplasia; EA: eosinophilic abscesses; SL: eosinophil surface layering; DIS: dilated intercellular spaces.

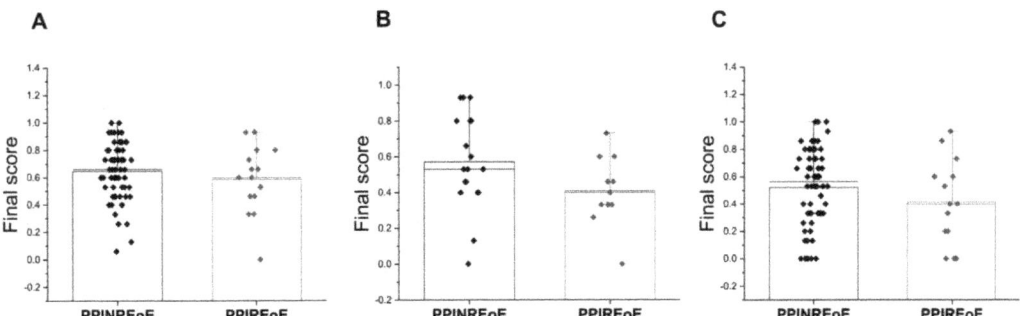

Figure 3. EoEHSS final score for stage of PPINREoE and PPIREoE; (A) EoEHSS final score of the distal esophagus; (B) EoEHSS final score of the middle esophagus; (C) EoEHSS final score of the proximal esophagus.

4. Discussion

The consistent increase in the incidence of EoE necessitates research regarding its etiology, pathogenesis, as well as the refinement of diagnostics and therapy. The primary objective of EoE treatment is not only to alleviate disease symptoms and enhance patients' quality of life but also to prevent potential complications, including those that could be life-threatening. Delay in treatment or application of inadequate therapy carries the risk of disease complications. The aim of this study is to predict the response to PPI therapy as the first-line treatment in patients with EoE, with the goal of initially selecting the therapy to which the patient will best respond. Additionally, there is still no method to predict the response to PPI therapy, which would enable selection of the appropriate treatment at the outset. Our study, encompassing 89 pediatric patients, provides valuable insights into the clinical and histological characteristics of EoE in relation to PPI responsiveness.

Taking into account the response to PPI therapy, our study showed a lower rate of response compared with most studies. However, there are also studies in the pediatric population that have shown a similar response rate [10]. Such findings can be explained by poorer compliance with therapy, considering that a significant number of adolescents were included in the study, where compliance with therapy is generally lower. Additionally, it has been demonstrated that the response to PPI therapy in the pediatric population is generally poorer compared with adults [11].

From a demographic perspective, our cohort predominantly comprised males, consistent with previous literature that has identified a male preponderance in EoE [12]. The age range of our study participants, spanning from 2 to 18 years, highlights the broad spectrum of pediatric ages at which EoE can manifest. Notably, the absence of significant age or gender differences between the PPIREoE and PPINREoE groups suggests that these demographic factors might not play a pivotal role in determining PPI responsiveness.

The clinical presentations of EoE are known to be diverse, and our study confirms this heterogeneity. While pain and dyspeptic complaints were more common in the PPIREoE group, regurgitation and food impaction were predominant in the PPINREoE group. This divergence in symptomatology could be attributed to variations in esophageal mucosal involvement, eosinophilic infiltration, or other inflammatory processes, which might be influenced by genetic, environmental, or immunological factors. The equal representation of vomiting and dysphagia in both groups, however, suggests that these symptoms might not be reliable indicators of PPI responsiveness. The exclusive presence of comorbidities in the non-responder group is intriguing and raises questions about potential associations between comorbid conditions and PPI resistance. Given that the comorbidities in our study group were highly diverse (asthma, epilepsy, Hashimoto's thyroiditis, kidney agenesis, cerebellar medulloblastoma, etc.), even after an extensive literature search, we were unable to find a connection with a lack of response to therapy. Therefore, further research on this topic is essential.

Although nearly fifty years have passed since EoE was first described, there are still no clear protocols regarding the number and localization of biopsies necessary for diagnosis [13,14]. While various studies emphasize the importance of performing a biopsy on both the proximal and distal segments of the esophagus for diagnosis [15], others highlight the significance of also sampling the middle segment of the esophagus [16,17]. The only point on which most researchers agree on is taking a larger number of biopsies from different locations (polytopic biopsies). Our study underscores the critical need for a standardized approach to biopsy protocols in EoE diagnosis. The ambiguity surrounding the optimal number and location of biopsies highlights a significant gap in the current understanding and approach to EoE diagnosis and management. The scores (grade and stage) for the distal and proximal segment did not show significant differences between the two groups. Even though they cannot be used to predict the response to PPI, biopsies of the distal and proximal esophageal segments are essential for the diagnosis of EoE and for differentiation from GERD. However, the middle segment of the esophagus emerged as a potential region of interest. In a recent study by Hiermath et al., it was shown that most histological features of EoE, except for DIS, are not uniformly represented in all parts of the esophagus, regardless of whether the EoE is active or in remission [18]. Lin et al. demonstrated that EoEHSS scores can significantly vary between the distal and middle segments of the esophagus in both the population of patients with active EoE and in patients in remission. Additionally, it has been shown that EoEHSS scores were not always higher in the distal segment of the esophagus, suggesting that such distribution might be associated with different types of EoE, varying symptomatology, and distinct therapeutic requirements and responses [17]. The significantly higher EoEHSS grade score for the PPINREoE group in the middle segment in our study suggests that this region might be more susceptible to severe eosinophilic infiltration, especially in non-responders to PPI therapy. The pronounced differences in individual components, particularly EA and SL, further emphasize the importance of performing a biopsy on the middle segment of the esophagus. Additionally, Lin et al. have shown that different segments of the esophagus do not undergo simultaneous repair, with the mid-esophagus, where changes related to damage have been observed to persist for a longer period [17]. Interestingly, despite the differences observed in the grade scores, the EoEHSS stage scores did not offer a clear distinction between the two groups across all esophageal segments. By analyzing individual score characteristics with respect to stage, a statistically significant difference between PPINREoE and PPIREoE was observed in the EA values of the middle segment and BZH values of the proximal segment, potentially indicating that the distribution of the disease may be significant in terms of response to therapy.

While this study brings new insights, it also has its limitations, primarily in terms of its retrospective nature, a small sample size and univariate analysis. Future studies should aim to validate our findings in larger cohorts and explore the underlying mechanisms driving the observed differences between PPI responders and non-responders.

Further research could employ immunohistochemistry to assess eosinophil activity, potentially highlighting differences between these groups. Molecular investigations are also essential for a more in-depth understanding. The role of genetic factors in determining the response to PPI therapy also cannot be overlooked. Genetic polymorphisms might influence the pharmacodynamics and pharmacokinetics of PPIs, thereby affecting the therapeutic outcomes. Understanding the genetic makeup of the patients could potentially aid in personalizing the treatment strategies, ensuring more effective and efficient management of EoE. Additionally, examining the intercellular connections in these two patient groups is crucial. The epithelium's permeability itself may be linked to the response to therapy, necessitating a comprehensive exploration in this aspect. Research on the esophageal microbiota could significantly contribute to understanding the pathogenesis and selection of therapy for EoE. It has been shown that the esophageal microbiota in EoE patients is altered, with an increase in Haemophilus and a decrease in Firmicutes [19–21]. Additionally, a study conducted by Parashette et al. demonstrated significant differences in microbiota among EoE patients in terms of their response to PPI therapy, particularly in the context of the *Bacteroidetes* phylum [22]. Therefore, further investigations of the microbiome may hold significance in predicting the response to PPI therapy.

5. Conclusions

The EoEHSS score was successfully applied for the first time in order to predict the response to PPI therapy in children with EoE. EoEHSS grade score of the middle esophageal segment in PPINREoE was significantly higher compared with PPIREoE. Although some authors recommend performing a biopsy of two regions of the esophagus (most commonly the proximal and distal segments), our study points to the need for all segments of the esophagus (proximal, middle and distal) to be examined, particularly the middle. This increases diagnostic precision and facilitates therapeutic personalization through prediction of PPI responsiveness. Additionally, besides assessing the response to various forms of therapy, EoEHSS can also be an excellent tool in predicting the response.

Author Contributions: Conceptualization, J.J. and R.J.; methodology, J.J. and V.P.; formal analysis, J.J., M.Ž. and V.P.; investigation, J.J., N.R., J.S. and R.J.; writing—original draft preparation, J.J., L.S., V.P., M.Ž., A.Ć., M.Đ., J.S., N.P. (Nevena Poljašević) and D.O.; writing—review and editing, J.J., R.J., N.R., I.M., M.R., N.P. (Nevena Popovac) and J.F.; supervision, R.J. and J.F. All authors have read and agreed to the published version of the manuscript.

Funding: This research received no external funding.

Institutional Review Board Statement: The study was conducted in accordance with the Declaration of Helsinki, and approved by the Ethics Committee of Faculty of Medicine, University of Belgrade (17/VI-5, 29 June 2023).

Informed Consent Statement: Patient consent was waived due to the fact that patients cannot be identified from the anonymized data used in the study.

Data Availability Statement: The data presented in this study are available in the article.

Conflicts of Interest: The authors declare no conflict of interest.

References

1. Dhar, A.; Haboubi, H.N.; Attwood, S.E.; Auth, M.K.H.; Dunn, J.M.; Sweis, R.; Morris, D.; Epstein, J.; Novelli, M.R.; Hunter, H.; et al. British Society of Gastroenterology (BSG) and British Society of Paediatric Gastroenterology, Hepatology and Nutrition (BSPGHAN) joint consensus guidelines on the diagnosis and management of eosinophilic oesophagitis in children and adults. *Gut* **2022**, *71*, 1459–1487. [CrossRef]
2. Dellon, E.S.; Erichsen, R.; Baron, J.A.; Shaheen, N.J.; Vyberg, M.; Sorensen, H.T.; Pedersen, L. The increasing incidence and prevalence of eosinophilic oesophagitis outpaces changes in endoscopic and biopsy practice: National population-based estimates from Denmark. *Aliment. Pharmacol. Ther.* **2015**, *41*, 662–670. [CrossRef]
3. Ristic, N.; Jankovic, R.; Dragutinovic, N.; Atanaskovic-Markovic, M.; Radusinovic, M.; Stevic, M.; Ristic, M.; Ristic, M.; Milovanovic, T. Diagnosis of Eosinophilic Esophagitis in Children: A Serbian Single-Center Experience from 2010 to 2017. *Med. Princ. Pract.* **2019**, *28*, 449–456. [CrossRef]
4. Straumann, A.; Bussmann, C.; Zuber, M.; Vannini, S.; Simon, H.U.; Schoepfer, A. Eosinophilic esophagitis: Analysis of food impaction and perforation in 251 adolescent and adult patients. *Clin. Gastroenterol. Hepatol.* **2008**, *6*, 598–600. [CrossRef]
5. Muir, A.; Falk, G.W. Eosinophilic Esophagitis: A Review. *JAMA* **2021**, *326*, 1310–1318. [CrossRef]
6. Lucendo, A.J.; Arias, Á.; Molina-Infante, J. Efficacy of Proton Pump Inhibitor Drugs for Inducing Clinical and Histologic Remission in Patients With Symptomatic Esophageal Eosinophilia: A Systematic Review and Meta-Analysis. *Clin. Gastroenterol. Hepatol.* **2016**, *14*, 13–22.e1. [CrossRef]
7. Franciosi, J.P.; Mougey, E.B.; Dellon, E.S.; Gutierrez-Junquera, C.; Fernandez-Fernandez, S.; Venkatesh, R.D.; Gupta, S.K. Proton Pump Inhibitor Therapy for Eosinophilic Esophagitis: History, Mechanisms, Efficacy, and Future Directions. *J. Asthma Allergy* **2022**, *15*, 281–302. [CrossRef]
8. Collins, M.H.; Martin, L.J.; Alexander, E.S.; Boyd, J.T.; Sheridan, R.; He, H.; Pentiuk, S.; Putnam, P.E.; Abonia, J.P.; Mukkada, V.A.; et al. Newly developed and validated eosinophilic esophagitis histology scoring system and evidence that it outperforms peak eosinophil count for disease diagnosis and monitoring. *Dis. Esophagus* **2017**, *30*, 1–8. [CrossRef]
9. Hirano, I.; Moy, N.; Heckman, M.G.; Thomas, C.S.; Gonsalves, N.; Achem, S.R. Endoscopic assessment of the oesophageal features of eosinophilic oesophagitis: Validation of a novel classification and grading system. *Gut* **2013**, *62*, 489–495. [CrossRef]
10. Schroeder, S.; Capocelli, K.E.; Masterson, J.C.; Harris, R.; Protheroe, C.; Lee, J.J.; Furuta, G.T. Effect of proton pump inhibitor on esophageal eosinophilia. *J. Pediatr. Gastroenterol. Nutr.* **2013**, *56*, 166–172. [CrossRef]
11. Molina-Infante, J.; Katzka, D.A.; Gisbert, J.P. Review article: Proton pump inhibitor therapy for suspected eosinophilic oesophagitis. *Aliment. Pharmacol. Ther.* **2013**, *37*, 1157–1164. [CrossRef]
12. Cruz, J.; Irvine, M.A.; Avinashi, V.; Chan, E.S.; Vallance, B.A.; Soller, L.; Bush, J.W. Application of the Eosinophilic Esophagitis Histology Scoring System Grade Scores in Patients at British Columbia Children's Hospital. *Fetal Pediatr. Pathol.* **2022**, *41*, 962–976. [CrossRef]
13. Dobbins, J.W.; Sheahan, D.G.; Behar, J. Eosinophilic gastroenteritis with esophageal involvement. *Gastroenterology* **1977**, *72*, 1312–1316. [CrossRef]
14. Koop, A.H.; Middleton, J.; Travers, P.M.; Ghoz, H.; Francis, D.; DeVault, K.R.; Pang, M. Number of bottles of esophageal biopsies in the evaluation of eosinophilic esophagitis and clinical outcomes. *Clin. Res. Hepatol. Gastroenterol.* **2023**, *47*, 102142. [CrossRef]
15. Yantiss, R.K.; Greenson, J.K.; Spechler, S. American registry of pathology expert opinions: Evaluating patients with eosinophilic esophagitis: Practice points for endoscopists and pathologists. *Ann. Diagn. Pathol.* **2019**, *43*, 151418. [CrossRef]
16. Dellon, E.S.; Speck, O.; Woodward, K.; Covey, S.; Rusin, S.; Shaheen, N.J.; Woosley, J.T. Distribution and variability of esophageal eosinophilia in patients undergoing upper endoscopy. *Mod. Pathol.* **2015**, *28*, 383–390. [CrossRef]

17. Lin, B.; Rabinowitz, S.; Haseeb, M.A.; Gupta, R. Usefulness of the Eosinophilic Esophagitis Histologic Scoring System in Distinguishing Active Eosinophilic Esophagitis From Remission and Gastroesophageal Reflux Disease. *Gastroenterol. Res.* **2021**, *14*, 220–226. [CrossRef]
18. Hiremath, G.; Sun, L.; Collins, M.H.; Bonis, P.A.; Arva, N.C.; Capocelli, K.E.; Chehade, M.; Davis, C.M.; Falk, G.W.; Gonsalves, N.; et al. Esophageal Epithelium and Lamina Propria Are Unevenly Involved in Eosinophilic Esophagitis. *Clin. Gastroenterol. Hepatol.* **2023**, *21*, 2807–2816.e3. [CrossRef]
19. Zhang, X.; Zhang, N.; Wang, Z. Eosinophilic esophagitis and esophageal microbiota. *Front. Cell Infect. Microbiol.* **2023**, *13*, 1206343. [CrossRef]
20. Angerami Almeida, K.; de Queiroz Andrade, E.; Burns, G.; Hoedt, E.C.; Mattes, J.; Keely, S.; Collison, A. The microbiota in eosinophilic esophagitis: A systematic review. *J. Gastroenterol. Hepatol.* **2022**, *37*, 1673–1684. [CrossRef]
21. Massimino, L.; Barchi, A.; Mandarino, F.V.; Spanò, S.; Lamparelli, L.A.; Vespa, E.; Passaretti, S.; Peyrin-Biroulet, L.; Savarino, E.V.; Jairath, V.; et al. A multi-omic analysis reveals the esophageal dysbiosis as the predominant trait of eosinophilic esophagitis. *J. Transl. Med.* **2023**, *21*, 46. [CrossRef] [PubMed]
22. Parashette, K.R.; Sarsani, V.K.; Toh, E.; Janga, S.C.; Nelson, D.E.; Gupta, S.K. Esophageal Microbiome in Healthy Children and Esophageal Eosinophilia. *J. Pediatr. Gastroenterol. Nutr.* **2022**, *74*, e109–e114. [CrossRef] [PubMed]

Disclaimer/Publisher's Note: The statements, opinions and data contained in all publications are solely those of the individual author(s) and contributor(s) and not of MDPI and/or the editor(s). MDPI and/or the editor(s) disclaim responsibility for any injury to people or property resulting from any ideas, methods, instructions or products referred to in the content.

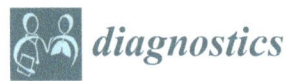

Review

Diagnosis and Management of Gastrointestinal Manifestations in Children with Cystic Fibrosis

Dana-Teodora Anton-Păduraru [1,2,†], Alina Mariela Murgu [1,2,*], Laura Iulia Bozomitu [1,2], Dana Elena Mîndru [1,2], Codruța Olimpiada Iliescu Halițchi [1], Felicia Trofin [3], Carmen Iulia Ciongradi [2,4], Ioan Sârbu [2,4], Irina Mihaela Eșanu [5,†] and Alice Nicoleta Azoicăi [1,2]

1. Department of Mother and Child Medicine, "Grigore T. Popa" University of Medicine and Pharmacy, 700115 Iași, Romania; dana.anton@umfiasi.ro (D.-T.A.-P.); laura.bozomitu@umfiasi.ro (L.I.B.); mindru.dana@umfiasi.ro (D.E.M.); olimpiada.iliescu@umfiasi.ro (C.O.I.H.); alice.azoicai@umfiasi.ro (A.N.A.)
2. "Sf. Maria" Children Emergency Hospital, 700309 Iasi, Romania; carmen.ciongradi@umfiasi.ro (C.I.C.); sarbu.ioan@umfiasi.ro (I.S.)
3. Department of Preventive Medicine and Interdisciplinarity–Microbiology, "Grigore T. Popa" University of Medicine and Pharmacy, 700115 Iași, Romania; felicia.trofin@umfiasi.ro
4. 2nd Department of Surgery, Pediatric Surgery and Orthopedics, "Grigore T. Popa" University of Medicine and Pharmacy, 700115 Iași, Romania
5. Medical Department, "Grigore T. Popa" University of Medicine and Pharmacy, 700115 Iași, Romania; irina.esanu@umfiasi.ro
* Correspondence: alina.murgu@umfiasi.ro
† These authors contributed equally to this work.

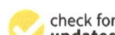

Citation: Anton-Păduraru, D.-T.; Murgu, A.M.; Bozomitu, L.I.; Mîndru, D.E.; Iliescu Halițchi, C.O.; Trofin, F.; Ciongradi, C.I.; Sârbu, I.; Eanu, I.M.; Azoicăi, A.N. Diagnosis and Management of Gastrointestinal Manifestations in Children with Cystic Fibrosis. *Diagnostics* 2024, 14, 228. https://doi.org/10.3390/diagnostics14020228

Academic Editor: Cristina Oana Marginean

Received: 15 December 2023
Revised: 16 January 2024
Accepted: 20 January 2024
Published: 22 January 2024

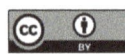

Copyright: © 2024 by the authors. Licensee MDPI, Basel, Switzerland. This article is an open access article distributed under the terms and conditions of the Creative Commons Attribution (CC BY) license (https://creativecommons.org/licenses/by/4.0/).

Abstract: Cystic fibrosis (CF) is primarily known for its pulmonary consequences, which are extensively explored in the existing literature. However, it is noteworthy that individuals with CF commonly display gastrointestinal (G-I) manifestations due to the substantial presence of the cystic fibrosis transmembrane conductance regulator (CFTR) protein in the intestinal tract. Recognized as pivotal nonpulmonary aspects of CF, G-I manifestations exhibit a diverse spectrum. Identifying and effectively managing these manifestations are crucial for sustaining health and influencing the overall quality of life for CF patients. This review aims to synthesize existing knowledge, providing a comprehensive overview of the G-I manifestations associated with CF. Each specific G-I manifestation, along with the diagnostic methodologies and therapeutic approaches, is delineated, encompassing the impact of innovative treatments targeting the fundamental effects of CF on the G-I tract. The findings underscore the imperative for prompt diagnosis and meticulous management of G-I manifestations, necessitating a multidisciplinary team approach for optimal care and enhancement of the quality of life for affected individuals. In conclusion, the authors emphasize the urgency for further clinical studies to establish a more robust evidence base for managing G-I symptoms within the context of this chronic disease. Such endeavors are deemed essential for advancing understanding and refining the clinical care of CF patients with G-I manifestations.

Keywords: cystic fibrosis; children; gastrointestinal manifestations; diagnosis; management

1. Introduction

Cystic fibrosis (CF) is an intricate multiorgan disorder affecting epithelial organs, including the respiratory tract, exocrine pancreas, intestine, hepatobiliary system, sweat glands, and, more recently, myeloid cells in secretory vesicle membranes [1–3]. It stands as the most prevalent autosomal recessive monogenic disease, exhibiting a chronic, progressive, and potentially fatal course in the Caucasian population. The condition involves a generalized dysfunction of the exocrine glands, particularly those producing mucus, resulting in the clinical triad of exocrine pancreatic insufficiency, chronic lung disease, and elevated chloride and sodium concentrations in sweat [4]. The gene responsible for encoding the cystic fibrosis transmembrane conductance regulator (CFTR) protein, a 1480-amino acid protein, was identified in 1989, with over 2000 mutations discovered to date and F508del representing 75% of mutations in Europe and North America [2].

Six pathogenic molecular mechanisms elucidate the extent of CFTR impairment, including protein-production defects (class I), processing defects (class II), regulatory defects (class III), conduction defects (class IV), reduced synthesis (class V), and decreased CFTR stability or impaired regulation of other channels (class VI) [2,4,5].

CF is predominantly renowned for its extensively studied pulmonary manifestations, yet it is noteworthy that these patients frequently experience gastrointestinal (G-I) problems due to the robust expression of the CFTR protein throughout the intestine [6,7]. The spectrum of G-I manifestations is diverse, encompassing exocrine pancreas involvement, meconium ileus, distal intestinal obstruction syndrome (DIOS), constipation, small intestinal bacterial overgrowth (SIBO), and intestinal inflammation. These manifestations significantly impact the quality of life and long-term prognosis [8], establishing them as the foremost nonpulmonary aspects of CF. Consequently, recognizing and effectively managing G-I manifestations hold paramount importance for maintaining health and enhancing the quality of life in CF patients.

The primary objectives of this study were to synthesize knowledge on G-I manifestations of CF, offering comprehensive insights into each G-I manifestation, the diagnostic methods, and the potential advancements in therapeutic strategies. This includes novel treatments addressing the fundamental effects of CF on the G-I tract and their outcomes.

2. Material and Methods

2.1. Search Strategy

This systematic review included 148 studies, identified through systematic database searches using "gastrointestinal manifestations" and "cystic fibrosis" on PubMed and Google Academic. After title screening, 12,745 articles were excluded due to title–research objective mismatch. Abstract examination excluded more articles based on relevance, publication date, accessibility, or pertinence. Thorough text analysis led to the exclusion of 218 articles due to relevance, methodological incongruity, scope misalignment, quality issues, or language barriers. The accompanying flowchart (Figure 1) illustrates the sequential progression of information through the review process, depicting the tally of records ascertained, incorporated, and eliminated.

2.2. Study Selection

The article selection and curation for our review adhered to strict criteria, including alignment with central research questions on G-I manifestations of CF in children, considering diagnosis and management. The criteria involved research objectives, publication year, scientific categorization, and presentation quality. Searches were precisely structured with keywords and Boolean operators.

After data extraction, selected articles underwent meticulous categorization and synthesis within a structured framework, forming the review's foundation. Qualitative analysis scrutinized scholarly adherence, clarity, brevity, citation frequency, sample size, data relevance, results articulation, and conclusions formulation. These facets were amalgamated into the final narrative synthesis.

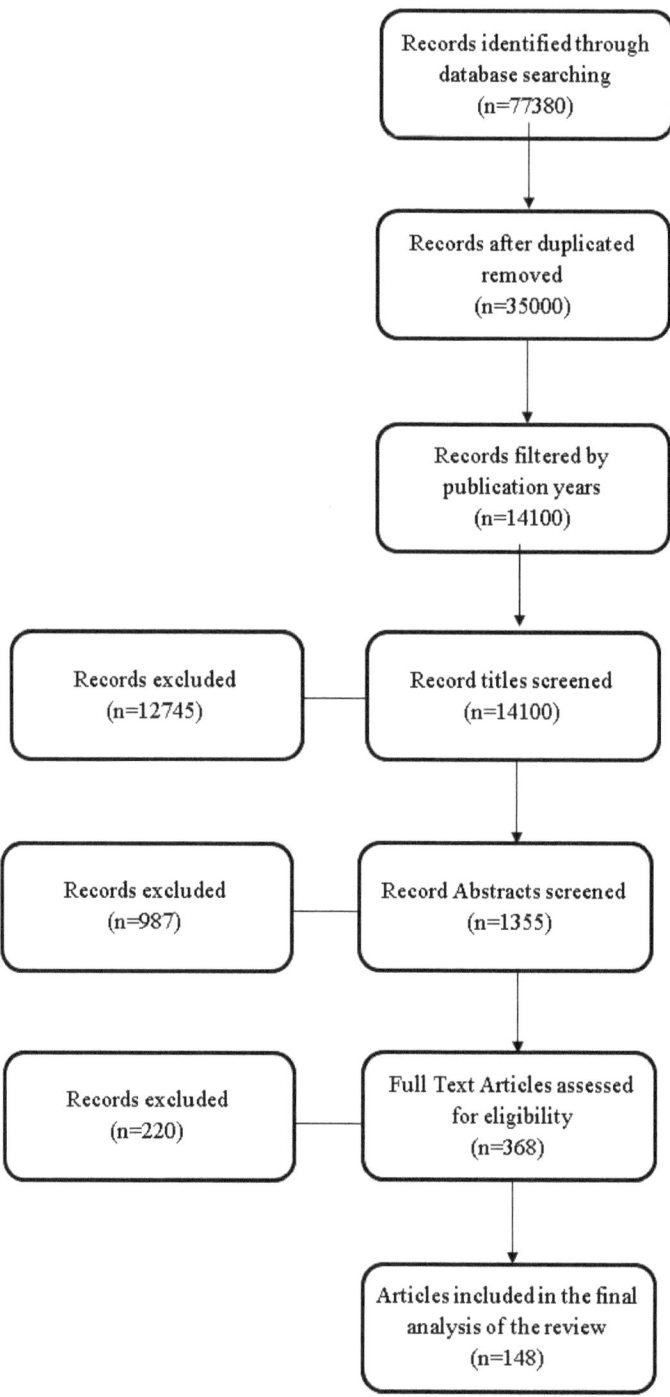

Figure 1. The review flowchart.

3. Results
3.1. Gastrointestinal Manifestations in CF—General Data

CF exerts its influence on the G-I tract from the uterine and neonatal stages, persisting throughout an individual's life [1,9]. G-I symptoms, observed in approximately 85% of cases, tend to be more prevalent in patients with severe disease or genotypes associated with moderate or severe abdominal involvement, potentially contributing to heightened morbidity and mortality among CF patients [10]. This phenomenon arises due to inadequate pancreatic enzyme release into the intestine, resulting in impaired food digestion. The multifactorial etiology of these manifestations involves CFTR dysfunction, a high-fat CF diet, and antibiotic use. Abdominal symptoms serve as a distinctive feature of multiorgan CF involvement, with patients undergoing intravenous antibiotic therapy often experiencing more pronounced G-I symptoms [11].

G-I impairment in CF is attributed to altered intestinal secretion, the absence of pancreatic fluids containing enzymes, dysbiosis, and intestinal inflammation. In the digestive tract, CFTR functionality is crucial for water and ion homeostasis, with a strong expression of the CFTR gene in the stomach and particularly in the intestinal tract. CFTR dysfunction adversely affects smooth-muscle contractility, leading to consequences such as pancreatic insufficiency, reduced bicarbonate, and fluid secretion, resulting in the formation of viscous secretions and fat malabsorption [12]. The CF gut operates within a deleterious cycle involving impaired luminal flux due to the viscous mucus layer, epithelial inflammation, infection, and/or dysbiosis [13]. The G-I damage observed in CF is attributed to the alteration of intestinal secretion, absence of pancreatic fluids containing enzymes, dysbiosis, and intestinal inflammation, as illustrated in Figure 2 [1,8,14,15].

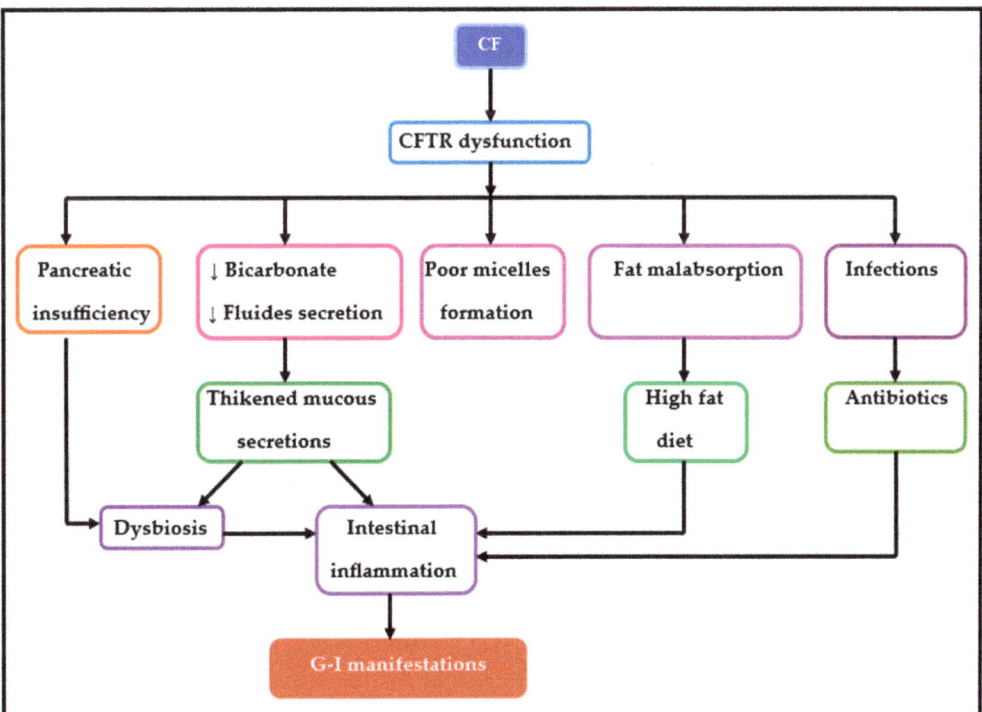

Figure 2. Etiology of G-I manifestations in CF (Legend: ↓ = decreased).

The dehydration of secretions leads to intraductal blockage, inflammation, fibrosis, and potential organic destruction in the presence of digestive enzymes [16–19]. Several studies report a reduction in β-cell area, ranging from 11% to 52%, while others indicate an unchanged number of pancreatic cells. In the proximal intestine, increased bicarbonate secretion fails to adequately neutralize gastric acid, contributing to imbalances. In pancreatic CF patients, low bicarbonate levels and secretion volume are observed, but the flow remains sufficient to support necessary enzyme secretion for digestion [14].

G-I symptoms in CF patients exhibit an inverse correlation with dietary fiber content. Studies on mice suggest that fiber reduces the paracellular permeability induced by oleic acid or reserpine, and elevated enzyme doses lead to intestinal eosinophilia and necrosis [20]. Emerging evidence highlights the significant role of intestinal inflammation in the manifestation of G-I symptoms in CF, with multifactorial causes contributing to inflammation.

Within the small intestine lumen of individuals with CF, elevated levels of inflammatory markers and morphological abnormalities, such as edema, erythema, ulceration, and destruction, are observed. Studies on mice indicate that intestinal inflammation correlates with reduced activity of ligand-dependent type-II nuclear receptors, impacting the metabolism and transport of fatty acids, sterols, bile acids, and xenobiotic acids. The modification of the intestinal microbial environment contributes to inflammation and the subsequent deterioration of the protective bacterial barrier in CF patients [21,22]. Inflammation further enhances *Escherichia coli* colonization of the intestinal mucosa. Conversely, *E. coli* can contribute to inflammation, impairing metabolism and lipid absorption, leading to malnutrition and symptom exacerbation [1]. Antibiotic use is recognized as an iatrogenic factor in CF associated with gut inflammation. Knoop et al. (2016) observed in a mouse study that oral antibiotic administration leads to increased inflammatory cytokines (IL-17, IFN-γ, and chemokine C-X-C motif ligand 1) alongside alterations in gut microbial composition [23]. Prolonged exposure to antibiotics in CF patients exacerbates the alteration of gut microbial composition [24–27]. During antibiotic treatments in CF, butyrate-producing strains, such as *Anaerostipes*, *Butyricicoccus*, and *Ruminococcus*, are diminished [21]. Regarding cumulative intravenous antibiotic use over one year, Bruzzese et al. (2014) reported a negative correlation between the number of intravenous antibiotic courses and gut microbiota diversity. The highest exposure to intravenous antibiotics was associated with the lowest proportions of *Bacteroidetes* and the highest proportions of *Firmicutes* [28].

In the short term, intestinal inflammation demonstrates an impact on nutritional status, as demonstrated by the correlation between calprotectin levels and Z-scores for weight and waistline. Over the long term, inflammation influences morbidity and mortality, particularly elevating the risk of colon cancer [29]. Chronic inflammation and perturbation of the gut microbiome are prevalent among individuals with CF. Research indicates heightened levels of inflammatory proteins in the intestine, increased fatty acids in stools, and endoscopic findings, revealing villous atrophy, edema, erythema, and mucosal ulceration. These histological manifestations are associated with elevated calprotectin levels in stools [13]. Nonetheless, although increased calprotectin levels in stools do not precisely predict intestinal inflammation in CF, their elevated values across both the pancreatic sufficiency and pancreatic insufficiency groups studied substantiate the concept of "enteropathy" in CF, irrespective of pancreatic status [30].

3.2. Gut Dysbiosis

In CF, gut dysbiosis manifests shortly after birth, impacting the intestine [14]. Dysbiosis arises from disruptions in microbiome cell density and diversity, antibiotic effects, and alterations in the luminal environment and small intestine physiology, as well as mucus and mucin accumulation. These factors influence both intestinal and extraintestinal manifestations [1,9,13,14]. Contributing factors to dysbiosis encompass hydro-electrolyte imbalances, intestinal exocrine dysfunction, slowed G-I transit time, impaired intestinal immunity, ingestion of infected mucus, severity of CFTR gene mutations, and a hypercaloric diet [29,31].

Alterations in the microbiome are associated with intestinal inflammation in CF, characterized by a deficit in species like *Bacteroides*, *Bifidobacterium adolescentis*, *Faecalibacterium prausnitzii*, and *Eubacterium* spp., accompanied by an increase in opportunistic bacteria such as *E. coli* and *Eubacterium biforme* [29,31–33]. Pediatric CF samples notably exhibited a higher *E. coli* prevalence compared to non-CF samples. Elevated *E. coli* concentrations in the colon correlate with inflammatory processes and carcinogenesis initiation in inflammatory bowel disease, suggesting a link between dysbiosis, particularly the overrepresentation of *E. coli*, and the development of chronic G-I pathology [34].

Intestinal motility and soluble mucins regulate bacterial load in the proximal intestine, while mucus adhesion and lubrication influence bacterial binding to complex oligosaccharides on mucin molecules. Abnormal colonization results from sticky mucus and slowed motility, leading to increased proinflammatory species (*E. coli*, *Enterobacteriacee*, *Bacteroides fragilis*, *Mycobacterium*, *Proteobacterii*, *Streptococcus*, and *Veillonella*) and reduced beneficial bacteria (bifidobacteria, *Akkermansia*, *Eggerthella*, and *Anostipes*). Specific microbial profiles are associated with distinct CF characteristics, such as elevated *E. coli* and *E. biforme* levels in F508del mutation carriers, increased *F. prausnitzii*, bifidobacteria, and *E. limosum* in those with moderate disease, and an altered *Firmicutes–Bacteroidetes* ratio in those with liver damage. An abundance of *Staphylococcus* and *Faecalibacterium* negatively correlates with body mass index (BMI) in CF patients, and increased Alistipes levels impact glucose homeostasis. Some CF patients harbor *Clostridioides difficile* in stool, often remaining asymptomatic or having nontoxigenic strains [9,13]. Notably, CF-associated loss of *Oxalobacter formigenes*, a microorganism metabolizing oxalates, increases the risk of hyperoxaluria and kidney stone formation [1,14]. Table 1 summarizes the findings from various studies regarding alterations in gut microbiota observed in individuals with CF.

Table 1. Gut microbiota changes in CF.

Study	Author	Year	Increased Level	Decreased Level	Reference
Gut and respiratory microbiome in CF in infants	Madan et al.	2012	*E. coli*	*Staphylococcus* spp.	[35]
			Parabacteroides spp.	*Clostridium* spp.	
			Veilonella spp.		
Microbiota composition of the CF patients	Fouhy et al.	2017	*Enterobacteriaceae* spp.	*Faecalibacterium prausnitzii*	[36]
			Clostridium spp.	*Actinobacteria* spp.	
			Enterococcus faecalis	*Bacteroidetes* spp.	
			Firmicutes spp.	*Proteobacteria* spp.	
Gut microbiota signatures in CF	Vernochi et al.	2018	*Propionibacterium* spp.	*Eggerthella* spp.	[37]
			Staphylococcus spp.	*Eubacterium* spp.	
			Clostridiaceae spp.	*Ruminococcus* spp.	
				Dorea spp.	
				Faecalibacterium prausnitzii	
				Lachnospiaceae spp.	
Microbiota disturbances in children with CF	Enaud et al.	2019	*E. coli*	*Bacteroides* spp.	[29]
			Eubacterium diforme	*Bifidobacterium adolescentis*	
				Faecalibacterium prausnitzii	
Gut microbiota in children with CF	Coffey et al.	2019	*Fusobacteria* spp.	*Verrucomicrobia* spp.	[38]
			Proteobacteria spp.	*Firmicutes* spp.	
				Ruminococcus spp.	
				Lachnospira spp.	

Table 1. Cont.

Study	Author	Year	Increased Level	Decreased Level	Reference
Impact of CF on gut microbiota	Kristensen et al.	2020	Enterococcus spp. Streptococcus spp. E.coli	Bacteroides spp. Bifidobacterium spp.	[26]
CF gut microbiome	van Dorst et al.	2022	Enterococcus spp. Veilonella spp. Enterobacter spp.	Bacteroidetes spp. Ruminococcacceae spp. Bifidobacterium spp. Roseburia spp.	[39]
Intestinal microbiome in CF	Price et al.	2023	Blautia spp.	Roseburia spp.	[40]

Several mechanisms intervene in the production of CF dysbiosis:

a. Mechanisms related to CFTR:
- Thick mucus due to chloride channel dysfunction;
- Deficient bicarbonate secretion that alters intestinal pH;
- Malabsorption due to pancreatic insufficiency;
- Intestinal dysmotility with prolonged transit time;
- Altered immune mechanisms in the mucosa;
- Increased inflammation;
- Damage to the intestinal barrier.

b. Acquired factors:
- Frequent use of antibiotics for recurrent respiratory infections;
- Hypercaloric, hyperlipidic diet;
- Use of other drugs (inhibitors of acid secretion, opioids, anticholinergics, immunosuppressants) [9].

Dysbiosis is associated with fat malabsorption, as evidenced by the heightened prevalence of *E. coli* in individuals with CF, indicating a positive correlation with intestinal inflammation and disturbances in lipid metabolism and absorption, further exacerbating malnutrition [41]. Identifying dysbiosis in infants and young children may offer an opportunity for intervention, enabling therapeutic modulation of their gut microbiota. Early onset of lung disease and intestinal dysbiosis mutually influence each other [9]. The clinical symptomatology observed in dysbiosis resembles that of bacterial overpopulation syndrome.

3.2.1. Diagnosis of Gut Dysbiosis

The tests that are useful for identifying gut dysbiosis are:
- Stool test that measures the amount of good and bad bacteria in the stool;
- Organic acid test that measures the number of organic acids in the urine, bacteria producing organic acids as by-products of metabolism;
- Hydrogen breath test that measures the amount of hydrogen exhaled after drinking a sugar solution and breathing into a test tube;
- DNA analysis tools for gut microbiota, used to identify and quantify disease severity [42].

New research methods on gut microbiota in CF patients include a multiomics approach, involving metagenomics, metatranscriptomics, metaproteomics, and metabolomics [43].

3.2.2. Treatment of Gut Dysbiosis

Methods of modulation of dysbiosis in CF are recommended:
- Change in the composition of macronutrients;
- Micronutrient supplementation;
- Administration of prebiotics, probiotics, symbiotics, postbiotics, and flavonoids [9].

Human-milk oligosaccharides contribute to elevated *Bifidobacterium* levels in the infant's gut, influencing acetate production and acting as a preventive measure against *E. coli* infection. Feeding infants with human milk enhances gut microbiome diversity and diminishes respiratory tract colonization [9]. In the context of CF, probiotics have demonstrated positive effects on gut motility, inhibition of bacterial colonization, enhancement of intestinal barrier function, improvement in metabolic processes, and modulation of immunity [44]. The administration of probiotics (specifically, *Lactobacillus rhamnosus* GG at one capsule/day, and *Lactobacillus reuteri* at five drops/day, continuously) proves beneficial in reducing markers of intestinal inflammation, as indicated by decreased fecal calprotectin and rectal nitric oxide levels, although such interventions are not yet part of routine prescription practices [9]. A recent study by Asensio-Grau et al. (2023) emphasized that supplementation with *Lacticaseibacillus rhamnosus*, *Limosilactobacillus reuteri*, and *Lactiplantibacillus plantarum* induced modifications in the colonic microbiota, reducing *Proteobacteria* and *Bacteroidota* levels while increasing *Firmicutes* abundance [45].

Nutritional factors impact the fecal microbiome, with nutritional supplements and high-calorie, high-fat, processed foods influencing the gut microbiota. However, it is essential to note that gut dysbiosis can also impact nutrient absorption. Treatment for *C. difficile* infection involves Metronidazole or Vancomycin administered for 10–14 days [13,46]. Furthermore, Ivacaftor (IVA) treatment has been associated with an elevation in *Akkermansia* species, known for mucosal protection, and this increase is negatively correlated with stool markers of inflammation [9].

3.3. Small Intestinal Bacterial Overgrowth (SIBO)

Impairment to peristalsis, antibacterial proteins, gastric acid, intestinal fluids, and the ileocaecal valve leads to bacterial overgrowth in the small intestine, representing a form of intestinal dysbiosis. This condition can advance to abdominal distension, flatulence, steatorrhea, weight loss, diarrhea, and macrocytic anemia. Concurrently, mucus accumulation, mucosal immune dysfunction, water and electrolyte imbalances, and malabsorption contribute to alterations in the nutrient pool within the G-I lumen [1]. The observed weight loss can be attributed to bacterial competition for ingested nutrients, the presence of inflammation, and the bacterial capacity to deconjugate bile acids, diminishing their efficacy in emulsifying fats [14].

SIBO is prevalent in approximately 30–40% of CF patients. It arises from the accumulation of thick mucus and the compromise of normal bacterial defenses, manifesting as the presence of over 10 colony-forming units/mL in the small intestine. The heightened bacterial load stimulates mucus secretion, perpetuating a detrimental cycle between mucus plaque formation and dysbiosis. SIBO may be linked to intestinal dysmotility and the malabsorption of essential nutrients, such as iron, vitamin D, vitamin B12, bile acids, and folates [13,47].

3.3.1. Diagnosis

SIBO encompasses a spectrum ranging from nonspecific abdominal manifestations (abdominal cramping or pain, steatorrhea, anemia, weight loss, abdominal distension, flatulence, fatigue, and poor concentration) to more severe outcomes like malnutrition and malabsorption [48,49].

The "gold standard" diagnostic method for SIBO involves an aspirate culture with a bacterial count of $\geq 10^3$ CFU/mL. However, due to its invasive nature, this method is not recommended for use in pediatric populations [49,50]. An alternative, noninvasive diagnostic approach employs the hydrogen breath test, with a positive outcome indicative of SIBO when hydrogen levels exceed 12 parts per million (ppm) [49,51]. In a study by Gabel et al. (2022), 73.7% of CF patients demonstrated a positive breath test, suggesting the presence of SIBO [52]. Another diagnostic alternative to the breath test involves the utilization of orally ingested capsule technology, which measures in vivo hydrogen and carbon levels following carbohydrate ingestion [49].

3.3.2. Treatment

Due to diagnostic limitations, empirical treatment is commonly employed for SIBO, with the resolution of clinical symptoms serving as confirmation for this syndrome.

Typically, SIBO treatment involves the administration of antibiotics, such as Metronidazole at a dosage of 20 mg/kg body weight/day, Rifaximin at 200 mg twice daily for children aged 3–11 years, and 550 mg twice daily for those over 12 years, Trimethoprim/Sulfamethoxazole at 12 mg/kg body weight/day, and Amoxicillin-clavulanate. A rotational strategy, alternating antibiotics every two weeks, is implemented to mitigate the risk of bacterial resistance development [13,47]. It is crucial to acknowledge that antibiotic usage impacts the normal commensal bacterial flora and may contribute to selective bacterial resistance. Additionally, antibiotic use raises the potential for *Clostridioides difficile* infection, triggering secretory diarrhea through the toxin-induced activation of CFTR-dependent chloride secretion [1].

Studies investigating the efficacy of probiotics in the context of SIBO have yielded conflicting outcomes. According to Dorsey et al. (2017), probiotics may serve as a viable treatment for SIBO, contributing to alterations in the fecal microbiome and a reduction in markers of inflammation [13]. Probiotic use in SIBO has been associated with a decrease in hydrogen (H2) levels and an elevation in decontamination rates. Zhong et al. (2017) suggest that probiotics are effective in diminishing the bacterial burden in SIBO, while the study by Husebye et al. (2001), conducted on rats, indicates that probiotics administered in SIBO exhibit prokinetic effects [53,54]. Dual therapy involving probiotics, such as *L. casei*, in conjunction with antibiotics, results in superior symptom improvement compared to the administration of antibiotics alone, as reported by Rosania et al. (2013), a finding corroborated by Khalighi et al. (2014), who assert that *Bacillus coagulan* probiotics administered during antibiotic therapy for SIBO can be beneficial in preventing complications [55,56]. It is noted that optimal outcomes are achieved by combining probiotics with rifaximin or minocycline [57]. However, the study by Rao et al. (2018) observes opposing effects, accentuating digestive symptoms following probiotic administration [58]. Aslan et al. (2023), in a study on rats treated with probiotics in conjunction with various essential oils (coconut, peppermint, lemon, and patchouli), demonstrated reduced proinflammatory cytokine levels (IL-1β, IL-6, and TNFα), histological improvement, and decreased inflammation [59]. The study by Kumar et al. (2018) concludes that the administration of *Bifidobacterium infantis* 35624 leads to an increase in methane levels in the breath test, while Zhong et al. (2017) determine that probiotic administration does not improve abdominal pain or stool frequency in SIBO patients [54,60]. Similarly, the results of the study by Khalighi et al. (2014), cited by Chen et al. (2014), indicate that probiotics do not significantly enhance pain, bloating, and diarrhea, with improvements in nausea, vomiting, and constipation similar to those observed in the control group. This study also reveals that the administration of symbiotics leads to the resolution of G-I symptoms in SIBO [61]. The study by Mitten et al. (2018) concludes that probiotic administration increases the risk of associating predominantly methanogenic SIBO forms with constipation [62].

The use of laxatives in the eradication of SIBO is posited to contribute to the normalization of intestinal transit [63]. In a study by Gabel et al. (2022), the administration of Lumacaftor/Ivacaftor (LUM/IVA), CFTR modulators, for one month did not result in significant changes in the breath test, with 65.8% of the patients still exhibiting a positive test [52].

Nutritional recommendations entail a reduction in fermented foods and the avoidance of fiber-rich products, polyols, sweeteners, and prebiotics [51]. The low fermentable oligosaccharides, disaccharides, monosaccharides, and polyols (FOODMAP) diet is considered optimal for individuals with SIBO, promoting the proliferation of less pathogenic bacteria [64]. Additionally, vegetarian and vegan diets appear to be more effective in managing SIBO [65].

3.4. Motility Disorders

The modulation of gut motility is orchestrated by the interplay among the gut luminal environment, immune system, enteric nervous system, and central nervous system. In individuals with CF, gastric motility may be impacted by a reduction in overall gastric secretion, leading to heightened viscosity and electrolyte concentration. Gut motility disorders observed in CF contribute to:

- Development of SIBO;
- Reducing the solubility of bile salts;
- Deconjugation of bile acids;
- Reducing intestinal absorption of bile acids;
- Excessive loss of bile acids in stools [66].

A correlation between dysbiosis and dysmotility exists, though it remains unclear whether dysbiosis serves as the cause or consequence [12]. Lewindon et al. (1998), as cited by Avelar-Rodriguez et al. (2019), observed a prolonged orocecal transit time in individuals with CF, potentially elevating the risk of SIBO [57]. SIBO, characterized by the presence of species such as *E. coli*, can contribute to intestinal dysmotility, leading to a deceleration of intestinal movements.

Within the initial 30 min following gastric evacuation, the small intestine exhibits abnormal acidity, facilitating the formation of mixed micelles with bile salts and lipid digestion products. This temporal window is crucial for the dissolution of pancreatic enzymes, influencing their efficacy. The administration of enzymes in the form of enteric-coated microcapsules ensures their passage through the acidic stomach lumen unaffected, subsequently dissolving in the less-acidic pH of the duodenum [1].

3.4.1. Diagnosis

In human investigations, Hedsund et al. (2012) utilized a radio-opaque marker and reported a significant prolongation in the orocecal transit time in individuals with CF compared to their healthy counterparts [67]. More recently, Ng et al. (2021) employed innovative magnetic resonance imaging (MRI) techniques, demonstrating prolonged orocecal transit times in CF patients, concurrently associated with an augmented colon volume [15]. Gastric emptying scans are considered the optimal diagnostic method for evaluating gastric emptying. Other contemporary methods facilitating the diagnosis of delayed gastric emptying include wireless luminal imaging, transit-time recording using the Pillcam or the Smart pill, and the 3D-Transit system [13]. Utilizing endoscopic capsules, Malagelada et al. (2020) observed a notable reduction in intestinal contractility, accompanied by increased retention of intraluminal content in individuals with CF compared to their healthy counterparts [68].

3.4.2. Treatment of Dysmotility

Given the interplay among the immune system, G-I secretions, microbiota, and fermentation byproducts in modulating gut motility, the utilization of probiotics appears promising for mitigating G-I dysmotility. Probiotics, such as *Lactobacillus rhamnosus* GG, exhibit potential in modulating mucosal and systemic immune barriers, consequently normalizing inflammation-related dysmotility, as evidenced by studies conducted by Guarino et al. (2008) and Isolauri et al. (2001) [69,70]. However, there is insufficient data regarding the role of prebiotics in G-I dysmotility. Dietary fiber consumption is reported to have a positive impact on stool consistency and frequency, as confirmed by other authors [71]. DeLisle et al. (2013) and Quigley et al. (2013) propose that probiotics positively influence the G-I tract by ameliorating visceral hypersensitivity, dysmotility, and permeability, albeit with limited impact on the intestinal microflora [14,72]. Studies conducted on mice have demonstrated that a novel molecule called "Oligo G" can reduce mucus levels and enhance intestinal transit [73].

3.5. Malabsorption Syndrome

Malabsorption in CF manifests as a severe and early-onset condition, exacerbated by the frequently observed delayed gastric evacuation in CF patients [74]. Maldigestion and lipid malabsorption are intensified by hyperacidity in the duodenum, typical in CF, along with pancreatic insufficiency-induced lipase deficiency and reduced bile acid resorption in the ileum [1]. Proteins and carbohydrates absorption and digestion seem to be less affected, with maltase and sucrase activities appearing unaltered, while lactase activity is notably lower or suppressed [75].

The multifactorial etiology involves dysfunction of the endocrine pancreas and liver, impaired bile acid metabolism, and intestinal resorption processes [76]. Nonetheless, pancreatic enzyme deficiency stands out as the primary cause of malabsorption. Contributing factors encompass bicarbonate deficiency, abnormalities in bile salt, disruptions in mucosal transport, various motility issues, abnormal intestinal mucus, structural anatomical changes, dysfunction in enteric circular muscles, defects in mucosal mechanisms leading to the abnormal release of lipoproteins into the bloodstream, intestinal bacterial overload, and inflammatory processes [74,75,77,78].

CF malabsorption manifests through impaired pancreatic enzyme release and intestinal damage, hindering nutrient absorption. Severe pancreatic damage in exocrine pancreatic insufficiency results in reliance on lingual and gastric lipase for lipolysis [79]. The factors contributing to persistent fat malabsorption in CF include:

a. Intestinal pH: CFTR dysfunction reduces bicarbonate secretion, leading to a lower pH. Improper mucin expansion due to disrupted bicarbonate secretion impedes lipid translocation, necessitating an increased pH for optimal fat absorption. Acid-suppressing treatments can enhance fat absorption but may induce SIBO and alter bile salt metabolism [13,79]. Cases of ongoing fat malabsorption despite enzyme-replacement treatment and low intestinal pH have been reported [80,81]. Stool pH correlates with fat absorption, possibly explaining enzyme-replacement ineffectiveness [81];

b. Intraluminal bile salts: CF patients exhibit increased bile salt loss in stools due to mucosal changes (thickened mucus, SIBO). An elevated glycine–taurine ratio and reduced bile solubilization capacity affect fat absorption and decrease the bile salt pool. Even CF patients without liver damage experience bile acid loss in stools, contributing to malabsorption [14,79,82];

c. Abnormalities of the gut mucosa: thick and adherent mucus, bacterial overgrowth, ileal hypertrophy, villous atrophy, increased permeability, and chronic inflammation contribute to fat malabsorption [79];

d. Reduced orocecal intestinal transit time: fat absorption is influenced by the duration that fats are in contact with the absorption surface [79];

e. Deficiency of essential fatty acids: low linoleic and docosahexaenoic acid levels, along with elevated arachidonic acid, can impede fat absorption, contributing to inflammation, mucus secretion, and smooth muscle relaxation [79].

3.5.1. Diagnosis

Clinical indicators of malabsorption in CF include inadequate weight and height gain in pediatric patients, while low BMI in adults may suggest malabsorption. Confirmatory laboratory assessments include stool fat evaluation, optical microscopy for fat droplets, acid steatocrit, and the 13C-mixed triglyceride breath test [83].

Traditional verification of fat malabsorption involves measuring fecal fat excretion over at least three days, assessing concurrent food intake, and quantifying fat intake and production for a percentage fat absorption calculation. An alternative, validated, semiquantitative method modifies the steatotrit technique through fecal homogenate acidification, requiring stool-specimen centrifugation [83].

The 13C-mixed triglyceride breath test provides a safe and repeatable, albeit costly and less accessible, means of assessing fat digestion [84,85]. Annual evaluations, combining clinical and laboratory methods, are recommended for all CF patients [86].

Histologically, most CF patients exhibit a normal brush-border appearance, but some may present ileal hypertrophy or partial villous atrophy in the small intestine due to acid aggression, chronic inflammation, or denutrition [87].

3.5.2. Treatment

Treatment of malabsorption syndrome has the following objectives:

- Control of symptoms;
- Correction of malabsorption;
- Obtaining a nutritional status and growth as close to normal as possible [77].

Effective enzyme-replacement therapy may enhance lipid absorption [74,88]. Despite treatment, lipid malabsorption persists in some cases, with absorption coefficients below 85–90% of dietary lipid intake [79]. The cause of persistent malabsorption extends beyond pancreatic insufficiency, involving abnormal interenterocytic events impacting plasma lipid transport [78]. Fat-balance measurement is the "gold standard" for enzyme-replacement therapy monitoring [82].

Supplementing with essential fatty acids (70 mg/kg body weight of docosahexaenoic acid for 6 weeks) and regular use of omega-3 fatty acids did not improve fat absorption and nutritional status [79]. Due to increased mucus viscosity in the CF intestinal epithelium, N-acetylcysteine administration, breaking disulfide bonds, may be beneficial [76].

3.6. Meconium Ileus

Observed in 10–20% of CF patients, it represents the earliest G-I manifestation [12,47,89,90]. Its pathophysiology, though not fully elucidated, is hypothesized to stem from CFTR dysfunction in the enteric nervous system, particularly affecting the ileal response to abnormal intraluminal content [12]. Common mutations include F508del, G542X, W1282X, R553X, and G551D [35], with approximately 67% survival [90].

3.6.1. Diagnostic

Manifestations emerge within the first 2 days, featuring signs of intestinal obstruction (abdominal distension, bile vomiting, delayed mucus elimination). Examination may reveal an abdominal mass in the right iliac fossa or supra pelvic region. Complicated cases may exhibit perforations, volvulus, or atresia [90,91]. Most cases involve pancreatic insufficiency [92]. Abdominal radiography shows dilated loops with hydro-aerial levels and an intra-abdominal mass, occasionally indicating meconial peritonitis [93].

3.6.2. Treatment

Treatment involves intravenous rehydration and barium enema with Gastrografin® or N-Acetylcysteine. Surgical intervention becomes necessary in cases with complications [90,94].

3.7. Rectal Prolapse

Rectal prolapse affects 3.5% of CF patients, with 3.6% of those experiencing prolapse having CF. Causes include constipation and heightened intra-abdominal pressure from coughing. Unexplained prolapse necessitates iontophoresis [95].

Treatment

Manual reduction, with the patient in the genupectoral position, constitutes the primary treatment. For recurrent cases, options include sclerotherapy or surgical intervention [93].

3.8. Intussusception

Intussusception is 10–20 times more prevalent in CF patients aged 9–12 years. Twenty-five percent of cases manifest as ileo-colonic forms. CFTR dysfunction, altered luminal environment, mucus clearance, abnormal bacterial colonization, dysbiosis, and appendiceal mucocele contribute to its etiology [1].

3.8.1. Diagnosis

Intussusception presents with severe cramp-like pain, vomiting, abdominal distension, dehydration, and lethargy. Palpation reveals a lower right quadrant mass, requiring differentiation from distal intestinal obstruction syndrome. Mechanically described as "telescoping", it commonly involves the ileum and cecum, with the mesentery's potential incorporation elevating the risk of ischemia and necrosis [96]. An unusual manifestation results from CF-induced constipation, demanding a thorough diagnostic evaluation to exclude other CF-associated G-I conditions [97].

3.8.2. Treatment

Management includes nasogastric tube placement for distension, intravenous electrolyte correction, nonopioid analgesics, and surgical intervention, if necessary [46]. Adewale et al. (2019) advocate conservative measures before surgery, emphasizing pancreatic enzyme use to prevent constipation and subsequent fecaloma formation, a potential trigger for intussusception [98].

3.9. Volvulus

Volvulus occurs in 15% of CF patients, causing 3–4 times proximal intestinal dilation. Meconium ileus complicated with volvulus poses a life-threatening scenario [99].

3.9.1. Diagnosis

Often diagnosed prenatally through ultrasound, it manifests as a hyperechoic intestine with ascites and abdominal distension. Decreased fetal movements and incidents like volvulus necessitate CF testing at birth [100].

3.9.2. Treatment

Intestinal volvulus is an urgent, life-threatening condition, particularly in confirmed or suspected CF cases. Emergency cesarean section and surgical resolution, involving intestinal resection, are imperative to mitigate absorption-function impairment [99].

3.10. Gastric and Duodenal Complications

Helicobacter pylori infection, inadequate gastric acidity neutralization, and prolonged antibiotic use contribute to gastroduodenal issues in CF [101,102]. *H. pylori* prevalence and cross reactivity with anti-*Pseudomonas* antibodies were explored in CF patients [103].

3.10.1. Diagnosis

Despite treatment, severe G-I symptoms persist in some patients, necessitating endoscopy with biopsy. Noninvasive *H. pylori* testing (fecal antigen test or urea breath test) may be warranted for those with dyspepsia or suspected peptic ulcer disease [104]. Gastroparesis prevalence rises with age in CF, with scintigraphy recommended for diagnosis [105].

3.10.2. Treatment

Gastroparesis treatment includes prokinetic agents, macrolides, gastrostomy, and gastro-jejunostomy tubes [78]. Inflammation on biopsy warrants immunomodulatory agents [106]. IVA and LUM/IVA modulators improve weight gain in CF, likely linked to reduced stool calprotectin and enhanced dietary-fat absorption [107,108]. IVA normalizes intestinal pH, decreases calprotectin, and increases *Akkermansia* abundance, resolving histopathological changes [40,47,107,109,110]. Modulator-induced intestinal inflammation mitigation may positively influence CF patient growth and nutrition [110].

3.11. Gastro-Esophageal Reflux (GER)

Less-specific GER symptoms are common in CF, particularly in youth [6,12]. CF patients with GERD experience worsened lung disease progression due to refluxed contents containing acid, enzymes, and bacteria [111]. Lower gastro-esophageal sphincter pressure reduction, elevated intra-abdominal pressure from chronic cough, and increased gastro-esophageal pressure gradient contribute to GER, which is intensified by higher negative intrathoracic pressure in CF [112,113].

This pressure difference may increase the gastroesophageal pressure gradient, leading to GER. Dysfunctional esophageal sphincter pressure contributes to increased proximal reflux, causing prolonged exposure to acidic contents, elevating GERD symptoms, and exacerbating lung issues [114,115].

3.11.1. Diagnosis

GER may cause pain and complications, requiring exploration of pepsin as an aspiration biomarker [115]. Esophageal manometry reveals coughing following reflux episodes [91]. For GER patients with Barrett's esophagus, endoscopy screening is recommended [111].

3.11.2. Treatment

No CF-specific GER treatment guideline exists; chronic PPI use correlates with a potential exacerbation risk [111,116,117]. PPIs improve esophageal acid exposure and the DeMeester Score [118]. Surgical intervention (Nissen fundoplication) is required for cases with unfavorable outcomes [91].

Zeybel et al. (2017) observed reduced GER symptoms during ivacaftor (IVA) administration over 52 weeks, with alkalization of the intestinal pH and improved enzyme functionality [118]. Ongoing studies assess Elexacaftor, Tezacaftor, and Ivacaftor (ETI) modulators, revealing improvements in GERD symptoms after 3 and 6 months of ETI administration [119,120].

3.12. Eosinophilic Esophagitis (EoE)

In CF, EoE, a chronic inflammatory disorder characterized by esophageal eosinophilic infiltration (≥ 15 eosinophils/field), presents with symptoms such as dysphagia, chest pain, burning sensation, abdominal pain, and growth difficulties [14,91,121]. The increased EoE prevalence in CF may result from factors like antibiotic exposure altering the G-I microbiome, higher GERD rates in CF patients, and associated PPI use, as well as an elevated prevalence of atopic manifestations [9,22,46,122].

3.12.1. Diagnosis

Diagnosis involves endoscopy and esophageal biopsy, with a crucial differential diagnosis from GER [14].

3.12.2. Treatment

Consensus guidelines propose three EoE treatment lines:

- Proton-pump inhibitor (PPI) use (20–50% success rate);
- Corticosteroid therapy (Budesonide, Fluticasone), with efficacy in 50–90% of cases;
- Dietary interventions (elimination of food allergens) [9,46,123–125].

3.13. Distal Intestinal Obstruction Syndrome (DIOS)

DIOS, a CF complication, results from the accumulation of viscous feces and mucus, causing obstruction in the terminal ileum and cecum [112]. Characterized by a complete or incomplete obstruction, it affects 10–22% of CF patients, with a higher incidence in older individuals and a 77% recurrence risk [90,126]. Risk factors include severe genotype, dehydration, meconial ileus history, and post-transplant complications, notably after lung transplantation [90].

3.13.1. Diagnosis

Acute onset includes periumbilical or lower right quadrant pain, distension, and bile vomiting. Differential diagnosis involves constipation, intussusception, inflammatory bowel disease, and fibrosing colonopathy [126].

3.13.2. General Treatment

- Laxatives;
    - Osmotic drugs (lactulose, Macrogol 3350, Diatrizoate);
    - Stimulants (Senna, Sodium docusate, Sodium picosulfate).
- Mucolytics: N-acetylcysteine (oral, diluted);
- Other agents: prokinetics (macrolides, Metoclopramide), Lubiprostone (Amitiza);
- Surgical procedures: considered for refractory cases [90,127].

Incomplete Forms Treatment:

- Oral rehydration, osmotic laxatives (PEG), magnesium citrate, or Gastrografin;
- Prokinetics are suggested in pseudo-obstructions or postoperatively [126,128].

Complete Forms Treatment:

- PEG in nonvomiting patients;
- Intestinal lavage;
- Rehydration (IV or Gastrografin enema);
- Cecum instillations (colonoscopy);
- Surgery (laparotomy, ileocecal resection) [126].

Prevention:

- Hydration;
- Laxatives;
- Adequate pancreatic enzymes;
- PEG 0.5–1 g/kg/day orally for 6–12 months [126].

CFTR Modulators:
Unclear impact; no specific studies conducted [129].

3.14. Constipation

Constipation, affecting over half of CF patients, is distinguished from DIOS, manifesting as gradual fecal impaction in the entire colon [90].

ESPGHAN working group definition:

1. Abdominal pain/distension;
    a. Reduced bowel movement frequency;
    b. Increased stool consistency.
2. Responds to laxatives [128].

Incidence is 1.5 times higher in pancreatic insufficiency. Contributing factors include meconium ileus history and fat malabsorption [111]. Colon barriers, vulnerable to compromise, may undergo destruction due to immune-cell infiltration and inflammation [1].

3.14.1. Diagnosis

The presence of defined symptoms constitutes diagnosis.

3.14.2. Treatment

There is no distinct CF approach; general-population treatments apply. Mineral oils are discouraged for those with lung disease [84]. The impact of CFTR modulators on constipation remains uncertain, with potential adverse events observed [130,131].

3.15. Colon Disease: Fibrosing Colonopathy

3.15.1. Fibrosing Colonopathy

Fibrosing colonopathy, a severe, yet infrequent, condition, typically emerges in patients aged 2–7 years. While its pathogenesis remains elusive, prolonged high-dose pancreatic enzyme therapy is implicated, though occurrences in untreated patients exist. Predisposing factors include youth, colitis history, meconium ileus, DIOS, bowel surgery, antioxidant deficiency, and drug use (laxatives, corticosteroids, dornase alpha, and H2 receptor antagonists) [132]. Primarily affecting the ascending colon, the disease may progress throughout the colon, histologically characterized by submucosal fibrosis and elevated calprotectin correlating with colonic inflammation [14,112].

Diagnosis

Often presenting as treatment-resistant intestinal obstruction resembling DIOS, symptoms include abdominal pain, distention, vomiting, and constipation. Diagnosis consideration arises when standard DIOS interventions prove ineffective. Submucosal concentric rings, muscular mucosa hypertrophy, inflammatory cell infiltration, and collagen deposition typify the disease, suggesting recurrent ischemic events and mucosal reparative mechanisms [133]. Excessive pancreatic enzyme doses (>50,000 U lipase/kg) show a significant correlation with increased fibrous colonopathy risk [134].

Treatment

Prevention involves limiting lipase to 10,000 IU/kg/day. Nonresponsive cases necessitate treatment-adherence review, enzyme-preparation adjustments, timing changes, gastric acidity reduction, and exclusion of other G-I diseases. Surgical intervention, such as right hemicolectomy, is occasionally warranted [75,135,136].

3.15.2. Crohn's Disease

Crohn's disease prevalence is 12.5 times higher in individuals with CF than in the general population. Genetic and environmental factors and immunological interactions with intestinal microbiota contribute to this heightened occurrence [1,14].

Diagnosis

In CF, elevated markers of intestinal inflammation (IL-8, IL-1β, neutrophilic elastase, eosinophilic cationic protein, and plasma proteins) and increased calprotectin in stool are observed [21,28]. Although serum biomarkers for inflammatory bowel disease may yield false values, a rectal biopsy is recommended to enhance diagnostic accuracy [1].

Treatment

Immunosuppressant use, particularly Infliximab, is infrequent in CF patients. Relative contraindications include bronchiectasis and *P. aeruginosa* colonization [137].

3.16. Celiac Disease

Celiac disease exhibits a prevalence 2–3 times higher in individuals with CF than in the general population. This association, first described in 1969, involves complex interactions, including CFTR as a molecular target of gluten, contributing to CD pathogenesis [138,139].

The heightened prevalence varies globally, with increased occurrences noted in certain countries, emphasizing geographic distinctions [138,140–142]. CFTR inhibition by gluten disrupts ion balance, autophagy, and proteostasis, mirroring the stress response observed in FC. CFTR dysfunction, linked to increased intestinal permeability and inflammation, may predispose individuals to CD. Exocrine pancreatic insufficiency intensifies the antigenic load and antibody response [138,142].

Studies reveal that gluten-derived peptides inhibit CFTR, causing local stress responses contributing to CD immunopathology. The correlation involves factors like undigested gluten proteins, intestinal mucosa destruction, and immunological reactions against wheat gluten. Chronic inflammation in CF increases susceptibility to osteoporosis and colorectal cancer [140,143].

CFTR loss escalates reactive oxygen species and activates transglutaminase, leading to NF-KB activation and proinflammatory cytokine release. Malabsorption, high-calorie diets, and shorter duration of natural diet increase the risk of CD in CF patients [144].

3.16.1. Diagnosis

CF and CD share malabsorption, clinical manifestations, and symptoms, posing challenges in differentiation. Liver damage, persistent anemia, and exocrine pancreatic insufficiency contribute to diagnostic complexities [115]. CF patients exhibit elevated antibodies, increased intestinal permeability, calprotectin levels, and microbiome alterations. Screening for CD is vital in CF patients with persistent symptoms, inappropriate growth, low BMD, and those requiring high pancreatic enzyme doses [14,99,138–140,145,146]. Pancreatic isoamylase activity distinguishes CF from CD in patients with steatorrhea [147].

3.16.2. Treatment

CFTR modulators, like VX-770 (IVA), mitigate gliadin's negative impact on CFTR function, reducing inflammation and inducing gluten tolerance in CD patients. CFTR modulators significantly enhance G-I symptoms and prognosis in both conditions [7].

3.17. Appendicular Disease

Appendicitis is uncommon in CF, presenting with atypical manifestations and a heightened risk of perforation and abscess formation.

3.17.1. Diagnosis

Diagnosing appendicitis in CF poses challenges, often characterized by an appendix diameter exceeding 6 mm due to luminal mucus. Delayed diagnosis, potentially confused with conditions like intussusception or DIOS, may lead to complications, such as appendicular abscess formation. Recognition of appendiceal mucocele involves identifying recurrent abdominal pain and palpable masses and confirmation through ultrasound examination [1,112,148].

3.17.2. Treatment

Appendectomy, involving appendix resection and cecal tip removal, is effective in preventing recurrence of appendicitis or appendiceal mucocele. However, studies suggest that asymptomatic cases may not necessitate surgical intervention. Noninvasive approaches, such as mucin distension of the appendix, emerge as potential methods to safeguard CF patients against appendicular inflammation [148].

4. Discussions

The diminished levels of bicarbonate and the absence of bicarbonate-rich pancreatic fluids, essential for food digestion, contribute to the emergence of G-I manifestations in CF. These manifestations significantly impact the patient's quality of life and long-term prognosis. While extensive research has been dedicated to pulmonary aspects, there is a notable scarcity of high-quality studies on G-I manifestations in CF. Therefore, further investigations are imperative to comprehensively assess the scope of G-I manifestations, the long-term risks associated with this pathology, and the potential impacts of emerging therapies specific to G-I manifestations.

Despite limited clinical studies on the efficacy of probiotics in managing CF patients, the presence of gut dysbiosis necessitates interventions targeting the gut microbiota. Probiotics such as *Lactobacillus reuteri* and *Lactobacillus rhamnosus* GG hold promise for conferring health benefits to CF patients. The heterogeneity in strains, doses, and treatment durations across existing studies underscores the need for large-scale investigations to elucidate the specific effects of these probiotics.

Given the early onset of G-I manifestations and the approval of CFTR modulators for older patients, it is crucial to explore their preventive effects on disease progression. Additionally, the discovery of novel CFTR modulators suitable for younger age groups warrants investigation. A worthwhile avenue for research involves examining the potential synergies between probiotics and CFTR modulators in alleviating CF G-I distress. Since existing studies primarily focus on the pulmonary effects of different CFTR modulators, future directions should encompass an exploration of their short-term and long-term impacts on G-I distress, including their role in preventing G-I cancer, along with considerations of optimal modulator-therapy timing.

5. Conclusions

Timely identification and intervention for gastrointestinal manifestations in cystic fibrosis hold significance not only in ameliorating symptoms but also in enhancing the nutritional status and overall survival of affected individuals. Given the intricate nature of G-I manifestations associated with CF, their effective management necessitates careful oversight and follow up, preferably administered through a collaborative effort involving a multidisciplinary healthcare team. This comprehensive approach is integral to optimizing care and elevating the quality of life for CF patients grappling with G-I complications.

Our contention underscores the imperative for further clinical investigations, aiming to establish a more robust and evidence-based framework for the management of G-I symptoms within the context of this chronic disease. Such scholarly endeavors are pivotal for advancing the understanding of the intricate interplay between CF and G-I manifestations, ultimately contributing to refined clinical strategies and improved outcomes for individuals facing these challenges.

Author Contributions: Conceptualization, D.-T.A.-P., I.M.E. and A.N.A.; methodology, A.N.A., C.I.C. and I.S.; software, I.S. and F.T.; validation, C.O.I.H., D.E.M. and C.I.C.; formal analysis, L.I.B. and A.M.M.; investigation, L.I.B. and A.M.M.; resources, C.O.I.H., D.E.M., F.T. and C.I.C.; data curation, C.O.I.H., D.E.M. and C.I.C.; writing—original draft preparation, D.-T.A.-P. and I.M.E.; writing—review and editing, D.-T.A.-P., I.M.E. and A.N.A.; visualization, I.S. and F.T.; supervision, D.-T.A.-P. and I.M.E.; project administration, D.-T.A.-P. All authors have read and agreed to the published version of the manuscript.

Funding: This research received no external funding.

Conflicts of Interest: The authors declare no conflicts of interest.

References

1. Adeyemo-Salami, O.A. Cystic Fibrosis in the Intestine and the Influence on Digestion. *J. Imunol. Sci.* **2020**, *4*, 22–32. [CrossRef]
2. Fiorotto, R.; Strazzabosco, M. Pathophysiology of Cystic Fibrosis Liver Disease: A Channelopathy Leading to Alterations in Innate Immunity and in Microbiota. *Cell. Mol. Gastroenterol. Hepatol.* **2019**, *8*, 197–207. [CrossRef]
3. Betapudi, B.; Aleem, A.; Kothadia, J.P. *Cystic Fibrosis and Liver Disease*; Stat Pearls Publishing: Treasure Island FL, USA, 2023.
4. Anton-Păduraru, D.T.; Trandafir, L. Fibroza chistică (mucoviscidoza). In *PEDIATRIE*; Miron, I., Ed.; "Gr.T. Popa", UMF: Iași, Romania, 2016; pp. 300–308.
5. Veit, G.; Avramescu, R.; Chiang, A.; Houck, S.; Cai, Z.; Peters, K.; Hong, J.S.; Pollard, H.B.; Guggino, W.B.; Balch, W.E.; et al. From CFTR biology toward combinatorial pharmacothetarpy: Expanded classification of cystic fibrosis mutations. *Mol. Biol. Cell* **2016**, *27*, 424–433. [CrossRef] [PubMed]
6. Galante, G.; Freeman, A.J. Gastrointestinal, Pancreatic, and Hepatic Manifestations of Cystic Fibrosis in the Newborn. *Neo Rev.* **2019**, *20*, e12–e24. [CrossRef] [PubMed]
7. Villella, V.; Venerando, A.; Cozza, G.; Esposito, S.; Ferrari, E.; Monzani, R.; Spinella, M.C.; Oikonomou, V.; Renga, G.; Tosco, A.; et al. A pathogenic role for CFTR in celiac disease. *EMBO J.* **2019**, *39*, e100101. [CrossRef] [PubMed]
8. Birimberg-Schwartz, L.; Wilschanski, M. Cystic Fibrosis Related Gastrointestinal Manifestations—Moving Forward. *J. Cyst. Fibros.* **2021**, *20*, 562–563. [CrossRef] [PubMed]
9. Thavamani, A.; Salem, I.; Sferra, T.; Sankararaman, S. Impact of Altered Gut Microbiota and Its Metabolites in Cystic Fibrosis. *Metabolites* **2021**, *11*, 123. [CrossRef]
10. Gabel, M.; Galante, G.; Freedman, S. Gastrointestinal and Hepatobiliary Disease in Cystic Fibrosis. *Semin. Resp. Crit. Care Med.* **2019**, *40*, 825–841. [CrossRef]

11. Tabori, H.; Arnold, C.; Jaudszus, A.; Mentzel, H.J.; Renz, D.; Reinsch, S.; Lorenz, M.; Michl, R.; Gerber, A.; Lehmann, T.; et al. Abdominal symptoms in cystic fibrosis and their relationship to genotype, history, clinical and laboratory findings. *PLoS ONE* **2017**, *12*, e0174463. [CrossRef]
12. Henen, S.; Denton, C.; Teckman, J.; Borowitz, D.; Patel, D. Review of Gastrointestinal Motility in Cystic Fibrosis. *J. Cyst. Fibros.* **2021**, *20*, 578–585. [CrossRef]
13. Dorsey, J.; Gonska, T. Bacterial overgrowth, dybiosis, inflammation, and dysmotility in the Cystic Fibrosis intestine. *J. Cyst. Fibros.* **2017**, *16*, S14–S23. [CrossRef]
14. DeLisle, R.; Borowitz, D. The Cystic Fibrosis Intestine. *Cold Spring Harb. Perspect. Med.* **2013**, *3*, a009753. [CrossRef]
15. Ng, C.; Dellschaft, N.; Hoad, C.; Marciani, L.; Ban, L.; Prayle, A.; Barr, H.L.; Jaudszus, A.; Mainz, J.G.; Spiller, R.C.; et al. Postprandial changes in gastrointestinal function and transit in cystic fibrosis assessed by Magnetic Resonance Imaging. *J. Cyst. Fibros.* **2021**, *20*, 591–597. [CrossRef]
16. Couce, M.; O'Brien, T.D.; Moran, A.; Roche, P.C.; Butler, P.C. Diabetes mellitus in cystic fibrosis is characterized by islet amyloidosis. *J. Clin. Endocrinol. Metab.* **1996**, *81*, 1267–1272. [CrossRef]
17. Bogdani, M.; Blackman, S.M.; Ridaura, C.; Bellocq, J.P.; Powers, A.C.; Aguilar-Bryan, L. Structural abnormalities in islets from very young children with cystic fibrosis may contribute to cystic fibrosis-related diabetes. *Sci. Rep.* **2017**, *7*, 17231. [CrossRef] [PubMed]
18. Hull, R.L.; Gibson, R.L.; McNamara, S.; Deutsch, G.H.; Fligner, C.L.; Frevert, C.W.; Ramsey, B.W.; Sanda, S. Islet interleukin-1beta immunoreactivity is an early feature of cystic fibrosis that may contribute to beta-cell failure. *Diabetes Care* **2018**, *41*, 823–830. [CrossRef] [PubMed]
19. Hart, N.J.; Aramandla, R.; Poffenberger, G.; Fayolle, C.; Thames, A.H.; Bautista, A.; Spigelman, A.F.; Babon, J.A.B.; DeNicola, M.E.; Dadi, P.K.; et al. Cystic fibrosis-related diabetes is caused by islet loss and inflammation. *JCI Insight* **2018**, *3*, e98240. [CrossRef]
20. Dodge, J.A. Fibrosing colonopathy. *Gut* **2000**, *46*, 152–153. [CrossRef]
21. Bruzzese, E.; Raia, V.; Gaudiello, G.; Polito, G.; Buccigrossi, V.; Formicola, V.; Guarino, A. Intestinal inflammation is a frequent feature of cystic fibrosis and is reduced by probiotic administration. *Aliment. Pharmacol. Ther.* **2004**, *20*, 813–819. [CrossRef]
22. Tam, R.Y.; van Dorst, J.M.; McKay, I.; Coffey, M.; Ooi, C.Y. Intestinal Inflammation and Alterations in the Gut Microbiota in Cystic Fibrosis: A Review of the Current Evidence, Pathophysiology and Future Directions. *J. Clin. Med.* **2022**, *11*, 649. [CrossRef]
23. Knoop, K.A.; McDonald, K.G.; Kulkarni, D.H.; Newberry, R.D. Antibiotics promote inflammation through the translocation of native commensal colonic bacteria. *Gut* **2016**, *65*, 1100–1109. [CrossRef] [PubMed]
24. Manor, O.; Levy, R.; Pope, C.E.; Hayden, H.S.; Brittnacher, M.J.; Carr, R.; Radey, M.C.; Hager, K.R.; Heltshe, S.L.; Ramsey, B.W.; et al. Metagenomic evidence for taxonomic dysbiosis and functional imbalance in the gastrointestinal tracts of children with cystic fibrosis. *Sci. Rep.* **2016**, *6*, 22493. [CrossRef] [PubMed]
25. Loman, B.R.; Shrestha, C.L.; Thompson, R.; Groner, J.A.; Mejias, A.; Ruoff, K.L.; O'Toole, G.A.; Bailey, M.T.; Kopp, B.T. Age and environmental exposures influence the fecal bacteriome of young children with cystic fibrosis. *Pediatr. Pulmonol.* **2020**, *55*, 1661–1670. [CrossRef] [PubMed]
26. Kristensen, M.; Prevaes, S.M.P.J.; Kalkman, G.; Tramper-Stranders, G.A.; Hasrat, R.; de Winter-de Groot, K.M.; Janssens, H.M.; Tiddens, H.A.; van Westreenene, M.; Sanders, E.A.M.; et al. Development of the gut microbiota in early life: The impact of cystic fibrosis and antibiotic treatment. *J. Cyst. Fibros.* **2020**, *19*, 553–561. [CrossRef] [PubMed]
27. Kotnala, S.; Dhasmana, A.; Kashyap, V.K.; Chauhan, S.C.; Yallapu, M.M.; Jaggi, M. A bird eye view on cystic fibrosis: An underestimated multifaceted chronic disorder. *Life Sci.* **2021**, *268*, 118959. [CrossRef]
28. Bruzzese, E.; Callegari, M.L.; Raia, V.; Viscovo, S.; Scotto, R.; Ferrari, S.; Morelli, L.; Buccigrossi, V.; Lo Vecchio, A.; Ruberto, E.; et al. Disrupted intestinal microbiota and intestinal inflammation in children with cystic fibrosis and its restoration with Lactobacillus GG: A randomised clinical trial. *PLoS ONE* **2014**, *9*, e87796. [CrossRef]
29. Enaud, R.; Hooks, K.; Barre, A.; Barnetche, T.; Hubert, C.; Massot, M. Intestinal Inflammation in Children with Cystic Fibrosis Is Associated with Crohn's-like Microbiota Disturbances. *J. Clin. Med.* **2019**, *8*, 645. [CrossRef] [PubMed]
30. Rumman, N.; Sultan, M.; El Chammas, K.; Goh, V.; Salzman, N.; Quintero, D.; Werlin, S. Calprotectin in Cystic Fibrosis. *BMC Pediatr.* **2014**, *14*, 133. [CrossRef]
31. Scanlan, P.; Buckling, A.; Kong, W.; Wild, Y.; Lynch, S.; Harrison, F. Gut dysbiosis in Cystic Fibrosis. *J. Cyst. Fibros.* **2012**, *11*, 454–455. [CrossRef]
32. Duytschaever, G.; Huys, G.; Bekaert, M.; Boulanger, L.; De Boeck, K.; Vandamme, P. Dysbiosis of bifidobacteria and Clostridium cluster XIVa in the cystic fibrosis fecal microbiota. *J. Cyst. Fibros.* **2013**, *12*, 206–215. [CrossRef]
33. Schippa, S.; Iebba, V.; Santangelo, F.; Gagliardi, A.; De Biase, R.V.; Stamato, A.; Bertasi, S.; Lucarelli, M.; Conte, M.P.; Quattrucci, S. Cystic fibrosis transmembrane conductance regulator (CFTR) allelic variants relate to shifts in faecal microbiota of cystic fibrosis patients. *PLoS ONE* **2013**, *8*, e61176. [CrossRef]
34. Arthur, J.C.; Perez-Chanona, E.; Mühlbauer, M.; Tomkovich, S.; Uronis, J.M.; Fan, T.J.; Campbell, B.J.; Abujamel, T.; Dogan, B.; Rogers, A.B.; et al. Intestinal inflammation targets cancer-inducing activity of the microbiota. *Science* **2012**, *338*, 120–123. [CrossRef] [PubMed]
35. Madan, J.C.; Koestler, D.C.; Stanton, B.A.; Davidson, L.; Moulton, L.A.; Housman, M.L.; Moore, J.H.; Guill, M.F.; Morrison, H.G.; Sogin, M.L.; et al. Serial analysis of the gut and respiratory microbiome in cystic fibrosis in infancy: Interaction between intestinal and respiratory tracts and impact of nutritional exposures. *mBio* **2012**, *3*, e00251-12. [CrossRef] [PubMed]

36. Fouhy, F.; Ronan, N.J.; O'Sullivan, O.; McCarthy, Y.; Walsh, A.M.; Murphy, D.M.; Daly, M.; Flanagan, E.T.; Fleming, C.; McCarthy, M.; et al. A pilot study demonstrating the altered gut microbiota functionality in stable adults with Cystic Fibrosis. *Sci. Rep.* **2017**, *7*, 6685. [CrossRef]
37. Vernocchi, P.; Del Chierico, F.; Russo, A.; Majo, F.; Rossitto, M.; Valerio, M.; Casadei, L.; La Storia, A.; De Filippis, F.; Rizzo, C.; et al. Gut microbiota signatures in cystic fibrosis: Loss of host CFTR function drives the microbiota enterophenotype. *PLoS ONE* **2018**, *13*, e0208171. [CrossRef]
38. Coffey, M.J.; Nielsen, S.; Wemheuer, B.; Kaakoush, N.O.; Garg, M.; Needham, B.; Pickford, R.; Jaffe, A.; Thomas, T.; Ooi, C.Y. Gut Microbiota in Children With Cystic Fibrosis: A Taxonomic and Functional Dysbiosis. *Sci. Rep.* **2019**, *9*, 18593. [CrossRef]
39. van Dorst, J.M.; Tam, R.Y.; Ooi, C.Y. What Do We Know about the Microbiome in Cystic Fibrosis? Is There a Role for Probiotics and Prebiotics? *Nutrients* **2022**, *14*, 480. [CrossRef]
40. Price, C.; Hampton, T.H.; Valls, R.A.; Barrack, K.E.; O'Toole, G.A.; Madan, J.C.; Coker, M.O. Development of the intestinal microbiome in cystic fibrosis in early life. *mSphere* **2023**, *8*, 4. [CrossRef]
41. Semova, I.; Carten, J.D.; Stombaugh, J.; Mackey, L.C.; Knight, R.; Farber, S.A.; Rawls, J.F. Microbiota regulate intestinal absorption and metabolism of fatty acids in the zebrafish. *Cell Host Microbe* **2012**, *12*, 277–288. [CrossRef]
42. Shah, A.; Talley, N.J.; Holtmann, G. Current and Future Approaches for Diagnosing Small Intestinal Dysbiosis in Patients with Symptoms of Functional Dyspepsia. *Front. Neurosci.* **2022**, *16*, 830356. [CrossRef]
43. Hardouin, P.; Chiron, R.; Marchandin, H.; Armengaud, J.; Grenga, L. Metaproteomics to Decipher CF Host-Microbiota Interactions: Overview, Challenges and Future Perspectives. *Genes* **2021**, *12*, 892. [CrossRef] [PubMed]
44. Anderson, J.L.; Miles, C.; Tierney, A.C. Effect of probiotics on respiratory, gastrointestinal and nutritional outcomes in patients with cystic fibrosis: A systematic review. *J. Cyst. Fibros.* **2017**, *16*, 186–197. [CrossRef] [PubMed]
45. Asensio-Grau, A.; Calvo-Lerma, J.; Ferriz-Jordán, M.; García-Hernández, J.; Heredia, A.; Andrés, A. Effect of Lactobacillaceae Probiotics on Colonic Microbiota and Metabolite Production in Cystic Fibrosis: A Comparative In Vitro Study. *Nutrients* **2023**, *15*, 3846. [CrossRef] [PubMed]
46. Hayden, H.; Eng, A.; Pope, C.; Brittnacher, M.; Vo, A.; Weiss, E.; Hager, K.R.; Martin, B.D.; Leung, D.H.; Heltshe, S.L.; et al. Fecal dysbiosis in infants with cystic fibrosis is associated with early linear growth failure. *Nat. Med.* **2020**, *26*, 215–221. [CrossRef] [PubMed]
47. Gelfond, D.; Heltshe, S.; Ma, C.; Rowe, S.M.; Frederick, C.; Uluer, A.; Sicilian, L.; Konstan, M.; Tullis, E.; Roach, C.R.N.; et al. Impact of CFTR Modulation on Intestinal pH, Motility, and Clinical Outcomes in Patients with Cystic Fibrosis and the G551D Mutation. *Clin. Transl. Gastroenterol.* **2017**, *8*, e81. [CrossRef] [PubMed]
48. Pimentel, M.; Saad, R.J.; Long, M.D.; Rao, S.S.C. ACG Clinical Guideline: Small Intestinal Bacterial Overgrowth. *Am. J. Gastroenterol.* **2020**, *115*, 165–178. [CrossRef] [PubMed]
49. Cho, Y.K.; Lee, J.; Paik, C.N. Prevalence, risk factors, and treatment of small intestinal bacterial overgrowth in children. *Clin. Exp. Pediatr.* **2023**, *66*, 377–383. [CrossRef]
50. Achufusi, T.O.; Sharma, A.; Zamora, E.A.; Manocha, D. Small Intestinal Bacterial Overgrowth: Comprehensive Review of Diagnosis, Prevention, and Treatment Methods. *Cureus* **2020**, *12*, e8860. [CrossRef]
51. Banaszak, M.; Górna, I.; Woźniak, D.; Przysławski, J.; Drzymała-Czyz, S. Association between Gut Dysbiosis and the Occurrence of SIBO, LIBO, SIFO and IMO. *Microorganisms* **2023**, *11*, 573. [CrossRef]
52. Gabel, M.E.; Wang, H.; Gelfond, D.; Roach, C.; Rowe, S.M.; Clancy, J.P.; Sagel, S.D.; Borowitz, D. Changes in Glucose Breath Test in Cystic Fibrosis Patients Treated with 1 Month of Lumacaftor/Ivacaftor. *J. Pediatr. Gastroenterol. Nutr.* **2022**, *75*, 42–47. [CrossRef]
53. Husebye, E.; Hellström, P.M.; Sundler, F.; Chen, J.; Midtvedt, T. Influence of microbial species on small intestinal myoelectric activity and transit in germ-free rats. *Am. J. Physiol. Gastrointest. Liver Physiol.* **2001**, *280*, G368–G380. [CrossRef] [PubMed]
54. Zhong, C.; Qu, C.; Wang, B.; Liang, S.; Zeng, B. Probiotics for preventing and treating small intestinal bacterial overgrowth: A meta-analysis and systematic review of current evidence. *J. Clin. Gastroenterol.* **2017**, *51*, 300–311. [CrossRef] [PubMed]
55. Rosania, R.; Giorgio, F.; Principi, M.; Amoruso, A.; Monno, R.; Di Leo, A.; Ierardi, E. Effect of probiotic or prebiotic supplementation on antibiotic therapy in the small intestinal bacterial overgrowth: A comparative evaluation. *Curr. Clin. Pharmacol.* **2013**, *8*, 169–172. [CrossRef]
56. Khalighi, A.R.; Khalighi, M.R.; Behdani, R.; Jamali, J.; Khosravi, A.; Kouhestani, S.; Radmanesh, H.; Esmaeelzadeh, S.; Khalighi, N. Evaluating the efficacy of probiotic on treatment in patients with small intestinal bacterial overgrowth (SIBO)—A pilot study. *Indian J. Med. Res.* **2014**, *140*, 604–608. [PubMed]
57. Avelar Rodriguez, D.; Ryan, P.M.; Toro Monjaraz, E.M.; Ramirez Mayans, J.A.; Quigley, E.M. Small Intestinal Bacterial Overgrowth in Children: A State-of-The-Art Review. *Front. Pediatr.* **2019**, *7*, 363. [CrossRef] [PubMed]
58. Rao, S.S.C.; Rehman, A.; Yu, S.; Andino, N.M. Brain fogginess, gas and bloating: A link between SIBO, probiotics and metabolic acidosis. *Clin Transl. Gastroenterol.* **2018**, *9*, 162. [CrossRef]
59. Aslan, I.; Tarhan Celebi, L.; Kayhan, H.; Kizilay, E.; Gulbahar, M.Y.; Kurt, H.; Cakici, B. Probiotic Formulations Containing Fixed and Essential Oils Ameliorates SIBO-Induced Gut Dysbiosis in Rats. *Pharmaceuticals* **2023**, *16*, 1041. [CrossRef] [PubMed]
60. Kumar, K.; Saadi, M.; Ramsey, F.V.; Schey, R.; Parkman, H.P. Effect of Bifidobacterium infantis 35624 (Align) on the lactulose breath test for small intestinal bacterial overgrowth. *Dig. Dis. Sci.* **2018**, *63*, 989–995. [CrossRef]
61. Chen, W.C.; Quigley, E.M. Probiotics, prebiotics & synbiotics in small intestinal bacterial overgrowth: Opening up a new therapeutic horizon! *Indian J. Med. Res.* **2014**, *140*, 582–584.

62. Mitten, E.; Goldin, A. S660: Recent probiotic use is independently associated with methane-positive breath test for small intestinal bacterial overgrowth. *Am. J. Gastroenterol.* **2018**, *113*, S660. [CrossRef]
63. De Lisle, R.C.; Roach, E.; Jansson, K. Effects of laxative and N-acetylcysteine on mucus accumulation, bacterial load, transit, and inflammation in the cystic fibrosis mouse small intestine. *Am. J. Physiol. Gastrointest. Liver Physiol.* **2007**, *293*, G577–G584. [CrossRef]
64. Brown, K.; Decoffe, D.; Molcan, E.; Gibson, D.L. Diet-induced dysbiosis of the intestinal microbiota and the effects on immunity and disease. *Nutrients* **2012**, *4*, 1095–1119. [CrossRef] [PubMed]
65. Zimmer, J.; Lange, B.; Frick, J.S.; Sauer, H.; Zimmermann, K.; Schwiertz, A.; Rusch, K.; Klosterhalfen, S.; Enck, P. A vegan or vegetarian diet substantially alters the human colonic faecal microbiota. *Eur. J. Clin. Nutr.* **2012**, *66*, 53–60. [CrossRef]
66. O'Brien, S.; Mulcahy, H.; Fenlon, H.; O'Broin, A.; Casey, M.; Burke, A.; FitzGerald, M.X.; Hegarty, J.E. Intestinal bile acid malabsorption in Cystic Fibrosis. *Gut* **1993**, *34*, 1137–1141. [CrossRef] [PubMed]
67. Hedsund, C.; Gregersen, T.; Joensson, I.M.; Olesen, H.V.; Krogh, K. Gastrointestinal transit times and motility in patients with cystic fibrosis. *Scand. J. Gastroenterol.* **2012**, *47*, 920–926. [CrossRef] [PubMed]
68. Malagelada, C.; Bendezú, R.; Seguí, S.; Vitrià, J.; Merino, X.; Nieto, A.; Sihuay, D.; Accarino, A.; Molero, X.; Azpiroz, F. Motor dysfunction of the gut in cystic fibrosis. *Neurogastroenterol. Motil.* **2020**, *32*, e13883. [CrossRef]
69. Guarino, M.P.; Altomare, A.; Stasi, E.; Marignani, M.; Severi, C.; Alloni, R.; Dicuonzo, G.; Morelli, L.; Coppola, R.; Cicala, M. Effect of acute mucosal exposure to Lactobacillus rhamnosus GG on human colonic smooth muscle cells. *J. Clin. Gastroenterol.* **2008**, *42 Pt 2* (Suppl. S3), S185–S190. [CrossRef] [PubMed]
70. Isolauri, E.; Sutas, Y.; Kankaanpaa, P.; Arvilommi, H.; Salminen, S. Probiotics: Effects on immunity. *Am. J. Clin. Nutr.* **2001**, *73* (Suppl. S2), 444S–450S. [CrossRef]
71. Van Biervliet, S.; Declercq, D.; Somerset, S. Clinical effects of probiotics in cystic fibrosis patients: A systematic review. *Clin. Nutr.* **2017**, *18*, 37–43. [CrossRef]
72. Quigley, E.M. Gut bacteria in health and disease. *Gastroenterol. Hepatol.* **2013**, *9*, 560–569.
73. Vitko, M.; Valerio, D.M.; Rye, P.D.; Onsøyen, E.; Myrset, A.H.; Dessen, A.; Drumm, M.L.; Hodges, C.A. A novel guluronate oligomer improves intestinal transit and survival in cystic fibrosis mice. *J. Cyst. Fibros.* **2016**, *15*, 745–751. [CrossRef] [PubMed]
74. Littlewood, J.M.; Wolfe, S.P. Control of malabsorption in cystic fibrosis. *Pediatr. Drugs* **2000**, *2*, 205–222. [CrossRef] [PubMed]
75. Li, L.; Somerset, S. Digestive system dysfunction in cystic fibrosis: Challenges for nutrition therapy. *Dig. Liver Dis.* **2014**, *46*, 865–874. [CrossRef] [PubMed]
76. Bouquet, J.; Sinaasappel, M.; Neijens, H.J. Malabsorption in cystic fibrosis: Mechanisms and treatment. *J. Pediatr. Gastroenterol.* **1988**, *7* (Suppl. S1), S30–S35. [CrossRef]
77. Littlewood, J.; Wolfe, S.; Conway, S. Diagnosis and treatment of intestinal malabsorption in cystic fibrosis. *Pediatr. Pulmonol.* **2006**, *41*, 35–49. [CrossRef] [PubMed]
78. Peretti, N.; Roy, C.; Drouin, E.; Seidman, E.; Brochu, P.; Casimir, G. Abnormal intracellular lipid processing contributes to fat malabsorption in cystic fibrosis patients. *Am. J. Physiol. Gastrointest. Liver Physiol.* **2006**, *290*, G609–G615. [CrossRef] [PubMed]
79. Wouthuyzen-Bakker, M.; Bodewes, F.A.J.A.; Verkade, H.J. Persistent fat malabsorption in cystic fibrosis; lessons from patients and mice. *J. Cyst. Fibros.* **2011**, *10*, 150–158. [CrossRef]
80. Bertolaso, C.; Groleau, V.; Schall, J.; Maqbool, A.; Mascarenhas, M.; Latham, N.; Dougherty, K.A.; Stallings, V.A. Fat Soluble Vitamins in Cystic Fibrosis and Pancreatic Insufficiency: Efficacy of a Nutrition Intervention. *J. Pediatr. Gastroenterol. Nutr.* **2014**, *58*, 443–448. [CrossRef]
81. Calvo-Lerma, J.; Roca, M.; Boon, M.; Colombo, C.; De Koning, B.; Fornes-Ferrer, V.; Masip, E.; Garriga, M.; Bulfamante, A.; Asensio-Grau, A.; et al. Association between faecal pH and fat absorption in children with Cystic Fibrosis on a controlled diet and enzyme supplements dose. *Pediatr. Res.* **2021**, *89*, 205–210. [CrossRef]
82. Kalivianakis, M.; Minich, D.; Bijleveld, C.; Van Aalderen, W.; Stellaard, F.; Laseur, M.; Vonk, R.J.; Verkade, H.J. Fat malabsorption in cystic fibrosis patients receiving enzyme replacement therapy is due to impaired intestinal uptake of long-chain fatty acids. *Am. J. Clin. Nutr.* **1999**, *69*, 127–134. [CrossRef]
83. Wagner, M.H.; Bowser, V.K.; Sherman, J.M.; Frachisco, M.P.; Theriaqued, D.; Novak, D.A. Comparison of steatocrit and fatabsorption in persons with cystic fibrosis. *J. Pediatr. Gastroenterol. Nutr.* **2002**, *35*, 202–205. [CrossRef] [PubMed]
84. Amarri, S.; Harding, M.; Coward, W.A.; Evans, T.J.; Weaver, L.T. 13carbon mixed triglyceride breath test and pancreatic supplementation in cystic fibrosis. *Arch. Dis. Child.* **1997**, *76*, 349–351. [CrossRef] [PubMed]
85. Ritz, M.A.; Fraser, R.J.; Di Mattteo, A.C.; Greville, H.; Butler, R.; Cmielewski, P.; Davidson, G. Evaluation of the 13C-triolein breath testsfor fat malabsorption in adult patients with cystic fibrosis. *J. Gastroenterol. Hepatol.* **2004**, *19*, 448–453. [CrossRef] [PubMed]
86. Standards for the Clinical Care of Children and Adults with Cystic Fibrosis in the UK. UK Cystic Fibrosis Trust Clinical Standardsand Accreditation Group. Cystic Fibrosis Trust. 2011. Available online: https://www.cysticfibrosis.org.uk/sites/default/files/2020-12/Cystic%20Fibrosis%20Trust%20Standards%20of%20care.pdf (accessed on 28 August 2023).
87. Peretti, N.; Marcil, V.; Dronin, E.; Levy, E. Mechanisms of lipid malabsorption in Cystic Fibrosis: The impact of essential fatty acids deficiency. *Nutr. Metab.* **2005**, *2*, 11. [CrossRef] [PubMed]
88. Olsen, M.F.; Kjøller-Svarre, M.S.; Møller, G.; Katzenstein, T.L.; Nielsen, B.U.; Pressler, T.; Lewis, J.I.; Mathiesen, I.H.; Mølgaard, C.; Faurholt-Jepsen, D. Correlates of Pancreatic Enzyme Replacement Therapy Intake in Adults with Cystic Fibrosis: Results of a Cross-Sectional Study. *Nutrients* **2022**, *14*, 1330. [CrossRef] [PubMed]

89. Green, J.; Gilchrist, F.; Carroll, W. Interventions for treating distal intestinal obstruction syndrome (DIOS) in Cystic Fibrosis. *Cochrane Database Syst. Rev.* **2018**, *8*, CD012798. [CrossRef]
90. Taylor, C.; Connolly, S. Gastrointestinal disease and nutrition. In *Cystic Fibrosis*, 2nd ed.; Horsley, A., Cunningham, S., Alistair, I., Eds.; Oxford University Press: Oxford, UK, 2015; pp. 73–84.
91. Cîrdei, E.; Anton, D. Mucoviscidoza (fibroza chistică de pancreas). In *Pediatrie—Patologie Digestivă, Nutrițională și Neurologică la Copil*; Burlea, M., Moraru, E., Cîrdei, E., Diaconu, G., Eds.; Editura Fundației Academice AXIS: Iași, Romania, 2008; pp. 62–77.
92. Kleinman, R. Nutrition in cystic fibrosis. In *Pediatric Nutrition Handbook*, 6th ed.; Kleinman, R., Ed.; American Academy of Pediatrics: Itasca, IL, USA, 2009; pp. 1001–1020.
93. Kliegman, R.; Geme, J.W.S.T.; Blum, N.J.; Shah, S.S.; Tasker, R.C.; Wilson, K.M.; Behrman, R.E.; Nelson, W.E. Cystic fibrosis. In *Nelson Textbook of Pediatrics*, 21st ed.; Elservier: Philadelphi, PA, USA, 2020; pp. 2282–2297.
94. Farrelly, P.J.; Charlesworth, C.; Lee, S.; Southern, K.W.; Baillie, C.T. Gastrointestinal surgery in cystic fibrosis: A 20-year review. *J. Pediatr. Surg.* **2014**, *49*, 280–283. [CrossRef]
95. El-Chammas, K.; Rumman, N.; Goh, V.L.; Quintero, D.; Goday, P. Rectal Prolapse and Cystic Fibrosis. *J. Pediatr. Gastroenterol. Nutr.* **2015**, *60*, 110–112. [CrossRef]
96. Baker, R.D. Acute abdominal pain. *Pediatr. Rev.* **2018**, *39*, 130–139. [CrossRef]
97. Adu, Y.; Wolkober, B.; Nesiama, E.; Thompson, L.; Laswi, M.; Obokhare, I. Adult intussusception of the small intestine caused by cystic fibrosis: A case report, review of the literature, and guide for management. *J. Surg. Case Rep.* **2023**, *2023*, rjad574. [CrossRef]
98. Adewale, A.T.; Rowe, S.M.; Solomon, G.M. Colocolonic intussusception in an adult cystic fibrosis patient. *J. Cyst. Fibros.* **2019**, *18*, e11–e13. [CrossRef] [PubMed]
99. Casaccia, G.; Trucchi, A.; Nahom, A.; Aite, L.; Lucidi, V.; Giorlandino, C.; Bagolan, P. The impact of cystic fibrosis on neonatal intestinal obstruction: The need for prenatal/neonatal screening. *Pediatr. Surg. Int.* **2003**, *19*, 75–78. [CrossRef] [PubMed]
100. Passos Ramos, A.F.; De Fucio, M.B.; Dias Moretzsohn, L.; Barbosa, A.J.A.; Do Carmo Friche Passos, M.; Said Carvalho, R.; Luiz Gonzaga, V.C. Cystic Fibrosis, gastroduodenal inflammation, duodenal ulcer, and Helicbascter pylori infection: The "Cystic Fibrosis paradox". *J. Cyst. Fibros.* **2013**, *12*, 2377–2383. [CrossRef]
101. Robertson, M.; Choe, K.; Joseph, P. Review of the abdominal manifestations of cystic fibrosis in the adult patient. *Radiographics* **2006**, *26*, 679–690. [CrossRef]
102. Marin, A.C.; Anton-Păduraru, D.T.; Cloșcă, N.B.; Mihăilă, D.; Burlea, M. Fibroza chistică și infecția cu Helicobacter pylori. *RJID* **2016**, *XIX*, 54–59. [CrossRef]
103. Drzymała-Czyż, S.; Kwiecień, J.; Pogorzelski, A.; Rachel, M.; Banasiewicz, T.; Pławski, A.; Szczawińska-Popłonyk, A.; Herzig, K.-H.; Walkowiak, J. Prevalence of Helicobacter pylori infection in patients with cystic fibrosis. *J. Cyst. Fibros.* **2013**, *12*, 761–765. [CrossRef]
104. Patel, D.; Baliss, M.; Saikumar, P.; Numan, L.; Teckman, J.; Hachem, C. A Gastroenterologist's Guide to Care Transitions in Cystic Fibrosis from Pediatrics to Adult Care. *Int. J. Mol. Sci.* **2023**, *24*, 15766. [CrossRef]
105. Corral, J.E.; Dye, C.W.; Mascarenhas, M.R.; Barkin, J.S.; Salathe, M.; Moshiree, B. Is Gastroparesis Found More Frequently in Patients with Cystic Fibrosis? A Systematic Review. *Scientifica* **2016**, *2016*, 2918139. [CrossRef]
106. Tan, H.L.; Shah, N.; Suri, R. The role of endoscopy and biopsy in the management of severe gastro-intestinal disease in Cystic Fibrosis patients. *Arch. Dis. Child.* **2011**, *96*, A20. [CrossRef]
107. Stallings, V.A.; Sainath, N.; Oberle, M.; Bertolaso, C.; Schall, J.I. Energy Balance and Mechanisms of Weight Gain with Ivacaftor Treatment of Cystic Fibrosis Gating Mutations. *J. Pediatr.* **2018**, *201*, 229–237.e4. [CrossRef]
108. Rowe, S.M.; Heltshe, S.L.; Gonska, T.; Donaldson, S.H.; Borowitz, D.; Gelfond, D.; Sagel, S.D.; Khan, U.; Mayer-Hamblett, N.; Van Dalfsen, J.M.; et al. Clinical Mechanism of the Cystic Fibrosis Transmembrane Conductance Regulator Potentiator Ivacaftor in G551D-mediated Cystic Fibrosis. *Am. J. Respir. Crit. Care Med.* **2014**, *190*, 175–184. [CrossRef] [PubMed]
109. Tétard, C.; Mittaine, M.; Bui, S.; Beaufils, F.; Maumus, P.; Fayon, M.; Burgel, P.-R.; Lamireau, T.; Delhaes, L.; Mas, E.; et al. Reduced Intestinal Inflammation with Lumacaftor/Ivacaftor in Adolescents with Cystic Fibrosis. *J. Pediatr. Gastroenterol. Nutr.* **2020**, *71*, 778–781. [CrossRef] [PubMed]
110. Gelfond, D.; Borowitz, D. Gastrointestinal Complications of Cystic Fibrosis. *Clin. Gastroenterol. Hepatol.* **2013**, *11*, 333–342. [CrossRef] [PubMed]
111. Lavelle, L.; McEvoy, S.; Gibney, R.; McMahon, C.; Heffernan, E.; Malone, D. Cystic Fibrosis below the Diaphragm: Abdominal Findings in Adult Patients. *Radio. Graph.* **2015**, *35*, 680–695. [CrossRef] [PubMed]
112. Pauwels, A.; Blondeau, K.; Dupont, L.; Sifrim, D. Mechanisms of Increased Gastroesophageal Reflux in Patients with Cystic Fibrosis. *Am. J. Gastroenterol.* **2012**, *107*, 1346–1353. [CrossRef] [PubMed]
113. Safe, M.; Cho, J.; Krishnan, U. Combined multichannel intraluminal impedance and pH measurement in detecting gastroesophageal reflux disease in children. *J. Pediatr. Gastroenterol. Nutr.* **2016**, *63*, e98–e106. [CrossRef]
114. Bongiovanni, A.; Manti, S.; Parisi, G.F.; Papale, M.; Mulè, E.; Rotolo, N.; Leonardi, S. Focus on gastroesophageal reflux disease in patients with cystic fibrosis. *World J. Gastroenterol.* **2020**, *26*, 6322–6334. [CrossRef]
115. Bongiovanni, A.; Parisi, G.; Scuderi, M.; Licari, A.; Brambilla, I.; Marseglia, G.; Leonardi, S. Gastroesophageal reflux and respiratory diseases: Does a real link exist? *Minerva Pediatr.* **2019**, *71*, 515–523. [CrossRef]
116. Dimango, E.; Walker, P.; Keating, C.; Berdella, M.; Robinson, N.; Langfelder-Schwind, E.; Levy, D.; Xinhua, L. Effect of esomeprazole versus placebo on pulmonary exacerbations in cystic fibrosis. *BMC Pulm. Med.* **2014**, *14*, 21. [CrossRef]

117. Brecelj, J.; Zidar, N.; Jeruc, J.; Orel, R. Morphological and functional assessment of oesophageal mucosa integrity in children with cystic fibrosis. *J. Pediatr. Gastroenterol. Nutr.* **2016**, *62*, 757–764. [CrossRef]
118. Zeybel, G.L.; Pearson, J.P.; Krishnan, A.; Bourke, S.J.; Doe, S.; Anderson, A.; Faruqi, S.; Morice, A.H.; Jones, R.; McDonnell, M.; et al. Ivacaftor and symptoms of extra-oesophageal reflux in patients with cystic fibrosis and G551D mutation. *J. Cyst. Fibros.* **2017**, *16*, 124–131. [CrossRef] [PubMed]
119. Sergeev, V.; Chou, F.; Lam, G.; Hamilton, C.M.; Wilcox, P.; Quon, B. The Extrapulmonary Effects of CFTR Modulators in Cystic Fibrosis. *Ann. Am. Thorac. Soc.* **2020**, *17*, 147–154. [CrossRef] [PubMed]
120. Shakir, S.; Echevarria, C.; Doe, S.; Brodlie, M.; Ward, C.; Bourke, S.J. Elexacaftor-tezacaftor-ivacaftor improve gastro-oesophageal reflux and sinonasal symptoms in advanced cystic fibrosis. *J. Cyst. Fibros.* **2022**, *21*, 807–810. [CrossRef] [PubMed]
121. Goralski, J.; Lercher, D.; Davis, S.; Dellon, E. Eosinophilic Esophagitis in Cystic Fibrosis: A Case Series and Review of the Literature. *J. Cyst. Fibros.* **2013**, *12*, 9–14. [CrossRef] [PubMed]
122. Capucilli, P.; Cianferoni, A.; Grundmeier, R.W.; Spergel, J.M. Comparison of comorbid diagnoses in children with and without eosinophilic esophagitis in a large population. *Ann. Allergy Asthma Immunol.* **2018**, *121*, 711–716. [CrossRef]
123. Dellon, E.S.; Liacouras, C.A.; Molina-Infante, J.; Furuta, G.T.; Spergel, J.M.; Zevit, N.; Spechler, S.J.; Attwood, S.E.; Straumann, A.; Aceves, S.S.; et al. Updated international consensus diagnostic criteria for eosinophilic esophagitis: Proceedings of the AGREE conference. *Gastroenterology* **2018**, *155*, 1022–1033.e10. [CrossRef]
124. Godwin, B.; Liacouras, C.; Mehta, V.; Eisenberg, J.; Agawu, A.; Brown-Whitehorn, T.; Ruffner, M.A.; Verma, R.; Cianferoni, A.; Spergel, J.M.; et al. A review of tertiary referrals for management of pediatric esophageal eosinophilia. *Front. Pediatr.* **2018**, *6*, 173. [CrossRef]
125. Gomez-Torrijos, E.; Garcia-Rodriguez, R.; Castro-Jimenez, A.; Rodriguez-Sanchez, J.; Mendez Diaz, Y.; Molina-Infante, J. The efficacy of step-down therapy in adult patients with proton pump inhibitor-responsive oesophageal eosinophilia. *Aliment. Pharmacol. Ther.* **2016**, *43*, 534–540. [CrossRef]
126. Colombo, C.; Ellemunter, H.; Houwen, R.; Munck, A.; Taylor, C.; Wilschanski, M. Guidelines for the diagnosis and management of distal intestinal obstruction syndrome in cystic fibrosis patients. *J. Cyst. Fibros.* **2011**, *10* (Suppl. S2), S24–S28. [CrossRef]
127. Subhi, R.; Ooi, R.; Finlayson, F.; Kotsimbos, T.; Wilson, J.; Lee, W.R.; Wale, R.; Warrier, S. Distal intestinal obstruction syndrome in cystic fibrosis: Presentation, outcome and management in a tertiary hospital (2007–2012). *ANZ J. Surg.* **2014**, *84*, 740–744. [CrossRef]
128. Abraham, J.; Taylor, C. Cystic Fibrosis & disorders of the large intestine: DIOS, constipation, and colorectal cancer. *J. Cyst. Fibros.* **2017**, *16*, S40–S49. [CrossRef] [PubMed]
129. Konrad, J.; Eber, E.; Stadlbauer, V. Changing paradigms in the treatment of gastrointestinal complications of cystic fibrosis in the era of cystic fibrosis transmembrane conductance regulator modulators. *Paediatr. Resp. Rev.* **2022**, *42*, 9–16. [CrossRef]
130. McNamara, J.J.; McColley, S.; Marigowda, G.; Liu, F.; Tian, S.; Owen, C.A.; Stiles, D.; Li, C.; Waltz, D.; Wang, L.T.; et al. Safety, pharmacokinetics, and pharmacodynamics of lumacaftor and ivacaftor combination therapy in children aged 2–5 years with cystic fibrosis homozygous for F508del-CFTR: An open-label phase 3 study. *Lancet Respir. Med.* **2019**, *7*, 325–335. [CrossRef] [PubMed]
131. Rosenfeld, M.; Wainwright, C.E.; Higgins, M.; Wang, L.T.; McKee, C.; Campbell, D.; Tian, S.; Schneider, J.; Cunningham, S.; Davies, J.C. Ivacaftor treatment of cystic fibrosis in children aged 12 to <24 months and with a CFTR gating mutation (ARRIVAL): A phase 3 single-arm study. *Lancet Respir. Med.* **2018**, *6*, 545–553. [CrossRef] [PubMed]
132. Șerban, D.S.; Florescu, P.; Miu, N. Fibrosing Colonopathy Revealing Cystic Fibrosis in a Neonate Before Any pancreatic Enzyme Supplementation. *J. Ped. Gastroenterol. Nutr.* **2002**, *35*, 356–359. [CrossRef]
133. Smyth, R.L.; Vanvelzen, D.; Smyth, A.R.; Lloyd, D.A.; Heaf, D.P. Strictures of ascending colon in cystic fibrosis and high-strength pancreatic-enzymes. *Lancet* **1994**, *343*, 85–86. [CrossRef]
134. Wilschanski, M.; Durie, P.R. Patterns of GI disease in adulthood associated with mutations in the CFTR gene. *Gut* **2007**, *56*, 1153–1163. [CrossRef]
135. Chaun, H. Colonic disorders in adult cystic fibrosis. *Can. J. Gastroenterol.* **2001**, *15*, 586–590. [CrossRef]
136. Moss, R.L.; Musemeche, C.A.; Feddersen, R.M. Progressive pan-colonic fibrosis secondary to oral administration of pancreatic enzymes. *Pediatr. Surg. Int.* **1998**, *13*, 168–170. [CrossRef]
137. Vincenzi, F.; Bizzarri, B.; Ghiselli, A.; de'Angelis, N.; Fornaroli, F.; de'Angelis, G.L. Cystic fibrosis and Crohn's disease: Successful treatment and long term remission with infliximab. *World J. Gastroenterol.* **2010**, *16*, 1924–1927. [CrossRef]
138. Emiralioglu, N.; Tural, D.A.; Hizarcioglu, G.H.; Ergen, Y.M.; Ozsezen, B.; Sunman, B.; Temizel, I.S.; Yalcin, E.; Dogru, D.; Ozcelik, U.; et al. Does Cystic Fibrosis make susceptible to celiac disease? *Eur. J. Ped.* **2021**, *180*, 2807–2813. [CrossRef] [PubMed]
139. Kostovski, A.; Zdraveska, N. Coagulopathy as initial manifestation of concomitant celiac disease and cystic fibrosis: A case report. *J. Med. Case Rep.* **2011**, *5*, 116. [CrossRef] [PubMed]
140. Fluge, G.; Olesen, H.V.; Gilljam, M.; Meyer, P.; Pressler, T.; Storrösten, O.T.; Karpati, F.; Hjelte, L. Co-morbidity of cystic fibrosis and celiac disease in Scandinavian cystic fibrosis patinets. *J. Cyst. Fibros.* **2009**, *8*, 198–202. [CrossRef] [PubMed]
141. Cystic Fibrosis and Celiac Disease. 2020. Available online: https://cystic-fibrosis.com/clinical/celiac-disease (accessed on 24 November 2023).

142. Walkowiak, J.; Blask-Osipa, A.; Lisowska, A.; Oralewska, B.; Pogorzelski, A.; Cichy, W.; Sapiejka, E.; Kowalska, M.; Korzon, M.; Szaflarska-Popławska, A. Cystic fibrosis is a risk factor for celiac disease. *Acta Biochim. Pol.* **2010**, *57*, 115–118. [CrossRef] [PubMed]
143. Maiuri, L.; Villella, V.; Piancentini, M.; Raia, V.; Kroemer, G. Defective proteostasis in celiac disease as a new therapeutic target. *Cell Death Dis.* **2019**, *10*, 114. [CrossRef]
144. Maiuri, L.; Villella, V.; Raia, V.; Kroemer, G. The gliadin—CFTR connection: New perspectives for the treatment of celiac disease. *Ital. J. Pediatr.* **2019**, *45*, 40. [CrossRef]
145. Putman, M.; Haagensen, A.; Neuringer, I.; Sicilian, L. Celiac Disease in Patients with Cystic Fibrosis-Related Bone Disease. *Hindawi Case Rep. Endocrinol.* **2017**, *2017*, 2652403. [CrossRef]
146. Hjelm, M.; Shaikhkhalil, A. Celiac Disease in Patients with Cystic Fibrosis on Ivacaftor: A Case Series. *J. Ped. Gastroenterol. Nutr.* **2020**, *71*, 257–260. [CrossRef]
147. Maillie, A.J.; Vaccaro, M.I.; Calvo, E.L.; Ruiz, J.A.; Emiliani, R.; Pivelta, O.H. Serum Isoamylase Activities in Cystic Fibrosis Patients, Determined by an Inhibitory Assay. *Scand. J. Gastroenterol.* **1986**, *21*, 941–944. [CrossRef]
148. Kelly, T.; Buxbaum, J. Gastrointestinal manifestations of cystic fibrosis. *Dig. Dis. Sci.* **2015**, *60*, 1903–1913. [CrossRef]

Disclaimer/Publisher's Note: The statements, opinions and data contained in all publications are solely those of the individual author(s) and contributor(s) and not of MDPI and/or the editor(s). MDPI and/or the editor(s) disclaim responsibility for any injury to people or property resulting from any ideas, methods, instructions or products referred to in the content.

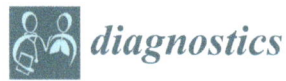

Article

Omicron in Infants—Respiratory or Digestive Disease?

Anca Cristina Drăgănescu [1,2], Victor Daniel Miron [1,*], Oana Săndulescu [1,2], Anuța Bilașco [2], Anca Streinu-Cercel [1,2], Roxana Gabriela Sandu [2], Adrian Marinescu [2], Deniz Gunșahin [1], Karina Ioana Hoffmann [1], Daria Ștefana Horobeț [1], Daniela Pițigoi [1,2], Adrian Streinu-Cercel [1,2] and Doina Anca Pleșca [1]

[1] Faculty of Medicine, Carol Davila University of Medicine and Pharmacy, 050474 Bucharest, Romania
[2] National Institute for Infectious Diseases "Prof. Dr. Matei Balș", 021105 Bucharest, Romania
* Correspondence: victor.miron@drd.umfcd.ro or mironvictordaniel@gmail.com

Abstract: The Omicron variant of SARS-CoV-2 has caused a large number of cases and hospitalizations in the pediatric population. Infants due to their age are susceptible to viral infections that may have a worse prognosis. Therefore, the aim of the current study has been to characterize the clinical features and the outcome of infants hospitalized with confirmed SARS-CoV-2 infection during the Omicron wave. We conducted a retrospective study of all consecutive infants hospitalized with symptomatic COVID-19 and no other co-infections, from January to September 2022 in one of the largest infectious diseases hospitals from Bucharest, Romania. A total of 613 infants were included in the analysis. The median age was 5 months (IQR: 3, 8 months). The clinical features were dominated by fever (96.4%), cough (64.8%) and loss of appetite (63.3%), and overall, respiratory symptoms were the most numerous (76.0%). Infants between 1-3 months old had a 1.5-fold increased risk of elevated alanine aminotransferase (ALT) values, and a longer length of hospitalization as compared to older infants. Infants between 7-9 months of age had 1.5-fold higher odds of loss of appetite, 1.7-fold more frequent cough and 1.6-fold more frequent digestive symptoms compared to infants in other age groups. The presence of digestive symptoms increased the probability of hepatic cytolysis (increased ALT) by 1.9-fold. Continued monitoring of COVID-19 among infants is very necessary, given the progressive character of SARS-CoV-2, in order to take correct and rapid therapeutic measures and to adapt to clinical changes driven by viral variant change.

Keywords: COVID-19; infants; children; Omicron; respiratory; digestive; SARS-CoV-2

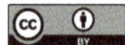

Citation: Drăgănescu, A.C.; Miron, V.D.; Săndulescu, O.; Bilașco, A.; Streinu-Cercel, A.; Sandu, R.G.; Marinescu, A.; Gunșahin, D.; Hoffmann, K.I.; Horobeț, D.Ș.; et al. Omicron in Infants—Respiratory or Digestive Disease? *Diagnostics* **2023**, *13*, 421. https://doi.org/10.3390/diagnostics13030421

Academic Editor: Cristina Oana Marginean

Received: 19 December 2022
Revised: 14 January 2023
Accepted: 19 January 2023
Published: 23 January 2023

Copyright: © 2023 by the authors. Licensee MDPI, Basel, Switzerland. This article is an open access article distributed under the terms and conditions of the Creative Commons Attribution (CC BY) license (https://creativecommons.org/licenses/by/4.0/).

1. Introduction

Infants are a particular group among children because of their age and specific anatomical and physiological characteristics [1,2]. The management of this type of patient during an acute infectious disease is based on a limited number of therapeutic resources and a careful follow-up of their clinical manifestations is necessary to prevent possible complications and an unfavorable course. Given the experiences with influenza viruses and respiratory syncytial virus for which infants are an at-risk group for hospitalization and potentially severe outcomes with respiratory failure [3–5], the onset of the COVID-19 pandemic has been regarded with concern [6] for this group of children.

However, somewhat unusually for a viral infection, children of all ages, including infants, have been significantly less affected than adults by COVID-19 since the beginning of the pandemic [7–9]. Factors hypothesized to have contributed to this initial trend included the non-pharmacological protective measures instituted, as well as the parental care for children [10,11], but different pathogenic mechanisms are also considered to have contributed to the different course of COVID-19 in children. Overall, children have had milder forms of the disease, with significantly lower rates of hospitalization and of severe disease compared to adults [7].

SARS-CoV-2 has undergone a number of changes in its viral structure so that the emergence of the Omicron variant caused an increase in the number of cases worldwide [12,13]. Omicron infection rates among children increased significantly, which has also resulted in an increase in hospitalizations for the pediatric population [13,14], but, fortunately, most cases have had a favorable outcome [13]. Although the first case of COVID-19 was identified in February 2020 [15], Romania experienced the largest wave of SARS-CoV-2 infections only after the first case of Omicron was identified [16] and the rate of confirmed cases of COVID-19 among children exceeded 10% [17].

The spectrum of clinical manifestations of COVID-19 in infants is highly heterogeneous, and each variant of SARS-CoV-2 has had a different impact on the clinical course in children [13,18]. Moreover, due to age, many subjective symptoms cannot be quantified and analyses on large groups of infants are needed to better characterize the impact of COVID-19 on this group of children. Therefore, we aimed at evaluating the spectrum of clinical symptoms of the omicron variant among infants hospitalized in one of the largest infectious disease hospitals in Romania.

2. Methods

We conducted a retrospective study among infants hospitalized with COVID-19 between 1 January and 30 September 2022 in the National Institute of Infectious Diseases "Prof. Dr. Matei Balș", Bucharest, (NIID), with the aim of characterizing the clinical features and outcome of infants with SARS-CoV-2 infection, Omicron variant. NIID is the largest tertiary infectious disease hospital in Romania and during the pandemic it was the main care center for patients with SARS-CoV-2 infection in the capital and the nearby metropolitan areas.

We included in the study all infants (under 1 year of age) consecutively hospitalized during the study period (1 January–30 September 2022) with symptomatic SARS-CoV-2 infection, confirmed by RT-PCR from nasopharyngeal swabs. We excluded from the analysis asymptomatic infants, those with confirmed respiratory, digestive, urinary tract or systemic co-infections, those with incomplete data in the medical charts, and those who had been transferred from another hospital after more than 24 h of previous hospitalization. Infants who, during hospitalization, turned 1 year of age were considered eligible and included in the final analysis.

Each infant according to the clinical presentation at the time of the hospital admission received investigations such as multiplex RT-PCR of the respiratory tract, rapid stool antigen testing, stool culture, multiplex RT-PCR of stool, urine culture and blood culture. Any positive result in one of these investigations was considered co-infection with SARS-CoV-2 and these patients were excluded from the final analysis.

Data for each patient were extracted from the patient medical charts by teams formed by two of the authors of this article. Cough, rhinorrhea or nasal obstruction and dyspnea were considered respiratory symptoms, and vomiting, diarrhea or constipation were considered digestive symptoms. Given the age of the patients analyzed, symptoms such as headache, sore throat, fatigue, or other subjective manifestations could not be analyzed. Fever and loss of appetite were analyzed as separate symptoms from respiratory and digestive symptoms. Chest imaging assessment was performed in a small number of infants, so we have not reported these data.

In 2022, a total number of 683 infants were hospitalized in NIID with confirmed SARS-CoV-2 infection. After applying eligibility criteria in the final analysis, 613 (89.8%) of the infants were included.

Data analysis was performed using IBM SPSS Statistics for Windows, version 25 (IBM Corp., Armonk, NY, USA). For a p-value of less than 0.05, data were considered to be statistically significant. Since our continuous variables were not normally distributed, we present the median and the interquartile range (IQR: 25th–75th percentile). Comparative analysis between this type of data was done using the Mann–Whitney U test and the

Kruskal–Wallis H test. For dichotomous variables we present frequencies and percentages and Chi-squared test values with odds ratios and 95%CI in the comparison analysis.

3. Results

3.1. General Data Analysis for the Whole Study Group On

A total of 613 infants were included in the analysis. The male sex was more numerous (n = 361, 58.9%), and the median age for the whole study group was 5 months (IQR: 3, 8 months), with a balanced distribution by age group (Table 1).

Table 1. Demographic and clinical characteristics for all infants included in the study.

Characteristic	Frequency, n	Percentage, %
Male sex	361	58.9
Age groups		
Newborn	14	2.3
1–3 months	182	29.7
4–6 months	160	26.1
7–9 months	149	24.3
10–12 months	108	17.6
Clinical features		
Fever	591	96.4
Loss of appetite	388	63.3
Respiratory symptoms	466	76.0
Cough	397	64.8
Rhinorrhea	295	48.1
Dyspnea	69	11.3
Digestive symptoms	309	49.6
Vomiting	148	24.1
Diarrhea	230	37.5
Constipation	21	3.4
Preterm	57	9.3
At least one chronic condition	69	11.3

The clinical presentation was dominated by fever (96.4%, n = 591), cough (64.8%, n = 397) and loss of appetite (63.3%, n = 388) (Table 1). Overall, respiratory symptoms were most common among infants with SARS-CoV-2 infection (76.0%, n = 466), and 11.3% (n = 69) had general manifestations only, such as fever and/or loss of appetite (Figure 1).

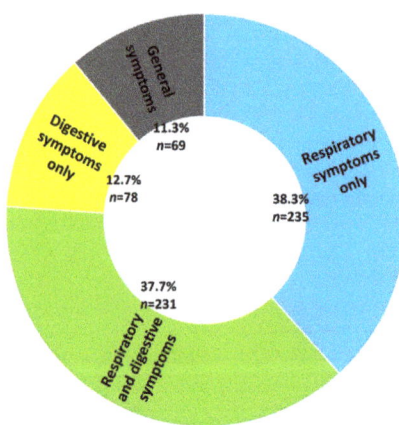

Figure 1. Distribution of symptom type in infants in the study.

White blood cell (WBC) counts showed no significant patterns, with a median of 6800 cells/µL (IQR: 4900, 9500 cells/µL); 24.6% (n = 151) showed increased WBC and 7.3% (n = 45) decreased WBC. A high number of infants, 82.9% (n = 508), had anemia at the time of hospitalization with median hemoglobin values of 10.9 g/dL (IQR: 10.2, 11.7 g/dL). Aspartate aminotransferase (AST) and lactate dehydrogenase (LDH) values were elevated in 80.1% (n = 491) and 83.8% (n = 514) of cases, respectively. In contrast, alanine aminotransferase (ALT) was abnormally high in 32.1% (n = 191) of patients. Increases in interleukin-6 (IL-6) were identified in 96.7% (n = 88/91) of infants, with a median of 177.7 pg/mL (IQR: 57.5, 1333.5 pg/mL) (Table 2).

Table 2. Laboratory findings in infants included in the study.

Laboratory Analysis	Results
WBC count, median (IQR)	6800 (4900, 9500) cells/µL
WBC increase, n (%)	151 (24.6)
WBC decrease, n (%)	45 (7.3)
Lymphocytes count, median (IQR)	3000 (1700, 5300) cells/µL
Lymphocytes decrease, n (%)	84 (13.7)
Hemoglobin, median (IQR)	10.9 (10.2, 11.7) g/dL
Anemia, n (%)	508 (82.9)
Platelets count, median (IQR)	278,000 (210,000, 356,000) cells/µL
Platelets increase, n (%)	11 (1.8)
Platelets decrease, n (%)	0 (0.0)
AST, median (IQR)	66 (53, 82) U/L
AST increase, n (%)	491 (80.1)
ALT, median (IQR)	32 (25, 45) U/L
ALT increase, n (%)	191 (31.2)
LDH, median (IQR)	350 (304, 406) U/L
LDH increase, n (%)	514 (83.8)
CRP, median (IQR) *	2.7 (0.9, 7.6) mg/L
CRP increase, n (%) *	182/509 (35.8)
IL-6, median (IQR) ×	177.7 (57.5, 1333.5) pg/mL
IL-6 increase, n (%) ×	88/91 (96.7)

WBC—white blood cells, ALT—alanine aminotransferase, AST—aspartate aminotransferase; LDH—lactate dehydrogenase; CRP—C-reactive protein; IL-6—interleukin 6; * Data available for 509 patients; × Data available for 91 patients.

The majority of infants were hospitalized within 1 day (IQR: 0, 2 days) of symptom onset and the median length of hospitalization was 4 days (IQR: 3, 5 days). A total of 11.3% (n = 6) of infants had a chronic condition and 9.3% (n = 57) were premature. However, these risk factors were not associated with an increased length of hospitalization ($p > 0.05$). All infants had a favorable outcome, and none required admission to intensive care.

3.2. Data Analysis by Age Group

The analysis of data by age group is highlighted in Table 3. Infants between 1–3 months had a 5.5-fold increased risk of anemia ($p < 0.001$, $\chi^2 = 27.07$, OR = 5.5, 95%CI: 2.7–11.2) and a 1.5-fold increased risk of liver cytolysis with increased ALT values ($p = 0.019$, $\chi^2 = 5.50$, OR = 1.5, 95%CI: 1.1–2.2). Similarly, infants between 4–6 months had a 1.5-fold increased risk of having increased ALT values ($p = 0.043$, $\chi^2 = 4.06$, OR = 1.5, 95%CI: 1.1–2.2). The 7–9 months age group had a 1.2-fold increased risk of loss of appetite ($p = 0.022$, $\chi^2 = 5.22$, OR = 1.5, 95%CI: 1.1–2.4), a 1.7-fold higher risk of cough ($p = 0.013$, $\chi^2 = 6.07$, OR = 1.7, 95%CI: 1.1–2.5) and 1.6-fold higher risk of having digestive symptoms ($p = 0.009$, $\chi^2 = 6.85$, OR = 1.6, 95%CI: 1.1–2.4). In terms of laboratory parameters, there was a 2.1-fold increased risk of elevated AST values in this age group ($p = 0.006$, $\chi^2 = 7.55$, OR = 2.1, 95%CI: 1.2–3.6). For infants between 10–12 months there was a 1.9-fold higher risk of vomiting ($p = 0.003$,

$\chi^2 = 8.73$, OR = 1.9, 95%CI: 1.2–3.1) and 1.7- and 2.1-fold higher risks of WBC ($p = 0.020$, $\chi^2 = 5.35$, OR = 1.7, 95%CI: 1.1–2.7) and C-reactive protein ($p = 0.001$, $\chi^2 = 9.66$, OR = 2.1, 95%CI: 1.3–3.3) increases, respectively.

Table 3. Data analysis according to age group.

Characteristics	Newborn N = 14	1–3 Months N = 182	4–6 Months N = 160	7–9 Months N = 149	10–12 Months N = 108	p-Value for Comparison between All Groups
Male sex, n (%)	10 (71.4)	93 (51.1)	96 (60.0)	96 (64.4)	66 (61.1)	0.105
Fever, n (%)	12 (85.7)	176 (96.7)	155 (96.9)	145 (97.3)	103 (95.4)	0.243
Loss of appetite, n (%)	11 (78.6)	109 (59.9)	93 (58.1)	106 (71.1)	69 (63.9)	0.093
Respiratory symptoms, n (%)	8 (57.1)	131 (72.0)	122 (76.3)	121 (81.2)	84 (77.8)	0.149
Cough, n (%)	3 (21.4)	106 (58.2)	111 (69.4)	109 (73.2) [+]	68 (63.0)	**<0.001**
Rhinorrhea, n (%)	6 (42.9)	80 (44.0)	76 (47.5)	84 (56.4)	84 (45.4)	0.211
Dyspnea, n (%)	2 (14.3)	15 (8.2)	23 (14.4)	15 (10.1)	14 (13.0)	0.433
Digestive symptoms, n (%)	5 (35.7)	76 (41.8)	84 (52.5)	89 (59.7) [+]	55 (50.9)	0.016
Vomiting, n (%)	2 (14.3)	20 (11.0)	39 (24.4)	49 (32.9)	38 (35.2) [+]	**<0.001**
Diarrhea, n (%)	4 (28.6)	59 (32.4)	68 (42.5)	65 (43.6)	34 (31.5)	0.083
Constipation, n (%)	0 (0.0)	7 (3.8)	7 (4.4)	2 (1.3)	5 (4.6)	0.484
Preterm, n (%)	4 (28.6)	17 (9.3)	17 (10.6)	10 (6.7)	9 (8.3)	0.099
Chronic conditions, n (%)	1 (7.1)	19 (10.4)	22 (13.8)	13 (8.7)	14 (13.2)	0.622
WBC increase, n (%)	3 (21.4)	29 (15.9)	41 (25.6)	42 (28.2)	36 (33.3) [+]	**0.011**
WBC decrease, n (%)	0 (0.0)	17 (9.3)	12 (7.5)	9 (6.0)	7 (6.5)	0.614
Lymphocytes decrease, n (%)	1 (7.1)	23 (12.6)	19 (11.9)	21 (14.1)	20 (18.5)	0.513
Anemia, n (%)	8 (57.1)	173 (95.1) [+]	132 (82.5)	119 (79.9)	76 (70.4)	**<0.001**
AST increase, n (%)	8 (57.1)	128 (70.3)	133 (83.1)	131 (87.9) [+]	91 (84.3)	**<0.001**
ALT increase, n (%)	3 (21.4)	69 (37.9) [+]	60 (37.5) [+]	37 (24.8)	22 (20.4)	**0.003**
LDH increase, n (%)	13 (92.9)	147 (80.8)	133 (83.1)	124 (83.2)	97 (89.9)	0.281
CRP increase *, n (%)	1/10 (10.0)	25/140 (17.9)	55/133 (41.4)	56/136 (41.2)	45/90 (50.0) [+]	**<0.001**
IL-6 increase [×], n (%)	1/1 (100)	18/18 (100)	21/21 (100)	30/32 (93.8)	18/19 (94.7)	0.656

WBC—white blood cells, ALT—alanine aminotransferase, AST—aspartate aminotransferase; LDH—lactate dehydrogenase; CRP—C-reactive protein; IL-6—interleukin 6; * Data available for 509 patients; [×] Data available for 91 patients; [+] Age group with statistical significance; In bold, data with statistical significance by comparing characteristics for all groups by $\chi^2(4)$.

The infants in the 1-3 months group presented earliest to the hospital (1 day (IQR: 0, 1 days)), and those in the 10–12 months group presented latest (1 day, (IQR: 1, 2.75 days)), $H(4) = 17.323$, $p = 0.002$, Figure 2. Also, the length of hospitalization was the highest in the 1–3 months group (4 days, (IQR: 3, 6 days)), $H(4) = 13.674$, $p = 0.008$, Figure 3.

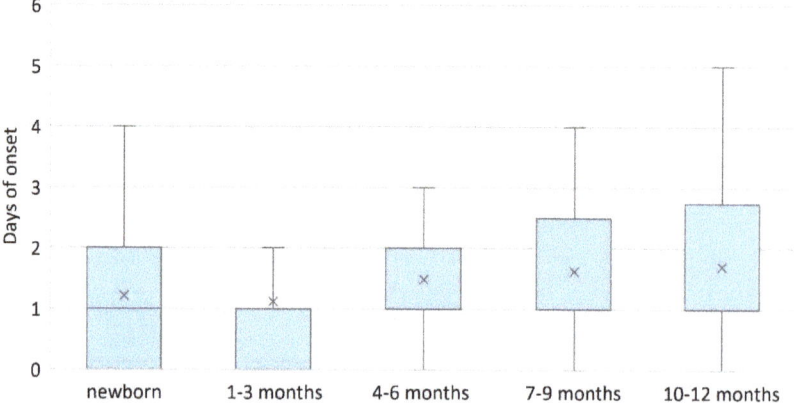

Figure 2. Number of days of onset of symptoms according to age group. Infants between 1–3 months presented to the hospital earliest after the onset of symptoms. In contrast, infants between 9–12 months presented the latest. Box and whiskers plot represent the 25th and 75th percentiles (box), the median (×) and the range (whiskers).

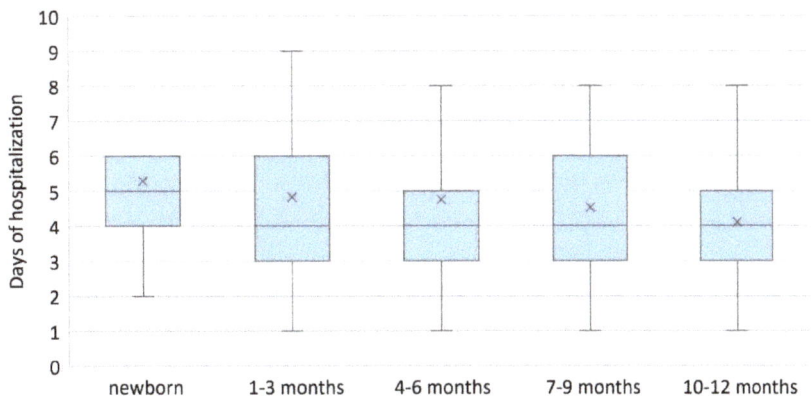

Figure 3. Number of days of hospitalization according to age group. The length of hospitalization was longer in infants between 1 and 3 months. Box and whiskers plot represent the 25th and 75th percentiles (box), the median (×) and the range (whiskers).

3.3. Analysis of Data by Type of Symptoms

The analysis of data by type of symptoms is presented in Table 4. The presence of combined respiratory and digestive symptoms was more common among males ($p = 0.028$, $\chi^2 = 4.82$, OR = 1.5, 95%CI: 1.1–2.0). In contrast, females were more likely to have digestive symptoms only ($p = 0.028$, $\chi^2 = 4.82$, OR = 1.5, 95%CI: 1.1–2.0). For infants in the 7–9 months age group, it was 1.9-fold more common ($p = 0.001$, $\chi^2 = 10.72$, OR = 1.9, 95%CI: 1.3–2.7) to have both respiratory and digestive manifestations during the COVID-19 episode as compared to the other age groups. ALT was significantly higher, 1.9-fold, among infants who experienced only digestive manifestations ($p = 0.011$, $\chi^2 = 6.44$, OR = 1.9, 95%CI: 1.1–3.0).

Table 4. Analysis of data according to the type of symptoms.

Characteristics	General Symptoms Only, N = 69	Respiratory Symptoms Only, N = 235	Respiratory and Digestive Symptoms, N = 231	Digestive Symptoms Only, N = 78	p-Value
Male	35 (50.7)	140 (59.6)	149 (64.5) [+]	37 (47.4)	0.027
Female	34 (49.3)	95 (40.4)	82 (35.5)	41 (52.6) [+]	
Newborn	3 (4.3)	6 (2.6)	2 (0.9)	3 (3.8)	
1–3 months	27 (39.1)	79 (33.6)	52 (22.5)	24 (29.7)	
4–6 months	15 (21.7)	61 (26.0)	61 (26.4)	23 (29.5)	0.049
7–9 months	12 (17.4)	48 (20.4)	73 (31.6) [+]	16 (20.5)	
10–12 months	12 (17.4)	41 (17.4)	43 (18.6)	12 (15.4)	
Preterm	2 (2.9)	24 (10.2)	28 (12.1)	3 (3.8)	0.056
At least one chronic condition	5 (7.2)	32 (13.6)	25 (10.8)	7 (9.0)	0.412
WBC increase	14 (20.3)	70 (29.8)	54 (23.4)	13 (16.7)	0.074
WBC decrease	5 (7.2)	17 (7.2)	16 (6.9)	7 (9.0)	0.947
Lymphocytes decrease	12 (17.4)	29 (12.3)	30 (13.0)	13 (16.7)	0.606
Anemia	60 (87.0)	187 (79.6)	193 (83.5)	68 (87.2)	0.295
AST increase	58 (84.1)	178 (75.7)	194 (84.0)	61 (78.2)	0.120
ALT increase	18 (26.1)	61 (26.0)	78 (34.2)	34 (42.3) [+]	**0.044**
LDH increase	54 (78.3)	198 (84.3)	198 (85.7)	64 (82.1)	0.494
CRP increase *	20/54 (37.0)	74/193 (38.3)	71/195 (36.4)	17/67 (25.4)	0.286
IL-6 increase [×]	7/7 (100)	42/44 (95.5)	32/33 (97.0)	7/7 (100)	0.873

WBC—white blood cells, ALT—alanine aminotransferase, AST—aspartate aminotransferase; LDH—lactate dehydrogenase; CRP—C-reactive protein; IL-6—interleukin 6; * Data available for 509 patients; [×] Data available for 91 patients; [+] Symptoms group with statistical significance; In bold, data with statistical significance by comparing characteristics for all groups by $\chi^2(3)$, and $\chi^2(12)$ for age groups.

The presence of general manifestations only (fever and/or loss of appetite) led to an earlier hospital presentation in infants with COVID-19, H(3) = 11.679, p = 0.009, Figure 4. Length of hospital stay was not influenced by the type of symptoms presented by infants, H(3) = 4.002, $p = 0.261$, Figure 5.

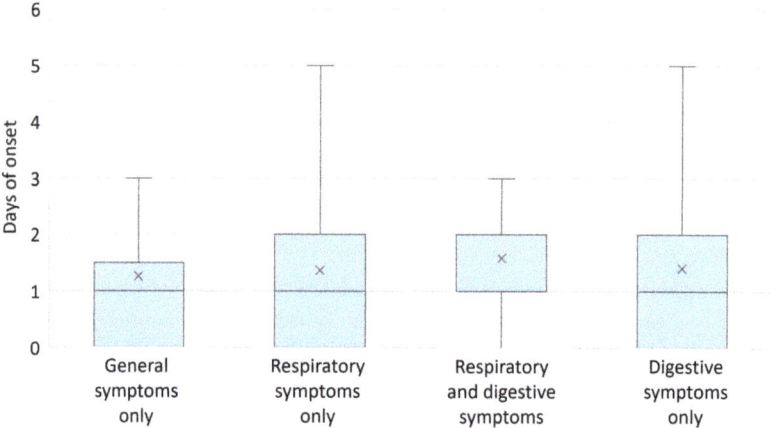

Figure 4. Number of days since onset of symptoms according to type of symptoms. The presence of general symptoms only (no digestive or respiratory symptoms) led to an earlier hospital presentation among infants. Box and whiskers plot represent the 25th and 75th percentiles (box), the median (×) and the range (whiskers).

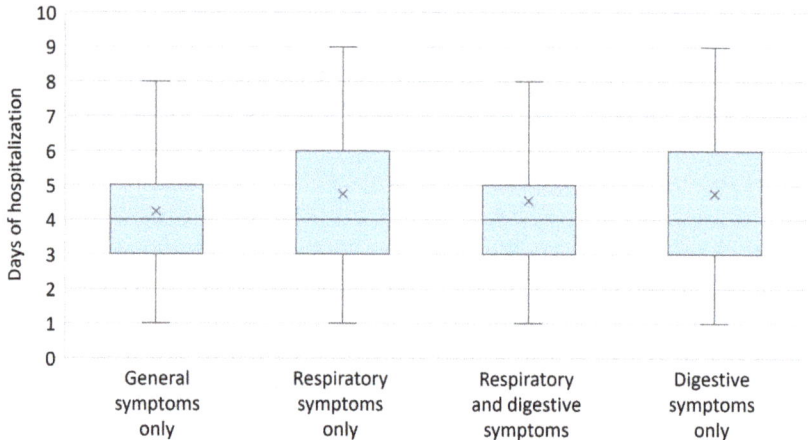

Figure 5. Number of days of hospitalization according to type of symptoms. The length of hospitalization was not influenced by the type of symptoms and was similar in all groups. Box and whiskers plot represent the 25th and 75th percentiles (box), the median (×) and the range (whiskers).

4. Discussion

In the present study we have conducted an extensive analysis of the demographic, clinical and laboratory characteristics of SARS-CoV-2 Omicron variant infection among infants hospitalized in a major infectious disease hospital in Romania. The number of children hospitalized for COVID-19 increased with the emergence of the omicron variant (65.0% of all children hospitalized in NIID since the onset of the pandemic), and infants represented an age group that required close medical monitoring during their COVID-19 episode. This trend is consistent with national [17] and international reports [13,19,20]; for example, in the USA, by early 2022 the proportion of children hospitalized with COVID-19 had increased four-fold from previous waves [21]. In a meta-analysis of pediatric cases of SARS-CoV-2 infection in 2020, Bhuiyan et al. showed that infants represented 53% of all pediatric COVID-19 hospitalizations, but most were asymptomatic [22]. During the

Delta variant circulation, epidemiological monitoring of SARS-CoV-2 infection showed an increase in pediatric cases and hospitalizations of infants, but these were associated with an increased incidence of COVID-19 in the adult population as well and were not due to increased Delta virulence in infants [23].

Fever (96.4%), cough (64.8%) and loss of appetite (63.3%) were the main symptoms of infants hospitalized with Omicron in our study. Overall, we showed that three out of four infants (76.0%) had a respiratory symptom and one out of two infants (49.6%) had a digestive symptom. Diarrhea was the main digestive manifestation in 37.5% of patients. In a report of 300 infants with COVID-19 from March to December 2020, fever and cough were also the two main symptoms present in different proportions, 77% and 40%, respectively [24]. In the same study, loss of appetite was reported in only 18% of infants, and digestive manifestations such as diarrhea (24%) and vomiting (10%) were also less frequent than in our study [24]. During the Delta variant, fever remained the main symptom in infants, but cough, rhinorrhea, diarrhea or vomiting were reported in lower percentages than in our study [13,23,25]. Both ours and most pediatric studies on COVID-19 highlighted the male sex as more likely to have symptomatic infection and hospitalization. In addition, we showed that female infants had a 1.7-fold higher risk of hospitalization when they had digestive manifestations only.

In the age group analysis, fever dominated in all age groups. Moreover, as significant clinical features we identified that loss of appetite, cough and digestive manifestations (of any type) were more common in those between 7–9 months of age, while vomiting was most common in infants between 10–12 months of age. We did not identify a similar analysis of COVID-19 manifestations by age group in existing field literature. Thus, this analysis is important in identifying clinical differences between infants, knowing that the rate of growth and development of infants is very rapid, and the therapeutic and management interventions of an infant are directly dependent on their age.

The clinical features of COVID-19 in children are similar to other viral infections, but their dominance varies widely by pediatric age group. Many symptoms are subjective and depend on children's ability to describe them. In many case reports fever was the most common symptom at presentation, followed by cough, rhinorrhea and sore throat for the entire pediatric population up to 18 years of age [26–30]. Additionally, Zhou et al. showed that nasal congestion/rhinorrhea, sore throat, abdominal pain, and digestive manifestations were commonly seen but did not have a strong association with COVID-19 in children [31]. This is of interest, but the analysis was performed on a heterogeneous age group of 0–18 years, therefore we believe that narrow age group analyses are essential for a comprehensive characterization of SARS-CoV-2 infection in children. Infants are a special group that cannot express certain symptoms, therefore our study focused only on the analysis of symptoms that could be quantified by the parent/physician.

Blood counts did not change significantly, but the increase in WBCs (24.6%) and decrease in lymphocytes (13.7%) were seen in higher proportions than in other studies with non-Omicron variants [32,33]. A high number of infants had anemia, a mild form (82.9%), especially in the 1–3 months age group. This finding should be interpreted with caution, as it may not be due to SARS-CoV-2 infection alone, particularly given the fact that some infants experience physiological anemia in the first months of life. We identified high percentages of infants with mild increases in AST and LDH, compared with reports from other studies [32–34]. These data are of great interest because they show that in infants Omicron infection presents a systemic involvement, not being limited to the respiratory or digestive tract. ALT, as a sign of hepatic cytolysis, was elevated in fewer infants and was significantly associated with a younger age (1–3, and 4–6 months), and only with the presence of digestive symptoms. These findings highlights the need for monitoring liver enzymes in clinical practice in infants under 6 months of age presenting with digestive manifestations only. The presence of inflammatory syndrome was evident in most infants, but IL-6 elevations were significant in all age groups at higher values than for non-Omicron variants, as reported in the literature (177.7 vs. 120.36 ng/mL) [34].

Newborns and infants between 1–3 months of age presented more quickly to the hospital after the onset of symptoms, compared to other infants. In addition, only the presence of general signs (fever and/or loss of appetite) also determined earlier hospital presentation. These aspects can be explained by parental worries and fears related to the very young infant, and the uncertainty of a diagnosis, without other symptoms, only in the presence of fever. Moreover, it is well known that infants under 3 months of age with signs of acute illness are a pediatric emergency. It is therefore important for parents to keep in close contact with their pediatrician and/or general practitioner to identify early alarm signs.

The median length of hospital stay was 4 days, comparable to other published reports for the Omicron variant [24,33], and young infants (1–3 months) required longer monitoring compared with other infants.

Overall, in our analysis we have shown that Omicron in infants has a very diverse spectrum of clinical manifestations with predominantly respiratory, but also intricate respiratory–digestive manifestations. Thus, clinical diagnosis can be difficult to establish based on symptoms alone, and testing for SARS-CoV-2 should remain a standard practice in emergency departments for rapid and targeted epidemiological and therapeutic measures.

Our study has several limitations mainly represented by the retrospective nature of the data and the absence of long-term follow-up of infants included in the study. The large number of infants included in the analysis with SARS-CoV-2 infection, however, provides a comprehensive overview of the burden that the Omicron variant has had in this pediatric group. The first year of every child's life is very important in physical, mental, and cognitive development. In this first year of life there are many stages of development, the newborn (0–28 days) being totally different from the young infant (1–3 months), and the latter being totally different from older infants (9–12 months). Infectious diseases among infants represent a big challenge, both for diagnosis (the clinical features are often atypical and vary according to the age groups mentioned above) and for treatment (each age group comes with certain treatment restrictions). If we analyze RSV or influenza viruses infection, we can see that infants are a group at risk of hospitalization and unfavorable outcomes. Therefore, we decided to perform an extensive analysis of infants hospitalized with Omicron. The Omicron variant is currently the dominant variant of SARS-CoV-2, and at the same time the variant that has caused the highest rates of morbidity and hospitalization among the pediatric population. We included a large number of infants in the study and performed an analysis of clinical and laboratory data. In addition, we conducted an analysis by age subgroups precisely to highlight the variability of these characteristics among infants. So far there are several reports on SARS-CoV-2 infection, including Omicron, among children, but none of them focus specifically on infants and age subgroups.

5. Conclusions

Infants are a pediatric group with very heterogeneous manifestations during SARS-CoV-2 infection, and these may be different even among them depending on age group. Age under 3 months was associated with earlier presentation to hospital and longer duration of hospitalization, and hepatic cytolysis was more common in infants with digestive manifestations only. Continued monitoring of COVID-19 among infants is highly necessary, given the evolving nature of SARS-CoV-2, in order to take accurate and rapid therapeutic and epidemiological measures, and to adapt to clinical changes driven by viral variant change.

Author Contributions: A.C.D., V.D.M., O.S., A.B., A.S.-C. (Anca Streinu-Cercel), R.G.S., A.M., D.G., K.I.H., D.Ș.H., D.P., A.S.-C. (Adrian Streinu-Cercel) and D.A.P. contributed equally to this article by participating in conceptualization, methodology, validation, formal analysis, data curation, writing—original draft preparation, writing-review and editing, supervision. All authors have read and agreed to the published version of the manuscript.

Funding: This research received no external funding.

Institutional Review Board Statement: The study was conducted in accordance with the Declaration of Helsinki and approved by the Institutional Review Board of National Institute for Infectious Diseases "Prof. Dr. Matei Balș", number C13797/09.12.2022.

Informed Consent Statement: Not applicable.

Data Availability Statement: The datasets generated and analysed during the current study are available from the corresponding author upon reasonable request.

Acknowledgments: Publication of this paper was supported by the University of Medicine and Pharmacy Carol Davila, through the institutional program Publish not Perish.

Conflicts of Interest: The authors declare no conflict of interest.

References

1. Stringer, M.D. Anatomy of the Infant and Child. *J. Pediatr. Surg. Gen. Princ. Newborn Surg.* **2020**, 83–101.
2. Phillips, B. Neonates are not little children. *Arch. Dis. Child.* **2019**, *104*, 1013. [CrossRef]
3. Miron, V.D.; Banica, L.; Sandulescu, O.; Paraschiv, S.; Surleac, M.; Florea, D.; Vlaicu, O.; Milu, P.; Streinu-Cercel, A.; Bilașco, A.; et al. Clinical and molecular epidemiology of influenza viruses from Romanian patients hospitalized during the 2019/20 season. *PLoS ONE* **2021**, *16*, e0258798. [CrossRef] [PubMed]
4. Hall, C.B.; Weinberg, G.A.; Blumkin, A.K.; Edwards, K.M.; Staat, M.A.; Schultz, A.F.; Iwane, M.K. Respiratory syncytial virus-associated hospitalizations among children less than 24 months of age. *Pediatrics* **2013**, *132*, e341–e348. [CrossRef]
5. McLaughlin, J.M.; Khan, F.; Schmitt, H.-J.; Agosti, Y.; Jodar, L.; Simões, E.A.F.; Swerdlow, D.L. Respiratory Syncytial Virus–Associated Hospitalization Rates among US Infants: A Systematic Review and Meta-Analysis. *J. Infect. Dis.* **2020**, *225*, 1100–1111. [CrossRef] [PubMed]
6. Săndulescu, O. COVID-19 and cold season preparedness. *Germs* **2020**, *10*, 149. [CrossRef] [PubMed]
7. Cruz, A.T.; Zeichner, S.L. COVID-19 in Children: Initial Characterization of the Pediatric Disease. *Pediatrics* **2020**, *145*, e20200834. [CrossRef]
8. Swann, O.V.; Pollock, L.; Holden, K.A.; Munro, A.P.S.; Bennett, A.; Williams, T.C.; Turtle, L.; Fairfield, C.J.; Drake, T.M.; Faust, S.N.; et al. Comparison of UK paediatric SARS-CoV-2 admissions across the first and second pandemic waves. *Pediatr Res.* **2022**, 1–10. [CrossRef]
9. Nijman, R.G. The impact of the COVID-19 pandemic on child health. *J. Lab. Med.* **2021**, *45*, 249–258. [CrossRef]
10. Perra, N. Non-pharmaceutical interventions during the COVID-19 pandemic: A review. *Phys. Rep.* **2021**, *913*, 1–52. [CrossRef]
11. Miron, V.D. COVID-19 in the pediatric population and parental perceptions. *Germs* **2020**, *10*, 294. [CrossRef] [PubMed]
12. Taylor, L. COVID-19: Omicron drives weekly record high in global infections. *BMJ* **2022**, *376*, o66. [CrossRef] [PubMed]
13. Marks, K.J.; Whitaker, M.; Agathis, N.T.; Anglin, O.; Milucky, J.; Patel, K.; Pham, H.; Kirley, P.D.; Kawasaki, B.; Meek, J.; et al. Hospitalization of Infants and Children Aged 0-4 Years with Laboratory-Confirmed COVID-19—COVID-NET, 14 States, March 2020-February 2022. *MMWR Morb. Mortal. Wkly. Rep.* **2022**, *71*, 429–436. [CrossRef]
14. Vladescu, C.; Ciutan, M.; Rafila, A. In-hospital admissions and deaths in the context of the COVID-19 pandemic, in Romania. *Germs* **2022**, *12*, 169–179. [CrossRef]
15. Streinu-Cercel, A.; Apostolescu, C.; Săndulescu, O.; Oțelea, D.; Streinu-Cercel, A.; Vlaicu, O.; Paraschiv, S.; Benea, O.E.; Bacruban, R.; Nițescu, M.; et al. SARS-CoV-2 in Romania—Analysis of the first confirmed case and evolution of the pandemic in Romania in the first three months. *Germs* **2020**, *10*, 132–134. [CrossRef] [PubMed]
16. Streinu-Cercel, A.; Sandulescu, O.; Miron, V.D.; Paraschiv, S.; Casangiu, C.; Hohan, R.; Bănică, L.; Surleac, M.; Streinu-Cercel, A. Undetected Omicron Transmission in Romania-Report of the First Detected Case of Locally Acquired Omicron Infection and Complete Epidemiological Investigation. *Diagnostics* **2022**, *12*, 348. [CrossRef] [PubMed]
17. Centrul Național de Supraveghere și Control al Bolilor Transmisibile. COVID-19 Raport săptămânal de Supraveghere—Date Raportate până la Data de 11 Decembrie 2022. Available online: https://www.cnscbt.ro/index.php/analiza-cazuri-confirmate-covid19/3370-raport-saptamanal-episaptamana49-2022 (accessed on 17 December 2022).
18. Maniu, I.; Maniu, G.; Totan, M. Clinical and Laboratory Characteristics of Pediatric COVID-19 Population—A Bibliometric Analysis. *J. Clin. Med.* **2022**, *11*, 5987. [CrossRef]
19. Cloete, J.; Kruger, A.; Masha, M.; du Plessis, N.M.; Mawela, D.; Tshukudu, M.; Manyane, T.; Komane, L.; Venter, M.; Jassat, W.; et al. Paediatric hospitalisations due to COVID-19 during the first SARS-CoV-2 omicron (B.1.1.529) variant wave in South Africa: A multicentre observational study. *Lancet Child Adolesc. Health* **2022**, *6*, 294–302. [CrossRef]
20. Torjesen, I. COVID-19: Omicron variant is linked to steep rise in hospital admissions of very young children. *BMJ* **2022**, *376*, o110. [CrossRef] [PubMed]
21. Kozlov, M. Does Omicron hit kids harder? *Nature* **2022**. [CrossRef]
22. Bhuiyan, M.U.; Stiboy, E.; Hassan, M.Z.; Chan, M.; Islam, M.S.; Haider, N.; Jaffe, A.; Homaira, N. Epidemiology of COVID-19 infection in young children under five years: A systematic review and meta-analysis. *Vaccine* **2021**, *39*, 667–677. [CrossRef] [PubMed]

23. Khemiri, H.; Ayouni, K.; Triki, H.; Haddad-Boubaker, S. SARS-CoV-2 infection in pediatric population before and during the Delta (B.1.617.2) and Omicron (B.1.1.529) variants era. *Virol. J.* **2022**, *19*, 144. [CrossRef] [PubMed]
24. Sobolewska-Pilarczyk, M.; Pokorska-Śpiewak, M.; Stachowiak, A.; Marczyńska, M.; Talarek, E.; Ołdakowska, A.; Kucharek, I.; Sybilski, A.; Mania, A.; Figlerowicz, M.; et al. COVID-19 infections in infants. *Sci. Rep.* **2022**, *12*, 7765. [CrossRef] [PubMed]
25. Ryu, B.-H.M.; Hong, S.I.M.; Lim, S.J.M.; Cho, Y.; Hong, K.-W.M.; Bae, I.-G.M.; Cho, O.-H.M. Features of COVID-19 among Children and Adolescents without Risk Factors before and after the Delta Variant Outbreak in South Korea. *Pediatr. Infect. Dis. J.* **2022**, *41*, e34–e35. [CrossRef]
26. Nikolopoulou, G.B.; Maltezou, H.C. COVID-19 in Children: Where do we Stand? *Arch. Med. Res.* **2022**, *53*, 1–8. [CrossRef]
27. Götzinger, F.; Santiago-García, B.; Noguera-Julián, A.; Lanaspa, M.; Lancella, L.; Carducci, F.; Gabrovska, N.; Velizarova, S.; Prunk, P.; Osterman, V.; et al. COVID-19 in children and adolescents in Europe: A multinational, multicentre cohort study. *Lancet Child. Adolesc. Health* **2020**, *4*, 653–661. [CrossRef]
28. King, J.A.; Whitten, T.A.; Bakal, J.A.; McAlister, F.A. Symptoms associated with a positive result for a swab for SARS-CoV-2 infection among children in Alberta. *CMAJ* **2021**, *193*, E1–E9. [CrossRef]
29. Zachariah, P.; Johnson, C.L.; Halabi, K.C.; Ahn, D.; Sen, A.I.; Fischer, A.; Banker, S.L.; Giordano, M.; Manice, C.S.; Diamond, R.; et al. Epidemiology, Clinical Features, and Disease Severity in Patients With Coronavirus Disease 2019 (COVID-19) in a Children's Hospital in New York City, New York. *JAMA Pediatr.* **2020**, *174*, e202430. [CrossRef]
30. Fleitas, P.E.; Paz, J.A.; Simoy, M.I.; Vargas, C.; Cimino, R.O.; Krolewiecki, A.J.; Aparicio, J.P. Clinical diagnosis of COVID-19. A multivariate logistic regression analysis of symptoms of COVID-19 at presentation. *Germs* **2021**, *11*, 221–237. [CrossRef] [PubMed]
31. Zhou, G.Y.; Penwill, N.Y.; Cheng, G.; Singh, P.; Cheung, A.; Shin, M.; Nguyen, M.; Mittal, S.; Burrough, W.; Spad, M.-A.; et al. Utility of illness symptoms for predicting COVID-19 infections in children. *BMC Pediatr.* **2022**, *22*, 655. [CrossRef]
32. Qi, K.; Zeng, W.; Ye, M.; Zheng, L.; Song, C.; Hu, S.; Duan, C.; Wei, Y.; Peng, J.; Zhang, W.; et al. Clinical, laboratory, and imaging features of pediatric COVID-19: A systematic review and meta-analysis. *Medicine* **2021**, *100*, e25230. [CrossRef] [PubMed]
33. Dona, D.; Montagnani, C.; Di Chiara, C.; Venturini, E.; Galli, L.; Lo Vecchio, A.; Denina, M.; Olivini, N.; Bruzzese, E.; Campana, A.; et al. COVID-19 in Infants Less than 3 Months: Severe or Not Severe Disease? *Viruses* **2022**, *14*, 2256. [CrossRef] [PubMed]
34. Lazova, S.; Alexandrova, T.; Gorelyova-Stefanova, N.; Atanasov, K.; Tzotcheva, I.; Velikova, T. Liver Involvement in Children with COVID-19 and Multisystem Inflammatory Syndrome: A Single-Center Bulgarian Observational Study. *Microorganisms* **2021**, *9*, 1958. [CrossRef] [PubMed]

Disclaimer/Publisher's Note: The statements, opinions and data contained in all publications are solely those of the individual author(s) and contributor(s) and not of MDPI and/or the editor(s). MDPI and/or the editor(s) disclaim responsibility for any injury to people or property resulting from any ideas, methods, instructions or products referred to in the content.

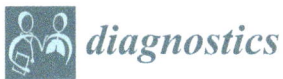

Review

Association between Childhood Onset Inflammatory Bowel Disease and Psychiatric Comorbidities in Adulthood

Andreea Sălcudean [1], Andreea Georgiana Nan [2,*], Cristina Raluca Bodo [3], Marius Cătălin Cosma [4], Elena Gabriela Strete [5,*] and Maria Melania Lica [1]

1. Department M2, Discipline of Bioethics, Social & Human Sciences, University of Medicine and Pharmacy, Sciences and Technology George Emil Palade of Targu Mures, 540142 Targu Mures, Romania
2. First Department of Psychiatry, Clinical County Hospital of Targu Mures, 540142 Targu Mures, Romania
3. Second Department of Psychiatry, Clinical County Hospital of Targu Mures, 540142 Targu Mures, Romania
4. Pediatric Cardiology Department, Institute of Cardiovascular Diseases and Cardiac Transplantation of Targu Mures, 540136 Targu Mures, Romania
5. Department M4, Discipline of Psychiatry, University of Medicine and Pharmacy, Sciences and Technology George Emil Palade of Targu Mures, 540142 Targu Mures, Romania
* Correspondence: nandree96@yahoo.com (A.G.N.); gabrielabuicu@yahoo.com (E.G.S)

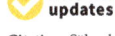

Citation: Sălcudean, A.; Nan, A.G.; Bodo, C.R.; Cosma, M.C.; Strete, E.G.; Lica, M.M. Association between Childhood Onset Inflammatory Bowel Disease and Psychiatric Comorbidities in Adulthood. *Diagnostics* 2023, *13*, 1868. https://doi.org/10.3390/diagnostics13111868

Academic Editor: Cristina Oana Marginean

Received: 14 December 2022
Revised: 17 May 2023
Accepted: 24 May 2023
Published: 26 May 2023

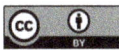

Copyright: © 2023 by the authors. Licensee MDPI, Basel, Switzerland. This article is an open access article distributed under the terms and conditions of the Creative Commons Attribution (CC BY) license (https://creativecommons.org/licenses/by/4.0/).

Abstract: Inflammatory bowel disease (IBD), which includes Crohn's disease, ulcerative colitis, and unspecified inflammatory bowel disease, is a chronic, unpredictable and immune-mediated condition of the gastrointestinal tract. In pediatric populations, the diagnosis of a chronic and debilitating pathology significantly reduces quality of life. Children diagnosed with IBD may cope with physical symptoms such as abdominal pain or fatigue, but mental and emotional well-being are also important for preventing and reducing the risk of developing psychiatric conditions. Short stature, growth delay and delayed puberty can contribute to poor body image and low self-esteem. Furthermore, treatment per se can alter psycho-social functioning due to the side effects of medication and surgical procedures such as colostomy. It is essential to acknowledge and treat early signs and symptoms of psychiatric distress in order to prevent the development of serious psychiatric disorders in adult life. The literature underlines the importance of incorporating psychological and mental health services as part of the management of inflammatory bowel disease. Diagnosing mental health problems in pediatric patients with IBD can improve their adherence to treatment and pathology course and, consequently, reduce long-term morbidity and mortality.

Keywords: pediatric inflammatory bowel disease; psychiatric comorbidities; gut–brain axis

1. Introduction

Inflammatory bowel disease (IBD) is a group of chronic inflammatory conditions of the gastrointestinal system with a remitting–relapsing evolutive character. Crohn's disease (CD), ulcerative colitis (UC) and unspecified IBD are subtypes described in the literature [1]. Patients frequently experience symptoms such as abdominal pain, diarrhea, weight loss, and delayed growth or fatigue [2,3]. The presenting symptoms of pediatric IBD are summarized in Table 1.

Table 1. Frequent presenting symptoms in pediatric IBD [4].

General	Gastrointestinal Tract
Weight loss	Abdominal pain
Fever	Diarrhea
Anorexia	Rectal bleeding
Delayed growth	Nausea/vomiting
Lethargy/fatigue	Constipation
	Perianal disease (CD)
	Mouth ulcers

Inflammatory bowel disease is often associated with extraintestinal manifestations (EIM) and complications (EIC) [5]. Reportedly, EIM occur in approximately 5–50% of patients [5]. The organs most commonly affected are joints, skin, ocular system and hepatobiliary tract, although nearly every system may be involved [6]. Table 2 summarizes the extraintestinal manifestations and complications (EIM and EIC) of IBD.

Table 2. Extraintestinal manifestations (EIM) and complications (EIC) of IBD.

System	Manifestation/Complication
Generalized	Fever [7], weight loss [8], fatigue [7,9], nausea/vomiting/appetite changing [7]
Ocular	Uveitis/episcleritis/iritis/conjunctivitis [6,10]
Oral	Cheilitis/stomatitis/oral ulcerations [6,11]
Pulmonary	Pulmonary vasculitis/fibrosing alveolitis [12,13]
Vascular	Vasculitis/thrombosis [14,15]
Hepatobiliary	Primary sclerosing cholangitis/fatty liver disease/granulomatous hepatitis/autoimmune liver disease/cholestasis/gallstone formation [6,16]
Pancreatic	Pancreatitis (acute, chronic, autoimmune) [17]
Renal/Urinary	Nephrolithiasis [18]/tubulointerstitial nephritis [19]/glomerulonephritis [20]/amyloidosis [21]
Hematologic	Iron deficiency/chronic anemia/thrombocytosis/vitamin B12 deficiency/autoimmune hemolytic anemia [6,22]
Endocrine	Decreased growth velocity/delayed sexual maturation [23,24]
Integumentary	Erythema nodosum/pyoderma gangrenosum/perianal disease/CD [6,25]
Musculoskeletal Neuropsychiatric	Osteopenia and osteoporosis/arthritis/arthralgias/ankylosing spondylitis/sacroiliitis [23,26] Venous and arterial thrombotic and thromboembolic events/demyelinating diseases/peripheral neuropathies/white matter lesion/psychiatric disorders [27]

The burden of living with various and multisystemic symptoms, and the need for implementing treatment has piqued considerable interest in the mental health management of patients with IBD [28].

The incidence of inflammatory bowel disease (IBD) appears to be more common in northern countries as well as in industrialized areas [29], and studies have shown that the risk for serious mental illness is generally higher in cities compared to rural areas [30]. Approximately 25% of patients diagnosed with IBD are younger than 18 years old. Although pediatric incidence is currently lower than that in adults, it continues to increase, and there is evidence that the illness can be chronic and has a very aggressive evolution in this particular group of patients [1,31,32].

2. Psychological Implications in Inflammatory Bowel Disease

2.1. Inflammatory Bowel Disease and Its Psychological Implications in Childhood and Young Adulthood

The pediatric manifestation of inflammatory bowel disease cannot be separated from its psychosocial context. Children and adolescents frequently feel embarrassed and ashamed by fecal incontinence and frequent bathroom visits and often experience social anxiety due to school absences, nutritional strategies such as exclusion diets and distorted body image perception related to short stature or other physical effects of gastrointestinal diseases [33,34]. Additional factors such as age, social support network, primarily represented by the family and coping mechanisms to stress may also influence how adolescents manage and react to their somatic burden [35]. Fatigue is a common symptom reported by children affected by IBD [36] and it refers to a subjectively overwhelming sense of tiredness associated with lack of energy and exhaustion that decreases the capacity for physical and mental activity, decreasing quality of life in similar ways as rheumatologic disease and cancer [37,38]. Fatigue, exhaustion, diminished physical activity and trouble sleeping are more common in children and adolescents with IBD than in their healthy counterparts. Fatigue is likely to be a multifactorial phenomenon and includes biological factors (such as disease activity), psycho-behavioral factors (such as anxiety, depression and family support) disorder [39]. The above-described factors can contribute to significant psychological and functional factors (such as decreased functional capacity) [37,38]. Moreover, fatigue represents a core symptom in major depressive burden that influences disease outcomes and patient's psychological development [40].

Moreover, inflammatory bowel disease is increasingly being recognized as a complex multifactorial and multisystemic disorder [6]. Alarmingly high rates of depression within the adolescent IBD population have been observed in the largest population-based study, which aimed to evaluate the burden of psychiatric disorders in children and young adults with IBD in USA, comprising a total of 11,316,450 patients aged between 5 and 24 years, including 58.020 patients with a diagnosis of IBD. The prevalence of psychiatric disorders was found to be 21.6% among IBD, and mainly comprised depression and anxiety disorders. The study's results also indicate that IBD is five times more likely to be associated with psychiatric disorders than controls ($p < 0.001$) [41]. Furthermore, studies on pediatric and adult populations show a significant relationship between depression and anxiety with IBD disease activity and evolution [42–44]. In 2018, Van den Brink et al. conducted a randomized controlled trial, concluding that active disease was a significant risk factor for depressive symptoms (OR 4.6, $p < 0.001$). Other significant risk factors for anxiety and/or depression included female gender (OR 1.7), active disease (OR 1.9), and a shorter disease duration (OR 1.4) (all $p < 0.025$) [43]. Furthermore, a meta-analytic review comprising a total of 1167 young people with IBD (M age = 14.33, 50% female) concluded that they had higher rates of depressive disorders and internalizing disorders than young people with other chronic conditions [45]. Extensive research has explored the idea that mental health comorbidities are only a direct result of the global burden of living with a chronic disease or complex mechanism involved in gut–brain interactions. Recent studies indicate that the relationship between IBD and mental illness can be bidirectional, evoking the systemic inflammation that damages the body's immune and nervous systems and is a possible mechanism for both IBD and mental illness, as well as complex gut–brain interactions [46–49]. Moreover, another management impairment is that patients with IBD and co-morbid depression and/or anxiety may be less likely to adhere to medical care procedures and therapeutic schemes, resulting in unnecessary escalation in therapy and complications [50–52]. The importance of family support and the coordination of the medical treatment are factors of pediatric IBD management that can impact psychological outcomes for children affected by the disease [53]. Younger and middle-aged adolescents benefitted from family support in the context of IBD care management according to Feldman et al.'s (2020) analysis conducted on 76 young IBD patients aged between 11 and 18 [51]. Dealing with a chronic illness and a lifelong management can be overwhelming for children [54]. As described in other chronic disease such as diabetes, poor treatment adherence can cause a high prevalence of psychiatric comorbidities [55]. Lifestyle changes sometimes occur unexpectedly due to disease exacerbation, impacting the lives of both patient and parents, resulting in disruptions to family life. According to a study comprising 87 patients and their parents, a worse disease course was directly associated with the increased distress of parents and indirectly with the lower health-related quality of life (HRQOL) of pediatric patients with IBD, emphasizing that parental distress should be considered in the management of pediatric IBD to improve HRQOL of children [56,57].

Anxiety symptoms may also be related to arising concerns about different lifestyles compared to other children and related to the unknown progression of the illness (relapse or complications of disease requiring surgical procedures or colostomy that can impact one's body-image perception and self-esteem) [34,58]. Social impairments may be caused by educational deficiencies due to school absences [59,60], as well as low self-esteem due to delayed development or a lack of satisfaction with one's physical appearance [61]. It is also important to acknowledge and prevent any educational impairments of children with IBD in order to prevent any delays in educational acquisitions. The financial burden of a chronic illness as well as familial sacrifices, repeated hospitalizations, and family issues are problems that a child with IBD may face [62].

Assessing the adaptation of pediatric patients to disease is an important component of long-term management of children with IBD. Existing models of assessment tools focus on evaluating a patient's social support network, coping mechanisms and skills, daily activities, and body image perception [56,57].

2.2. Critic Period: Transition from Pediatric to Adult Inflammatory Bowel Disease Care

While the pediatric management of chronic illnesses includes the benefit provided by the patients' family support, the transition from children to adult life mandates the development of abilities of self-management and self-care. This transition can be facilitated by gradually increasing the patient's responsibility and participation in their care plan. Older adolescents should be taught to recognize the warning signs of an emergency and be able to appropriately describe the manifestations and seek immediate treatment, as well as being familiar with administered medication. It is well documented that any discontinuity in patients with IBD care during the transition from a pediatric to adult patient can result in severe adverse outcomes, unfavorable evolution and higher medical costs [53]. Because most patients with pediatric-onset inflammatory bowel disease progress into adulthood, the chances of disease's long- and short-term complications increase, and burdens of IBD are also increased by psychosocial factors including poor coping ability and other obstacles regarding medical management, as described above. The economic burden and financial impact of a chronic illness must be taken into account in patients experiencing chronic and debilitating symptoms, especially regarding the current evidence for an impaired quality of working life in IBD patients [63]. Regarding work impairments, concentration problems (72%), low working pace (78%) and delayed work productivity (50%) were the most prevalent IBD-related work difficulties described in a questionnaire-based study including 202 IBD patients [64].

It is ideal for the transition from pediatric to adult care to happen when young adults already have a basic understanding of IBD, as well as its therapeutic schemes, prognosis and evolution in both the presence and absence of specific treatments [65,66]. Somatic disease course is beneficial for young adults who have stable mental health, sufficient self-efficacy and are willing to communicate regarding self-care behaviors, developing a beneficial patient–healthcare worker relationship [66,67]. On the other hand, it is widely known that self-management skills may be undermined by the onset of mental illnesses or other psychosocial problems; therefore, it is critical to efficiently diagnose and treat any mental-health-related disturbances.

Findings from a pilot study conducted in the United States of America aimed to understand disease transitions from a broader psychosocial perspective. The results show that transition barriers include disease uncertainty and lack of control, psychological distress, and disruptions to daily life [33]. Facilitators such as mental health support, adequate social support and adequate communication ease the transition process for young patients. Furthermore, the study highlights certain particular and adaptable interventions for facilitating the transition to adulthood IBD care and management, as presented in Table 3 [33,68–70].

Table 3. Interventions considered to facilitate IBD care transition [33].

Adaptable Intervention	Elements/Examples
Develop a disease narrative	What is IBD and what symptoms are most prominent for you day-to-day? What are some of the challenges that you might experience related to having IBD (e.g., managing medications, medical procedures, dietary or activity restrictions)? In what ways have you grown through the challenges of living with IBD?
Practice gratitude	Write a gratitude letter Keep a gratitude journal
Pay it forward	Engagement with the IBD community Voluntary Mentorship
Set SMART Goals	Specific Measurable Achievable Relevant Time-sensitive goals
Master the gut–brain axis	Optimizing education about the complex interactions of the gut and brain axis Understanding relationship stress symptoms Useful questions: What do you notice about how your stress levels influence your IBD symptoms? Conversely, when you begin to experience the onset of IBD symptoms, how does that impact your mental state?

Although we present several interventions/facilitators, additional research is needed to evaluate the impact of incorporating these exercises into psychosocial programs and to discover further targeted interventions designed to facilitate the transition process.

Finally, these interventions can be introduced to patients at any age and in any order following the opinion of a healthcare professional regarding the most appropriate treatment for the patient and their particularities. However, if not previously initiated, the pediatric-to-adult transition may benefit from the inclusion of these interventions in care management.

The above-mentioned interventions are recommendations that can be implemented during the pediatric IBD care management or as part of transitioning process. The interventions are based on positive psychology and cognitive–behavioral principles, which may be associated with improved disease outcomes across the spectrum of digestive disorders [71].

These facilitating interventions can be introduced to patients at any age and include the following recommendations:

- Develop a disease narrative to develop ways to talk about IBD with those who are not familiar with the disease. Before transitioning to adult care, pediatric patients may benefit from establishing their own disease narrative. By discussing how the disease has affected the patient's life experiences in a positive way can encourage patients to adopt an optimistic point of view, be self-efficient, and advocate for themselves. This method of communication strengthens mechanisms of growth and learning abilities and was previously associated with happiness, gratefulness, as well as reduced stress and depressive symptoms [72].

- Practicing gratitude has the benefit of enhancing support and strengthening existing connections and social support networks. Examples of gratitude activities include writing letters (in which the patient expresses their gratitude to the persons that helped them during difficult times) and writing a gratitude journal (logging disease symptoms and subsequent emotions that can be easily accessed to help patients focus on the positive aspects of their lives) [33,73].
- Paying it forward means to engage in IBD community activities such as volunteering and mentorship for the newly diagnosed patients. These interventions can boost self-efficacy and are associated with increased satisfaction, well-being and happiness [74].
- Setting SMART goals is a means to divide up large and sometimes difficult goals into smaller and more achievable targets. Setting SMART goals for IBD management can allow adolescent patients and their caregivers to prioritize the goals of interest, focusing on optimizing their chances of successfully completing the tasks, consequently building efficacy that prepares patients to reach the disease management independency.

SMART is an acronym that highlights the key features of the goal:
- Specific: what, where, and when will we work toward on this goal?
- Measurable: how can we evaluate if we have achieved the goal or not?
- Achievable: is this goal within the realm of possibility?
- Relevant to larger goals: does this goal fit into my value system?
- Time-sensitive: at what point will we check in on progress to determine whether we have reached the goal? [75]
- Mastering the gut–brain axis means to optimize education about the complex interactions of the gut–brain axis that may help pediatric patients to better manage their disease. Helping patients differentiate between their symptoms can help reduce concerns for those who may feel that stress-induced symptoms are not important. It is therefore mandatory for doctors to identify certain concerning symptoms and establish multidisciplinary approaches with qualified mental health professionals (psychologists and psychiatrists) [33,76].

2.3. Anatomopathology and Reported Pathogenesis of Psychiatric Implications in Patients with Inflammatory Bowel Disease

The complexity of the gut–brain axis has sparked significant interest from researchers over the last twenty years [49,77,78]. The gut–brain axis is a complex bidirectional communication system driven by neural, hormonal, metabolic, immunological, and microbial signals [77,78]. Signaling events from the gut can modulate brain function, and recent evidence suggests that the gut–brain axis may play a pivotal role in linking gastrointestinal and neuropsychiatric pathologies [78,79]. In a review article, RK Masanetz et al. explored a series of cascade events along the gut–immune–brain axis, initiated by the evasion of chronic intestinal inflammation, that pass through the epithelial–vascular barrier in the gut and cause systemic inflammation [79]. Moreover, the malfunctioning of the gut–brain axis described in IBD patients includes structural and functional abnormalities of the enteric nervous system (ENS) and induced abnormal, innate, and adaptive immunological responses, affecting intestinal barrier integrity and leading to systemic fallout [80]. It has been postulated that neuroinflammation-induced depression in IBD involves peripheral inflammatory mediators originating from the inflammation in the gastrointestinal system, penetrating the blood–brain barrier and activating the resident macrophage-like microglial cells within the central nervous system [46,81,82].

It has been reported that neuroinflammation can induce the dysregulation of the hypothalamus–pituitary–adrenal (HPA) axis [83] and decrease serotonin levels [84], as well as altering the hippocampus [85], mechanisms involved in major depressive disorder (MDD) [81]. In a previous study, low serum serotonin levels were correlated with depressive symptoms [86] and in a small study, plasmatic serotonin level was used as a screening marker for anxiety and depression in patients with type 2 diabetes [87]. Further studies are essential for evaluating the use of serum serotonin as a predictor of depression.

Bonaz BL (2013) suggested a dysfunction of brain–gut interactions in the pathogenesis of IBD, evidenced by the dysfunctionality of the autonomic nervous system and abnormal functioning of the hypothalamic–pituitary–adrenal axis. Their study is supported by [77], which found similar results for the cholinergic anti-inflammatory pathway [88]. The harmful effect of stress, abnormal association of the prefrontal cortex–amygdala, and an abnormal microbiota–brain relationship were found in pro-inflammatory models [83,88].

In Neurogastroenterology and Motility, Agostini et al. (2013) evaluated patients with Crohn's disease for brain volumetric alterations, and the results indicate decreased gray matter volumes in the dorsolateral prefrontal cortex and anterior midcingulate cortex. Illness time evolution was negatively correlated with volumetric measures in the subgenual anterior cingulate cortex, posterior midcingulate cortex, ventral posterior cingulate, and parahippocampal cortex [89]. The anterior midcingulate cortex was responsible for feedback-mediated decision making [90]. The gray matter volume in the subgenual anterior cingulate cortex was found to be abnormally reduced in subjects with major depressive disorder and bipolar disorder [91,92]. The ventral posterior cingulate cortex plays a role in self-monitoring the personal relevance of somatosensory stimuli. It is also involved in spatial processing, actions in space, and some types of memory pathways [93] that may be interrupted by posterior cingulate cortex atrophy, as discovered in small studies of Crohn's disease [89,94]. Moreover, a systematic multi-database study comparing adult IBD patients versus healthy controls ($n = 687$) concluded that IBD patients had significant deficits in attention, executive function, and working memory compared with healthy controls, suggesting that cognitive impairment is a potential extraintestinal manifestation of IBD [95]. Another small comparative study on a pediatric population found that patients with IBD and cystic fibrosis performed more poorly than healthy controls in attention and memory tests [96].

Moreover, white matter alterations have also been observed in IBD patients compared to controls in a small number of studies on nervous system imaging in patients with IBD. The lesions were clinically asymptomatic and potentially associated with IBD, and whether these structural changes represent a unique extraintestinal manifestation of the disease remains unclear and further studies must be conducted [97]. In contrast, a study with a relatively small sample size did not find an increased rate of white matter lesions among patients with IBD when compared to healthy controls [98]. Conflicting data and small studies regarding white matter lesions mandate further studies.

Inflammatory bowel disease has been associated with a higher risk of cerebrovascular accidents [99] according to a study including 261,890 IBD patients compared to non-IBD patients (6.24% vs. 0.48%, $p < 0.0001$) [100]. The hypercoagulability [14] state present in IBD could be a mechanism by which the presence of IBD might lead to the development of cerebrovascular accidents.

2.4. Mental Disorders Associated with Inflammatory Bowel Disease

In patients with IBD, several studies have described an increased frequency of various mental disorders, ranging from mild depression to severe forms of schizophrenia and serious dementia, but the prevalence of mental disorders depends on the study, as described below.

Upon examining the literature, depression and anxiety disorders were the most studied mental health disorders, both in pediatric and adult IBD patients [41,101,102].

IBD patients often suffer from anxiety and depression that may influence the course of disease via the complexity of the gut–brain axis [101]. In a systematic review, Mickoka et al. (2016) demonstrated that the prevalence of anxiety and depression is higher in patients with IBD and even higher in the active phase of the disease [101]. A review and meta-analysis of 60.114 adult and pediatric IBD patients identified high prevalence of: mood disorders, 10%; anxiety disorders, 12%; substance misuse, 3%; psychotic disorders, 2%; behavioral disorders, 1%; personality disorders, 3%; developmental disorders, 1%; and behavioral and emotional disorders with onset usually during childhood, 1% [102].

Thavamani et al. conducted a retrospective case–control analysis, including 58,020 IBD pediatric patients, of which 12,540 were diagnosed with psychiatric disorders. Depression, anxiety and adjustment disorder contributed to about 95% of all psychiatric disorders. Among the screened psychiatric disorders, IBD patients had an increased risk of associated anxiety, depression, panic disorder, phobias and dysthymias [41]. The study results are presented in Table 4.

Table 4. Association between psychiatric disorders and inflammatory bowel disease in pediatric population and young adults (<24 years) (adapted following Thavamani et al.) [41].

Mental Health Disorder	Odds Ratio (OR)	Lower CI-Upper CI	p-Value
Bipolar disorder	3.5	3.3–3.73	<0.001
Depression	3.94	3.82–4.06	<0.001
Anxiety disorder	4.05	3.96–4.16	<0.001
Any mental health disorder	3.83	3.75–3.91	<0.001

Comparatively, Bernstain et al. conducted a retrospective matched-control study analyzing the incidence and prevalence of psychiatric disorders in an adult IBD cohort compared with a matched cohort without IBD [103]. The results are presented in Table 5.

Table 5. Association between psychiatric disorders and inflammatory bowel disease in young adult (18–24 years) and adult populations (>24 years) (adapted following [103]).

Mental Health Disorder	IRR Incidence Rate Ratio in IBD Patients	IRR in Match Cohort	p Value
Depression	1.58 (>)	1.0	$p < 0.05$
Anxiety disorder	1.39 (>)	1.0	$p < 0.05$
Bipolar disorder	1.82 (>)	1.0	$p < 0.05$
Schizophrenia	1.64 (>)	1.0	$p > 0.05$

Various researchers studied the risk factors of depression among patients with IBD and concluded that age, severe disease, flare ups, disability, unemployment, socioeconomic impairment [104] and coronavirus disease 2019 isolation due to extensive lockdown measures are factors responsible for developing depressive symptoms [105]. Various studies highlight the increased risk of suicide among IBD patients [106–108].

There is conflicting research data regarding the association between bipolar disorder and inflammatory bowel disease. A population-based, cross-sectional study from Taiwan demonstrated that patients with IBD were more likely to have bipolar disorder. Moreover, a national cohort study conducted in Denmark presented a higher risk of bipolar disorder only in patients with CD [109,110]. Thavamani et al. observed a high odds ratio (OR) of bipolar disorder in an IBD pediatric population [41]. In 2022, Wang et al. found a significant, positive association for genetically predicted bipolar disorder with the risk for IBD and ulcerative colitis (per log/odds ratio increase; odds ratios: 1.18 and 1.19, respectively) [111].

Regarding comorbid IBD–schizophrenia, studies show inconsistent results. While a population-based cohort study conducted in Taiwan (2020) demonstrated a significant association between schizophrenia and subsequent IBD development (1.14% vs. 0.25% in non-IBD population), other studies failed to demonstrate any association between somatic and mental illnesses [112,113]. In pediatric populations, rare and isolated cases of medication-induced psychosis are described in the literature [114,115]

Recent evidence suggests there is a possible association between IBD and eating disorders, although the exact mechanisms involved in its ethio-pathogenesis are not fully understood. This association may lead to worse prognosis [108,116,117].

Table 6 presents the association between childhood-onset inflammatory bowel disease and mental health disorders in adulthood as well as the specific adaptation hazard ratios as found by Butwicka et al. (2019) [108].

Table 6. Association between childhood-onset IBD and psychiatric comorbidities [108].

Psychiatric Pathology in Patients with Childhood-Onset Inflammatory Bowel Disease						
Psychiatric Pathology	Ulcerative Colitis		Crohn's Disease		IBD—Unclassified	
	HR (85% CI)	p Value	HR (85% CI)	p Value	HR (85% CI)	p Value
Psychotic disorders	0.9 (0.5–1.5)	0.58	1.3 (0.8–2.2)	0.27	0.8 (0.2–3.1)	0.7
Mood disorder	1.4 (1.3–1.7)	<0.001	1.6 (1.4–1.9)	<0.001	1.8 (1.3–2.4)	<0.001
Anxiety disorders	1.6 (1.4–1.8)	<0.001	2.2 (1.9–2.4)	<0.001	2.4 (1.9–3.0)	<0.001
Eating disorders	1.3 (0.9–1.8)	0.13	1.9 (1.4–2.6)	<0.001	2.4 (1.3–4.3)	0.005
Substance misuse	1.1 (0.9–1.3)	0.33	1.2 (0.9–1.4)	0.16	0.7 (0.4–1.1)	0.12
Personality disorders	1.4 (1.0–2.0)	0.03	1.2 (0.8–1.8)	0.44	2.0 (1.0–3.9)	0.04
Behavioral disorders	0.8 (0.3–1.9)	0.64	2.0 (1.0–3.9)	<0.05	1.4 (0.3–5.8)	0.62
ADHD	1.2 (1.0–1.5)	0.07	1.2 (0.9–1.5)	0.13	1.1 (0.6–1.7)	0.8
Autism spectrum disorders	1.5 (1.1–2.1)	0.01	1.2 (0.8–1.7)	0.42	1.6 (0.8–3.3)	0.19
Intellectual disability	1.1 (0.7–1.9)	0.62	0.9 (0.4–1.7)	0.68	2.7 (1.2–5.7)	0.01
All psychiatric disorders	1.4 (1.3–1.5)	<0.001	1.7 (1.6–1.9)	<0.001	1.8 (1.5–2.1)	<0.001
Suicide attempts	1.2 (0.9–1.6)	0.23	1.5 (1.1–2.0)	0.01	2.3 (1.4–3.8)	0.001

Abbreviations: HR—hazard ratio, IBD—inflammatory bowel disease.

Moreover, suicide represents a serious global public health burden. According to the WHO (World Health Organization), approximately 703,000 people per year die from suicide worldwide [118]. In 2019, suicide accounted for more than 1 out of 100 deaths, and 58% of suicides occurred before age 50. Mental disorders are the leading cause of disability worldwide, accounting for one in six cases of disability [119]. Patients diagnosed with severe mental health conditions die on average 10–20 years earlier than the general population. Sexual molesting and bullying are major causes of depression in children, and bullying should not be overlooked in pediatric IBD patients, especially in those who lack confidence in their physical appearance [119].

The most severe outcome in patients with depression is suicide, but the risk of suicide in patients with IBD is not entirely clear. A systematic review based on 28 studies concluded that patients with inflammatory bowel disease were associated with an increased risk of suicide attempts (relative risk= 1.39; 95% CI, 1.08–1.79) and deaths from suicide (relative risk= 1.25; 95% CI, 1.09–1.43) compared to controls. The review also concluded that Crohn's disease subtypes, female patients, childhood-onset IBD, young-adult IBD, and short-duration IBD characteristics are factors that carry a high risk of suicide [106]. Another case–control study regarding the Danish population highlights the necessity to correctly assess the risk of suicide among IBD patients. The results indicate increased rates of suicide among participants with CD (odds ratio = 1.6, 95%) and UC (OR = 1.9, 95%) [120]. Butwicka et al. observed an increased hazard ratio (HR = 1.2, respectively 1.5) in UC and childhood-onset CD [108].

Regarding these findings, healthcare providers should consider a multidisciplinary approach that includes medical and psychological factors. Psychological factors should always be considered via assessments of depressive symptomology and the co-occurrence of suicide risk, especially if patients with IBD present co-occurring factors, such as active disease phase or high pain levels, that increase the risk of suicide [59]. The identification and treatment of mental health conditions such as depression in IBD populations is essential for reducing the high number of patients at risk of suicide [121]. Childhood traumas must also be assessed, as certain traumatic events may increase suicide risk [122].

3. Conclusions

To our knowledge, childhood-onset inflammatory bowel disease has an impact on more than just the gastrointestinal tract; patients often have psychological comorbidities and mental health implications further in adult life. Although the pathogenetic mechanisms between inflammatory bowel disease and mental illnesses are not fully elucidated, genetic factors and the gut–brain interaction seem to contribute to the increased prevalence of mental disorders in patients with IBD, and further studies must be established in order to describe and elucidate the complex mechanisms. Childhood-onset inflammatory bowel disease tends to have a more severe evolutive course than IBD diagnosed in adulthood, and mental health burden adds to the overall low quality of life rates described in this particular group of patients. Psychiatric comorbidities are independent predictors of the severity of IBD symptoms, not only negatively impacting a patient's quality of life, but also increasing healthcare utilization and economic burden. The importance of family support and the coordination of the medical treatment is a particularity that can impact psychological outcomes for children affected by inflammatory bowel disease. Addressing mental health problems in pediatric patients with IBD can improve their medication adherence and somatic disease course, reducing overall morbidity and mortality. Specific measurable variables such as serum serotonin levels may become useful tools in assessing a patients' risk of developing psychiatric comorbidities such as depression, but further larger research studies are required.

Understanding the need to implement various transition mechanisms of psychological support from childhood to adulthood care in patients with IBD is important for both healthcare providers and insurance payers, as it has a direct impact on medical care and disease outcomes. It is ideal for the transition from child to adult care to happen when young adults already have a good general understanding of their disease. Social and educational impairments in pediatric patients require special attention regarding the management of inflammatory bowel disease patients because adaptation difficulties can underlie the development of serious mental health problems in adult life and decrease the global functionality.

Somatic disease courses may benefit patients who are stable in terms of their mental health and have sufficient self-efficacy and willingness to communicate regarding self-care behaviors.

The increased frequency of psychiatric comorbidities in childhood-onset inflammatory bowel disease, as described in the literature, especially mood and anxiety disorders, demonstrates that early interventions can prevent and attenuate the development of serious psychiatric pathologies; however, further studies and investigations are mandatory for developing the best approaches and multidisciplinary protocols to manage mental health implications in pediatric inflammatory bowel disease. We believe that further prospective follow-up studies on the prevalence of psychiatric disorders in childhood-onset IBD populations would be greatly valuable and of considerable interest to researchers.

Author Contributions: Conceptualization, A.S., E.G.S. and M.M.L.; methodology, A.S., E.G.S., A.G.N. and M.C.C.; validation, A.S. and E.G.S.; investigation, A.S., A.G.N., M.C.C. and C.R.B.; writing—original draft preparation, A.S. and A.G.N.; writing—review and editing, A.S., A.G.N., C.R.B., E.G.S., M.C.C. and M.M.L.; supervision, A.S. All authors have read and agreed to the published version of the manuscript.

Funding: This study was funded by George Emil Palade University of Medicine, Pharmacy, Sciences and Technology of Targu Mures, Research Grant Number 164/25/10.01.2023.

Institutional Review Board Statement: Not applicable.

Data Availability Statement: Not applicable.

Conflicts of Interest: The authors declare no conflict of interest.

Abbreviations

CD	Crohn's disease
CI	Confidence interval
EIM	Extraintestinal manifestations
EIC	Extraintestinal complications
HPA	Hypothalamus–pituitary–adrenal axis
HRQOL	Health-related quality of life
IBD	Inflammatory bowel disease
MDD	Major depressive disorder
OR	Odds ratio
IRR	Incidence rate ratio
UC	Ulcerative colitis
WHO	World Health Organization

References

1. Conrad, M.A.; Rosh, J.R. Pediatric Inflammatory Bowel Disease. *Pediatr. Clin. N. Am.* **2017**, *64*, 577–591. [CrossRef] [PubMed]
2. Diefenbach, K.A.; Breuer, C.K. Pediatric inflammatory bowel disease. *World J. Gastroenterol.* **2006**, *12*, 3204–3212. [CrossRef] [PubMed]
3. Murch, S.H.; Baldassano, R.; Buller, H.; Chin, S.; Griffiths, A.M.; Hildebrand, H.; Jasinsky, C.; Kong, T.; Moore, D.; Orsi, M. Inflammatory Bowel Disease: Working Group Report of the Second World Congress of Pediatric Gastroenterology, Hepatology, and Nutrition. *J. Pediatr. Gastroenterol. Nutr.* **2004**, *39* (Suppl. S2), S647–S654. [CrossRef]
4. Rosen, M.J.; Dhawan, A.; Saeed, S.A. Inflammatory Bowel Disease in Children and Adolescents. *JAMA Pediatr.* **2015**, *169*, 1053–1060. [CrossRef]
5. Malik, T.F.; Aurelio, D.M. Extraintestinal Manifestations of Inflammatory Bowel Disease. In *StatPearls*; StatPearls Publishing: Tampa, FL, USA, 2022.
6. Aloi, M.; Cucchiara, S. Extradigestive manifestations of IBD in pediatrics. *Eur. Rev. Med. Pharmacol. Sci.* **2009**, *13* (Suppl. S1), 23–32.
7. Singh, S.; Blanchard, A.; Walker, J.R.; Graff, L.A.; Miller, N.; Bernstein, C.N. Common Symptoms and Stressors Among Individuals with Inflammatory Bowel Diseases. *Clin. Gastroenterol. Hepatol.* **2011**, *9*, 769–775. [CrossRef] [PubMed]
8. Moeeni, V.; Day, A.S. Impact of Inflammatory Bowel Disease upon Growth in Children and Adolescents. *ISRN Pediatr.* **2011**, *2011*, 365712. [CrossRef] [PubMed]
9. Jelsness-Jørgensen, L.-P.; Bernklev, T.; Henriksen, M.; Torp, R.; Moum, B.A. Chronic fatigue is more prevalent in patients with inflammatory bowel disease than in healthy controls. *Inflamm. Bowel Dis.* **2011**, *17*, 1564–1572. [CrossRef]
10. Troncoso, L.L.; Biancardi, A.L.; de Moraes, H.V., Jr.; Zaltman, C. Ophthalmic manifestations in patients with inflammatory bowel disease: A review. *World J. Gastroenterol.* **2017**, *23*, 5836–5848. [CrossRef]
11. Klichowska-Palonka, M.; Komsta, A.; Pac-Kożuchowska, E. The condition of the oral cavity at the time of diagnosis of inflammatory bowel disease in pediatric patients. *Sci. Rep.* **2021**, *11*, 21898. [CrossRef]
12. Ji, X.-Q.; Wang, L.-X.; Lu, D.-G. Pulmonary manifestations of inflammatory bowel disease. *World J. Gastroenterol.* **2014**, *20*, 13501–13511. [CrossRef]
13. Olpin, J.D.; Sjoberg, B.P.; Stilwill, S.E.; Jensen, L.E.; Rezvani, M.; Shaaban, A.M. Beyond the Bowel: Extraintestinal Manifestations of Inflammatory Bowel Disease. *Radiographics* **2017**, *37*, 1135–1160. [CrossRef] [PubMed]
14. Zezos, P.; Kouklakis, G.; Saibil, F. Inflammatory bowel disease and thromboembolism. *World J. Gastroenterol.* **2014**, *20*, 13863–13878. [CrossRef]
15. Arvanitakis, K.D.; Arvanitaki, A.D.; Karkos, C.D.; Zintzaras, E.A.; Germanidis, G.S. The risk of venous thromboembolic events in patients with inflammatory bowel disease: A systematic review and meta-analysis. *Ann. Gastroenterol.* **2021**, *34*, 680–690. [CrossRef] [PubMed]
16. Yarur, A.J.; Czul, F.; Levy, C. Hepatobiliary manifestations of inflammatory bowel disease. *Inflamm. Bowel Dis.* **2014**, *20*, 1655–1667. [CrossRef] [PubMed]
17. Fousekis, F.S.; Theopistos, V.I.; Katsanos, K.H.; Christodoulou, D.K. Pancreatic Involvement in Inflammatory Bowel Disease: A Review. *J. Clin. Med. Res.* **2018**, *10*, 743–751. [CrossRef] [PubMed]
18. Ganji-Arjenaki, M.; Nasri, H.; Rafieian-Kopaei, M. Nephrolithiasis as a common urinary sys-tem manifestation of inflamma-tory bowel diseases; A clinical review and meta-analysis. *J. Nephropathol.* **2017**, *6*, 264–269. [CrossRef]
19. Tokuyama, H.; Wakino, S.; Konishi, K.; Hashiguchi, A.; Hayashi, K.; Itoh, H. Acute interstitial nephritis associated with ulcerative colitis. *Clin. Exp. Nephrol.* **2010**, *14*, 483–486. [CrossRef]
20. Ambruzs, J.M.; Walker, P.D.; Larsen, C.P. The Histopathologic Spectrum of Kidney Biopsies in Patients with Inflammatory Bowel Disease. *Clin. J. Am. Soc. Nephrol.* **2014**, *9*, 265–270. [CrossRef]
21. Elaziz, M.M.A.; Fayed, A. Patterns of renal involvement in a cohort of patients with inflammatory bowel disease in Egypt. *Acta Gastro Enterol. Belg.* **2018**, *81*, 381–385.

22. Shizuma, T. Coexistence of Crohn's Disease and Autoimmune Hemolytic Anemia. *Austin. J. Gastroenterol.* **2015**, *2*, 1043.
23. Jin, H.-Y.; Lim, J.-S.; Lee, Y.; Choi, Y.; Oh, S.-H.; Kim, K.-M.; Yoo, H.-W.; Choi, J.-H. Growth, puberty, and bone health in children and adolescents with inflammatory bowel dis-ease. *BMC Pediatr.* **2021**, *21*, 35. [CrossRef] [PubMed]
24. Amaro, F.; Chiarelli, F. Growth and Puberty in Children with Inflammatory Bowel Diseases. *Biomedicines* **2020**, *8*, 458. [CrossRef]
25. Stephan, R.V.; Schoepfer, A.; Scharl, M.; Lakatos, P.L.; Navarini, A.; Rogler, G. Extraintestinal Manifestations of Inflammatory Bowel Disease. *Inflamm. Bowel Dis.* **2015**, *21*, 1982–1992. [CrossRef]
26. Fornaciari, G.; Salvarani, C.; Beltrami, M.; Macchioni, P.L. Muscoloskeletal manifestations in inflam-matory bowel disease. *Can. J. Gastroenterol.* **2001**, *15*, 399–403. [CrossRef]
27. Plata-Bello, J.; Acosta-López, S. Neurological Manifestations of Inflammatory Bowel Disease. In *New Concepts in Inflammatory Bowel Disease*; Intechopen: London, UK, 2018. [CrossRef]
28. Umar, N.; Harvey, P.; King, D.; Chandan, J.S.; Nirantharakumar, K.; Adderley, N.; Haroon, S.; Trudgill, N. O33 The association between IBD and mental ill health: A retrospective primary care cohort studyGut. *BJM* **2022**, *71*, A20–A21.
29. Cui, G.; Liu, H.; Xu, G.; Laugsand, J.-B.; Pang, Z. Exploring Links Between Industrialization, Urbanization, and Chinese Inflammatory Bowel Disease. *Front. Med.* **2021**, *8*, 757025. [CrossRef]
30. Gruebner, O.; Rapp, M.A.; Adli, M.; Kluge, U.; Galea, S.; Heinz, A. Cities and Mental Health. *Dtsch. Arztebl. Int.* **2017**, *114*, 121–127. [CrossRef]
31. Kuenzig, M.E.; Fung, S.G.; Marderfeld, L.; Mak, J.W.; Kaplan, G.G.; Ng, S.C.; Wilson, D.C.; Cameron, F.; Henderson, P.; Kotze, P.G.; et al. Twenty-first Century Trends in the Global Epidemiology of Pediatric-Onset Inflammatory Bowel Disease: Systematic Review. *Gastroenterology* **2022**, *162*, 1147–1159.e4. [CrossRef]
32. Mamula, P.; Markowitz, J.E.; Baldassano, R.N. Inflammatory bowel disease in early childhood and adolescence: Special considerations. *Gastroenterol. Clin. N. Am.* **2003**, *32*, 967–995. [CrossRef]
33. Mendiolaza Michelle, L.; Feingold Jordyn, H.; Kaye-Kauderer Halley, P.; Dubinsky Marla, C.; Gorbenko Ksenia, O.; Keefer Laurie, A. Transitions from pediatric to adult IBD care: Incorporating lessons from psychogastroenterology. *Front. Gastroenterol.* **2022**, *1*, 037421. [CrossRef]
34. Kum, D.J.; Bang, K.-S. Body image, self-esteem, and quality of life in children and adolescents with inflammatory bowel disease in a tertiary hospital in South Korea. *Child Health Nurs. Res.* **2021**, *27*, 181–189. [CrossRef]
35. Murray, C.D.R.; Flynn, J.; Ratcliffe, L.; Jacyna, M.R.; Kamm, M.A.; Emmanuel, A.V. Effect of acute physical and psychological stress on gut autonomic innervation in irri-table bowel syndrome. *Gastroenterology* **2004**, *127*, 1695–1703. [CrossRef]
36. Van De Vijver, E.; Van Gils, A.; Beckers, L.; Van Driessche, Y.; Moes, N.D.; Van Rheenen, P.F. Fatigue in children and adolescents with inflammatory bowel disease. *World J. Gastroenterol.* **2019**, *25*, 632–643. [CrossRef]
37. van Langenberg, D.R.; Gibson, P.R. Systematic review: Fatigue in inflammatory bowel dis-ease. *Aliment. Pharmacol. Ther.* **2010**, *32*, 131–143. [CrossRef] [PubMed]
38. Marcus, S.B.; Strople, J.A.; Neighbors, K.; Weissberg–Benchell, J.; Nelson, S.P.; Limbers, C.; Varni, J.W.; Alonso, E.M. Fatigue and Health-Related Quality of Life in Pediatric Inflammatory Bowel Disease. *Clin. Gastroenterol. Hepatol.* **2009**, *7*, 554–561. [CrossRef] [PubMed]
39. Ghanean, H.; Ceniti, A.K.; Kennedy, S.H. Fatigue in Patients with Major Depressive Disorder: Prevalence, Burden and Pharmacological Approaches to Management. *CNS Drugs* **2018**, *32*, 65–74. [CrossRef] [PubMed]
40. Mackner, L.M.; Greenley, R.N.; Szigethy, E.; Herzer, M.; Deer, K.; Hommel, K.A. Psychosocial issues in pediatric inflammatory bowel disease: Report of the north American society for pediatric gastroen-terology, hepatology, and nutrition. *J. Pediatr. Gastroenterol. Nutr.* **2013**, *56*, 449–458. [CrossRef]
41. Thavamani, A.; Umapathi, K.K.; Khatana, J.; Gulati, R. Burden of Psychiatric Disorders among Pediatric and Young Adults with Inflammatory Bowel Disease: A Population-Based Analysis. *Pediatr. Gastroenterol. Hepatol. Nutr.* **2019**, *22*, 527–535. [CrossRef]
42. Brink, G.V.D.; Stapersma, L.; Vlug, L.; Rizopolous, D.; Bodelier, A.; Van Wering, H.; Hurkmans, P.; Stuyt, R.; Hendriks, D.; Van Der Burg, J.; et al. P205 Prevalence and risk factors for anxiety and depressive symptoms in children, adolescents and young adults with inflammatory bowel disease. *J. Crohn's Colitis* **2018**, *12* (Suppl. S1), S202–S203. [CrossRef]
43. Brink, G.V.D.; Stapersma, L.; Vlug, L.E.; Rizopolous, D.; Bodelier, A.G.; van Wering, H.; Hurkmans, P.C.W.M.; Stuyt, R.J.L.; Hendriks, D.M.; van der Burg, J.A.T.; et al. Clinical disease activity is associated with anxiety and depressive symptoms in adolescents and young adults with inflammatory bowel disease. *Aliment. Pharmacol. Ther.* **2018**, *48*, 358–369. [CrossRef]
44. Szigethy, E.; Levy-Warren, A.; Whitton, S.; Bousvaros, A.; Gauvreau, K.; Leichtner, A.M.; Beardslee, W.R. Depressive Symptoms and Inflammatory Bowel Disease in Children and Adolescents: A Cross-Sectional Study. *J. Pediatr. Gastroenterol. Nutr.* **2004**, *39*, 395–403. [CrossRef] [PubMed]
45. Greenley, R.N.; Hommel, K.A.; Nebel, J.; Raboin, T.; Li, S.H.; Simpson, P.; Mackner, L. A meta-analytic review of the psychosocial adjust-ment of youth with inflammatory bowel disease. *J. Pediatr. Psychol.* **2010**, *35*, 857–869. [CrossRef]
46. Craig, C.F.; Filippone, R.T.; Stavely, R.; Bornstein, J.C.; Apostolopoulos, V.; Nurgali, K. Neuroinflammation as an etiological trigger for depression comorbid with inflammatory bowel disease. *J. Neuroinflamm.* **2022**, *19*, 4. [CrossRef] [PubMed]
47. Keefer, L.; Kane, S.V. Considering the bidirectional pathways between depression and IBD: Recommendations for comprehensive IBD care. *Gastroenterol. Hepatol.* **2017**, *13*, 164–169.
48. Gracie, D.J.; Ford, A.C. Psychological Comorbidity and Inflammatory Bowel Disease Activity: Cause or Effect? *Clin. Gastroenterol. Hepatol.* **2016**, *14*, 1061–1062. [CrossRef]

49. Appleton, J. The Gut-Brain Axis: Influence of Microbiota on Mood and Mental Health. *Integr. Med.* **2018**, *17*, 28–32.
50. Keethy, D.; Mrakotsky, C.; Szigethy, E. Pediatric inflammatory bowel disease and depression: Treatment implications. Current opinion in pediatrics. *Curr. Opin. Pediatr.* **2014**, *26*, 561–567. [CrossRef]
51. Feldman, E.C.; Durkin, L.K.; Greenley, R.N. Family Support is Associated with Fewer Adherence Barriers and Greater Intent to Adhere to Oral Medications in Pediatric IBD. *J. Pediatr. Nurs.* **2021**, *60*, 58–64. [CrossRef]
52. Spekhorst, L.M.; Hummel, T.Z.; Benninga, M.A.; van Rheenen, P.F.; Kindermann, A. Adherence to Oral Maintenance Treatment in Adolescents with Inflammatory Bowel Disease. *J. Pediatr. Gastroenterol. Nutr.* **2016**, *62*, 264–270. [CrossRef]
53. Abraham, B.P.; Kahn, S.A. Transition of Care in Inflammatory Bowel Disease. *Gastroenterol. Hepatol.* **2014**, *10*, 633–640.
54. Turkel, S.; Pao, M. Late Consequences of Chronic Pediatric Illness. *Psychiatr. Clin. N. Am.* **2007**, *30*, 819–835. [CrossRef] [PubMed]
55. Lica, M.; Papai, A.; Salcudean, A.; Crainic, M.; Covaciu, C.; Mihai, A. Assessment of Psychopathology in Adolescents with Insulin-Dependent Diabetes (IDD) and the Impact on Treatment Management. *Children* **2021**, *8*, 414. [CrossRef] [PubMed]
56. Day, A.; Whitten, K.; Bohane, T. Childhood inflammatory bowel disease: Parental concerns and expectations. *World J. Gastroenterol.* **2005**, *11*, 1028–1031. [CrossRef]
57. Diederen, K.; Haverman, L.; Grootenhuis, M.A.; Benninga, M.A.; Kindermann, A. Parental Distress and Quality of Life in Pediatric Inflammatory Bowel Disease: Implications for the Outpatient Clinic. *J. Pediatr. Gastroenterol. Nutr.* **2018**, *66*, 630–636. [CrossRef] [PubMed]
58. De Boer, M.; Grootenhuis, M.; Derkx, B.; Last, B. Health-related quality of life and psychosocial functioning of adolescents with inflammatory bowel disease. *Inflamm. Bowel. Dis.* **2005**, *11*, 400–406. [CrossRef] [PubMed]
59. Assa, A.; Ish-Tov, A.; Rinawi, F.; Shamir, R. School Attendance in Children with Functional Abdominal Pain and Inflammatory Bowel Diseases. *J. Pediatr. Gastroenterol. Nutr.* **2015**, *61*, 553–557. [CrossRef]
60. Eloi, C.; Foulon, G.; Bridoux-Henno, L.; Breton, E.; Pelatan, C.; Chaillou, E.; Grimal, I.; Darviot, E.; Carré, E.; Gastineau, S.; et al. Inflammatory Bowel Diseases and School Absenteeism. *J. Pediatr. Gastroenterol. Nutr.* **2019**, *68*, 541–546. [CrossRef]
61. Engström, I. Mental Health and Psychological Functioning in Children and Adolescents with Inflammatory Bowel Disease: A Comparison with Children having Other Chronic Illnesses and with Healthy Children. *J. Child Psychol. Psychiatry* **1992**, *33*, 563–582. [CrossRef]
62. Manzari, Z.S.; Mohsenizadeh, S.M.; Vosoghinia, H.; Ebrahimipour, H. Family caregivers' burden in inflammatory bowel diseases: An integrative review. *J. Educ. Health Promot.* **2020**, *9*, 289. [CrossRef]
63. van Gennep, S.; de Boer, N.K.H.; Gielen, M.E.; Rietdijk, S.T.; Gecse, K.B.; Ponsioen, C.Y.; Duijvestein, M.; D'Haens, G.R.; Löwenberg, M.; de Boer, A.G.E.M. Impaired Quality of Working Life in Inflammatory Bowel Disease Patients. *Dig. Dis. Sci.* **2020**, *66*, 2916–2924. [CrossRef] [PubMed]
64. De Boer, A.G.; Evertsz', F.B.; Stokkers, P.C.; Bockting, C.L.; Sanderman, R.; Hommes, D.W.; Sprangers, M.A.; Frings-Dresen, M.H. Employment status, difficulties at work and quality of life in inflammatory bowel disease patients. *Eur. J. Gastroenterol. Hepatol.* **2016**, *28*, 1130–1136. [CrossRef] [PubMed]
65. Karve, S.; Candrilli, S.; Kappelman, M.D.; Tolleson-Rinehart, S.; Tennis, P.; Andrews, E. Healthcare Utilization and Comorbidity Burden among Children and Young Adults in the United States with Systemic Lupus Erythematosus or Inflammatory Bowel Disease. *J. Pediatr.* **2012**, *161*, 662–670.e2. [CrossRef] [PubMed]
66. Click, B.; Rivers, C.R.; Koutroubakis, I.; Babichenko, D.; Anderson, A.; Hashash, J.G.; Dunn, M.A.; Schwartz, M.; Swoger, J.; Baidoo, L.; et al. Demographic and Clinical Predictors of High Healthcare Use in Patients with Inflammatory Bowel Disease. *Inflamm. Bowel Dis.* **2016**, *22*, 1442–1449. [CrossRef] [PubMed]
67. Carlsen, K.; Haddad, N.; Gordon, J.; Phan, B.L.; Pittman, N.; Benkov, K.; Dubinsky, M.C.; Keefer, L. Self-efficacy and Resilience Are Useful Predictors of Transition Readiness Scores in Adolescents with Inflammatory Bowel Diseases. *Inflamm. Bowel Dis.* **2017**, *23*, 341–346. [CrossRef]
68. Regueiro, M.D.; McAnallen, S.E.; Greer, J.B.; Perkins, S.E.; Ramalingam, S.; Szigethy, E. The Inflammatory Bowel Disease Specialty Medical Home: A new model of patient-centered care. *Inflamm. Bowel Dis.* **2016**, *22*, 1971–1980. [CrossRef]
69. Gray, W.N.; Holbrook, E.; Morgan, P.J.; Saeed, S.A.; Denson, L.A.; Hommel, K.A. Transition readiness skills acquisition in adolescents and young adults with inflammatory bowel disease: Findings from integrating assessment into clinical practice. *Inflamm. Bowel Dis.* **2015**, *21*, 1125–1131. [CrossRef] [PubMed]
70. Klostermann, N.R.; McAlpine, L.; Wine, E.; Goodman, K.J.; Kroeker, K.I. Assessing the Transition Intervention Needs of Young Adults with Inflammatory Bowel Diseases. *J. Pediatr. Gastroenterol. Nutr.* **2018**, *66*, 281–285. [CrossRef]
71. Feingold, J.; Murray, H.B.; Keefer, L. Recent Advances in Cognitive Behavioral Therapy for Digestive Disorders and the Role of Applied Positive Psychology Across the Spectrum of GI Care. *J. Clin. Gastroenterol.* **2019**, *53*, 477–485. [CrossRef]
72. Scheier, M.F.; Carver, C.S. Optimism, coping, and health: Assessment and implications of generalized outcome expectancies. *Health Psychol.* **1985**, *4*, 219–247. [CrossRef]
73. Komase, Y.; Watanabe, K.; Hori, D.; Nozawa, K.; Hidaka, Y.; Iida, M.; Imamura, K.; Kawakami, N. Effects of gratitude intervention on mental health and well-being among workers: A systematic review. *J. Occup. Health* **2021**, *63*, e12290. [CrossRef]
74. Thoits, P.A.; Hewitt, L.N. Volunteer Work and Well-Being. *J. Health Soc. Behav.* **2001**, *42*, 115–131. [CrossRef]
75. Bailey, R.R. Goal Setting and Action Planning for Health Behavior Change. *Am. J. Lifestyle Med.* **2017**, *13*, 615–618. [CrossRef]
76. Keefer, L.; Palsson, O.S.; Pandolfino, J.E. Best Practice Update: Incorporating Psychogastroenterology Into Management of Digestive Disorders. *Gastroenterology* **2018**, *154*, 1249–1257. [CrossRef]

77. Ge, L.; Liu, S.; Li, S.; Yang, J.; Hu, G.; Xu, C.; Song, W. Psychological stress in inflammatory bowel disease: Psychoneuroimmunological insights into bidirectional gut–brain communications. *Front. Immunol.* **2022**, *13*, 1016578. [CrossRef] [PubMed]
78. Günther, C.; Rothhammer, V.; Karow, M.; Neurath, M.F.; Winner, B. The Gut-Brain Axis in Inflammatory Bowel Disease—Current and Future Perspectives. *Int. J. Mol. Sci.* **2021**, *22*, 8870. [CrossRef]
79. Masanetz, R.K.; Winkler, J.; Winner, B.; Günther, C.; Süß, P. The Gut–Immune–Brain Axis: An Important Route for Neuropsychiatric Morbidity in Inflammatory Bowel Disease. *Int. J. Mol. Sci.* **2022**, *23*, 11111. [CrossRef] [PubMed]
80. Zhang, Y.Z.; Li, Y.Y. Inflammatory bowel disease: Pathogenesis. *World J. Gastroenterol.* **2014**, *20*, 91–99. [CrossRef]
81. Troubat, R.; Barone, P.; Leman, S.; Desmidt, T.; Cressant, A.; Atanasova, B.; Brizard, B.; El Hage, W.; Surget, A.; Belzung, C.; et al. Neuroinflammation and depression: A review. *Eur. J. Neurosci.* **2021**, *53*, 151–171. [CrossRef]
82. Brites, D.; Fernandes, A. Neuroinflammation and Depression: Microglia Activation, Extracellular Microvesicles and microRNA Dysregulation. *Front. Cell. Neurosci.* **2015**, *9*, 476. [CrossRef] [PubMed]
83. Bonaz, B. Inflammatory bowel diseases: A dysfunction of brain-gut interactions? *Minerva Gastroenterol. Dietol.* **2013**, *59*, 241–259. [CrossRef]
84. Sublette, M.E.; Postolache, T.T. Neuroinflammation and depression: The role of indoleamine 2,3-dioxygenase (IDO) as a mo-lecular pathway. *Psychosom. Med.* **2012**, *74*, 668–672. [CrossRef] [PubMed]
85. Eisch, A.J.; Petrik, D. Depression and hippocampal neurogenesis: A road to remission? *Science* **2012**, *338*, 72–75. [CrossRef] [PubMed]
86. Trujillo-Hernández, P.E.; Sáenz-Galindo, A.; Saucedo-Cárdenas, O.; Villarreal-Reyna, M.D.L.; Salinas-Santander, M.A.; Carrillo-Cervantes, A.L.; Torres-Obregón, R.; Esparza-González, S.C. Depressive Symptoms are Associated with low Serotonin Levels in Plasma but are not 5–HTTLPR Genotype Dependent in Older Adults. *Span. J. Psychol.* **2021**, *24*, e28. [CrossRef] [PubMed]
87. Moroianu, L.-A.; Cecilia, C.; Ardeleanu, V.; Stoian, A.P.; Cristescu, V.; Barbu, R.-E.; Moroianu, M. Clinical Study of Serum Serotonin as a Screening Marker for Anxiety and Depression in Patients with Type 2 Diabetes. *Medicina* **2022**, *58*, 652. [CrossRef]
88. Bonaz, B.L.; Bernstein, C.N. Brain-Gut Interactions in Inflammatory Bowel Disease. *Gastroenterology* **2013**, *144*, 36–49. [CrossRef] [PubMed]
89. Agostini, A.; Benuzzi, F.; Filippini, N.; Bertani, A.; Scarcelli, A.; Farinelli, V.; Marchetta, C.; Calabrese, C.; Rizzello, F.; Gionchetti, P.; et al. New insights into the brain involvement in patients with Crohn's disease: A voxel-based morphometry study. *Neurogastroenterol. Motil.* **2012**, *25*, 147-e82. [CrossRef] [PubMed]
90. Vogt, B.A. Midcingulate cortex: Structure, connections, homologies, functions and diseases. *J. Chem. Neuroanat.* **2016**, *74*, 28–46. [CrossRef]
91. Drevets, W.C.; Savitz, J.; Trimble, M. The Subgenual Anterior Cingulate Cortex in Mood Disorders. *CNS Spectr.* **2008**, *13*, 663–681. [CrossRef]
92. Drevets, W.C.; Price, J.L.; Simpson, J.R., Jr.; Todd, R.D.; Reich, T.; Vannier, M.; Raichle, M.E. Subgenual prefrontal cortex abnormalities in mood disorders. *Nature* **1997**, *386*, 824–827. [CrossRef]
93. Rolls, E.T. The cingulate cortex and limbic systems for action, emotion, and memory. *Handb. Clin. Neurol.* **2019**, *166*, 23–37. [CrossRef] [PubMed]
94. Bao, C.H.; Liu, P.; Liu, H.R.; Wu, L.Y.; Shi, Y.; Chen, W.F.; Qin, W.; Lu, Y.; Zhang, J.Y.; Jin, X.M.; et al. Alterations in Brain Grey Matter Structures in Patients With Crohn's Disease and Their Correlation With Psychological Distress1. *J. Crohn's Colitis* **2015**, *9*, 532–540. [CrossRef] [PubMed]
95. Hopkins, C.W.; Powell, N.; Norton, C.; Dumbrill, J.L.; Hayee, B.; Moulton, C.D. Cognitive Impairment in Adult Inflammatory Bowel Disease: A Systematic Review and Meta-Analysis. *J. Acad. Consult.-Liaison Psychiatry* **2021**, *62*, 387–403. [CrossRef] [PubMed]
96. Piasecki, B.; Stanisławska-Kubiak, M.; Strzelecki, W.; Mojs, E. Attention and Memory Impairments in Pediatric Patients with Cystic Fibrosis and Inflammatory Bowel Disease in Comparison to Healthy Controls. *J. Investig. Med.* **2017**, *65*, 1062–1067. [CrossRef]
97. Chen, M.; Lee, G.; Kwong, L.N.; Lamont, S.; Chaves, C. Cerebral White Matter Lesions in Patients with Crohn's Disease. *J. Neuroimaging* **2010**, *22*, 38–41. [CrossRef]
98. Dolapcioglu, C.; Guleryuzlu, Y.; Uygur-Bayramicli, O.; Ahishali, E.; Dabak, R. Asymptomatic Brain Lesions on Cranial Magnetic Resonance Imaging in Inflammatory Bowel Disease. *Gut Liver* **2013**, *7*, 169–174. [CrossRef]
99. Horta, E.; Burke-Smith, C.; Megna, B.W.; Nichols, K.J.; Vaughn, B.P.; Reshi, R.; Shmidt, E. Prevalence of cerebrovascular accidents in patients with ulcerative colitis in a single academic health system. *Sci. Rep.* **2022**, *12*, 18668. [CrossRef]
100. Ghoneim, S.; Shah, A.; Dhorepatil, A.; Butt, M.U.; Waghray, N. The Risk of Cerebrovascular Accidents in Inflammatory Bowel Disease in the United States: A Population-Based National Study. *Clin. Exp. Gastroenterol.* **2020**, *13*, 123–129. [CrossRef]
101. Mikocka-Walus, A.; Knowles, S.R.; Keefer, L.; Graff, L. Controversies Revisited: A Systematic Review of the Comorbidity of Depression and Anxiety with Inflammatory Bowel Diseases. *Inflamm. Bowel Dis.* **2016**, *22*, 752–762. [CrossRef]
102. Arp, L.; Jansson, S.; Wewer, V.; Burisch, J. Psychiatric Disorders in Adult and Paediatric Patients with Inflammatory Bowel Diseases—A Systematic Review and Meta-Analysis. *J. Crohn's Colitis* **2022**, *16*, 1933–1945. [CrossRef]
103. Bernstein, C.N.; Hitchon, C.A.; Walld, R.; Bolton, J.M.; Sareen, J.; Walker, J.R.; Graff, L.A.; Patten, S.B.; Singer, A.; Lix, L.M.; et al. Increased Burden of Psychiatric Disorders in Inflammatory Bowel Disease. *Inflamm. Bowel Dis.* **2018**, *25*, 360–368. [CrossRef] [PubMed]

104. Nahon, S.; Lahmek, P.; Durance, C.; Olympie, A.; Lesgourgues, B.; Colombel, J.-F.; Gendre, J.-P. Risk factors of anxiety and depression in inflammatory bowel disease. *Inflamm. Bowel Dis.* **2012**, *18*, 2086–2091. [CrossRef]
105. Sempere, L.; Bernabeu, P.; Cameo, J.; Gutierrez, A.; Laveda, R.; Garcia, M.F.; Aguas, M.; Zapater, P.; Jover, R.; Ruiz-Cantero, M.T.; et al. Evolution of the emotional impact in patients with early inflammatory bowel disease during and after COVID-19 lockdown. *Gastroenterol. Hepatol.* **2021**, *45*, 123–133. [CrossRef]
106. Xiong, Q.; Tang, F.; Li, Y.; Xie, F.; Yuan, L.; Yao, C.; Wu, R.; Wang, J.; Wang, Q.; Feng, P. Association of inflammatory bowel disease with suicidal ideation, suicide attempts, and suicide: A systematic review and meta-analysis. *J. Psychosom. Res.* **2022**, *160*, 110983. [CrossRef] [PubMed]
107. Sánta, A.; Szántó, K.J.; Sarlós, P.; Miheller, P.; Farkas, K.; Molnár, T. Letter: Suicide risk among adult inflammatory bowel disease patients. *Aliment. Pharmacol. Ther.* **2020**, *51*, 1213–1214. [CrossRef] [PubMed]
108. Butwicka, A.; Olén, O.; Larsson, H.; Halfvarson, J.; Almqvist, C.; Lichtenstein, P.; Serlachius, E.; Frisén, L.; Ludvigsson, J.F. Association of Childhood-Onset Inflammatory Bowel Disease with Risk of Psychiatric Disorders and Suicide Attempt. *JAMA Pediatr.* **2019**, *173*, 969–978. [CrossRef]
109. Eaton, W.W.; Pedersen, M.G.; Nielsen, P.R.; Mortensen, P.B. Autoimmune diseases, bipolar disorder, and non-affective psychosis. *Bipolar Disord.* **2010**, *12*, 638–646. [CrossRef]
110. Kao, L.-T.; Lin, H.-C.; Lee, H.-C. Inflammatory bowel disease and bipolar disorder: A population-based cross-sectional study. *J. Affect. Disord.* **2019**, *247*, 120–124. [CrossRef]
111. Wang, Z.; Wang, X.; Zhao, X.; Hu, Z.; Sun, D.; Wu, D.; Xing, Y. Causal relationship between bipolar disorder and inflammatory bowel disease: A bidirectional two-sample mendelian randomization study. *Front. Genet.* **2022**, *13*, 970933. [CrossRef] [PubMed]
112. Sung, K.; Zhang, B.; Wang, H.E.; Bai, Y.; Tsai, S.; Su, T.; Chen, T.; Hou, M.; Lu, C.; Wang, Y.; et al. Schizophrenia and risk of new-onset inflammatory bowel disease: A nationwide longitudinal study. *Aliment. Pharmacol. Ther.* **2022**, *55*, 1192–1201. [CrossRef]
113. West, J.; Logan, R.F.; Hubbard, R.B.; Card, T.R. Risk of schizophrenia in people with coeliac disease, ulcerative colitis and Crohn's disease: A general population-based study. *Aliment. Pharmacol. Ther.* **2006**, *23*, 71–74. [CrossRef]
114. Kim, J.W.; Kang, K.S.; Kang, N.R. Steroid-induced Psychosis in Adolescent Patient with Crohn's Disease. *Soach'ongsonyon Chongsin Uihak J. Child Adolesc. Psychiatry* **2020**, *31*, 161–164. [CrossRef] [PubMed]
115. Locher, M.R.; Alam, A. Acute Psychosis in an Adolescent Treated with Infliximab for Crohn's Disease. *Prim. Care Companion J. Clin. Psychiatry* **2015**, *17*, 4. [CrossRef] [PubMed]
116. Galmiche, M.; Déchelotte, P.; Lambert, G.; Tavolacci, M.P. Prevalence of eating disorders over the 2000-2018 period: A sys-tematic literature review. *Am. J. Clin. Nutr.* **2019**, *109*, 1402–1413. [CrossRef] [PubMed]
117. Kuźnicki, P.; Neubauer, K. Emerging Comorbidities in Inflammatory Bowel Disease: Eating Disorders, Alcohol and Narcotics Misuse. *J. Clin. Med.* **2021**, *10*, 4623. [CrossRef]
118. World Health Organization. Suicide Worldwide in 2019: Global Health Estimates. Available online: https://www.who.int/publications/i/item/9789240026643 (accessed on 8 December 2022).
119. World Health Organization. Report Urges Mental Health Decision Makers and Advocates to Step Up Commitment and Action to Change Attitudes, Actions and Approaches to Mental Health, Its Determinants and Mental Health Care. Available online: https://www.who.int/news/item/17-06-2022-who-highlights-urgent-need-to-transform-mental-health-and-mental-health-care (accessed on 8 December 2022).
120. Gradus, J.L.; Qin, P.; Lincoln, A.K.; Miller, M.; Lawler, E.; Sørensen, H.T.; Lash, T.L. Inflammatory bowel disease and completed suicide in Danish adults. *Inflamm. Bowel Dis.* **2010**, *16*, 2158–2161. [CrossRef]
121. Mihajlovic, V.; Tripp, D.A.; Jacobson, J.A. Modelling symptoms to suicide risk in individuals with inflammatory bowel disease. *J. Health Psychol.* **2020**, *26*, 2143–2152. [CrossRef]
122. Moulton, C.; Pavlidis, P.; Norton, C.; Norton, S.; Pariante, C.; Hayee, B.; Powell, N. Depressive symptoms in inflammatory bowel disease: An extraintestinal manifestation of inflammation? *Clin. Exp. Immunol.* **2019**, *197*, 308–318. [CrossRef]

Disclaimer/Publisher's Note: The statements, opinions and data contained in all publications are solely those of the individual author(s) and contributor(s) and not of MDPI and/or the editor(s). MDPI and/or the editor(s) disclaim responsibility for any injury to people or property resulting from any ideas, methods, instructions or products referred to in the content.

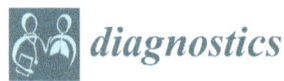

Review

The Crosstalk between Vitamin D and Pediatric Digestive Disorders

Cristina Oana Mărginean [1], Lorena Elena Meliț [1,*], Reka Borka Balas [1], Anca Meda Văsieșiu [2] and Tudor Fleșeriu [3]

1. Department of Pediatrics I, "George Emil Palade" University of Medicine, Pharmacy, Science, and Technology of Târgu Mureș, Gheorghe Marinescu Street No 38, 540136 Târgu Mureș, Romania
2. Department of Infectious Disease, "George Emil Palade" University of Medicine, Pharmacy, Science, and Technology of Târgu Mureș, Gheorghe Marinescu Street No 38, 540136 Târgu Mureș, Romania
3. Department of Infectious Disease, County Clinical Hospital Târgu Mureș, Gheorghe Doja Street No 89, 540394 Târgu Mureș, Romania
* Correspondence: lory_chimista89@yahoo.com

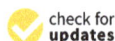

Citation: Mărginean, C.O.; Meliț, L.E.; Borka Balas, R.; Văsieșiu, A.M.; Fleșeriu, T. The Crosstalk between Vitamin D and Pediatric Digestive Disorders. *Diagnostics* 2022, 12, 2328. https://doi.org/10.3390/diagnostics12102328

Academic Editor: Costin Teodor Streba

Received: 31 August 2022
Accepted: 23 September 2022
Published: 27 September 2022

Publisher's Note: MDPI stays neutral with regard to jurisdictional claims in published maps and institutional affiliations.

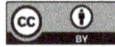

Copyright: © 2022 by the authors. Licensee MDPI, Basel, Switzerland. This article is an open access article distributed under the terms and conditions of the Creative Commons Attribution (CC BY) license (https://creativecommons.org/licenses/by/4.0/).

Abstract: Vitamin D is a cyclopentane polyhydrophenanthrene compound involved mainly in bone health and calcium metabolism but also autophagy, modulation of the gut microbiota, cell proliferation, immune functions and intestinal barrier integrity. The sources of vitamin D include sunlight, diet and vitamin D supplements. Vitamin D3, the most effective vitamin D isoform is produced in the human epidermis as a result of sunlight exposure. Vitamin D undergoes two hydroxylation reactions in the liver and kidney to reach its active form, 1,25-dihydroxyvitamin D. Recent studies highlighted a complex spectrum of roles regarding the wellbeing of the gastrointestinal tract. Based on its antimicrobial effect, it was recently indicated that vitamin D supplementation in addition to standard eradication therapy might enhance *H. pylori* eradication rates. Moreover, it was suggested that low levels of vitamin D might also be involved in the acquisition of *H. pylori* infection. In terms of celiac disease, the negative effects of vitamin D deficiency might begin even during intrauterine life in the setting of maternal deficiency. Moreover, vitamin D is strongly related to the integrity of the gut barrier, which represents the core of the pathophysiology of celiac disease onset, in addition to being correlated with the histological findings of disease severity. The relationship between vitamin D and cystic fibrosis is supported by the involvement of this micronutrient in preserving lung function by clearing airway inflammation and preventing pathogen airway colonization. Moreover, this micronutrient might exert anticatabolic effects in CF patients. Inflammatory bowel disease patients also experience major benefits if they have a sufficient level of circulating vitamin D, proving its involvement in both induction and remission in these patients. The findings regarding the relationship between vitamin D, food allergies, diarrhea and constipation remain controversial, but vitamin D levels should be monitored in these patients in order to avoid hypo- and hypervitaminosis. Further studies are required to fill the remaining gaps in term of the complex impact of vitamin D on gastrointestinal homeostasis.

Keywords: vitamin D; digestive disorders; children

1. Introduction

Vitamin D belongs to the group of fat-soluble vitamins, which can be found in two compounds: cholecalciferol (vitamin D2) and ergocalciferol (vitamin D3). This vitamin can be obtained from a pro-vitamin of the skin in the presence of ultraviolet B rays from the sun by conversion in cholecalciferol or from alimentation by consumption of fish, mushrooms, dairy products or some supplements [1]. Vitamin D undergoes two hydroxylation reactions, first at the level of the liver, where it is transformed into 25(OH)D (25-hydroxyvitamin D), which is also the main circulation form, and then at the level of the kidneys, where it is further converted into 25-(OH)2D (1,25-dihydroxyvitamin D), also known as calcitriol, the active form of the vitamin (Figure 1). The functions of calcitriol in the body are mediated by the nuclear vitamin D receptor (VDR), expressed in various tissues such as the skin, adipocytes, small intestine, colon, parathyroid, etc. VDR and the retinoic acid receptor (RXR) form a heterodimer, which, at the level of the nucleus, binds to the vitamin D response element (VDRE), which involved in nuclear transcription regulation [1–3]. VDRE is found in multiple genes, explaining certain vitamin D-associated activities, such as autophagy [4], modulation of the gut microbiota [4–6], cell proliferation [7], immune functions and the intestinal barrier role [8,9]. Nevertheless, regulation of bone health and governance of calcium homeostasis remain the most important and well-documented roles of vitamin D [2,3,5]. Thus, vitamin D is essential for bone mineralization and bone mass development (Figure 1).

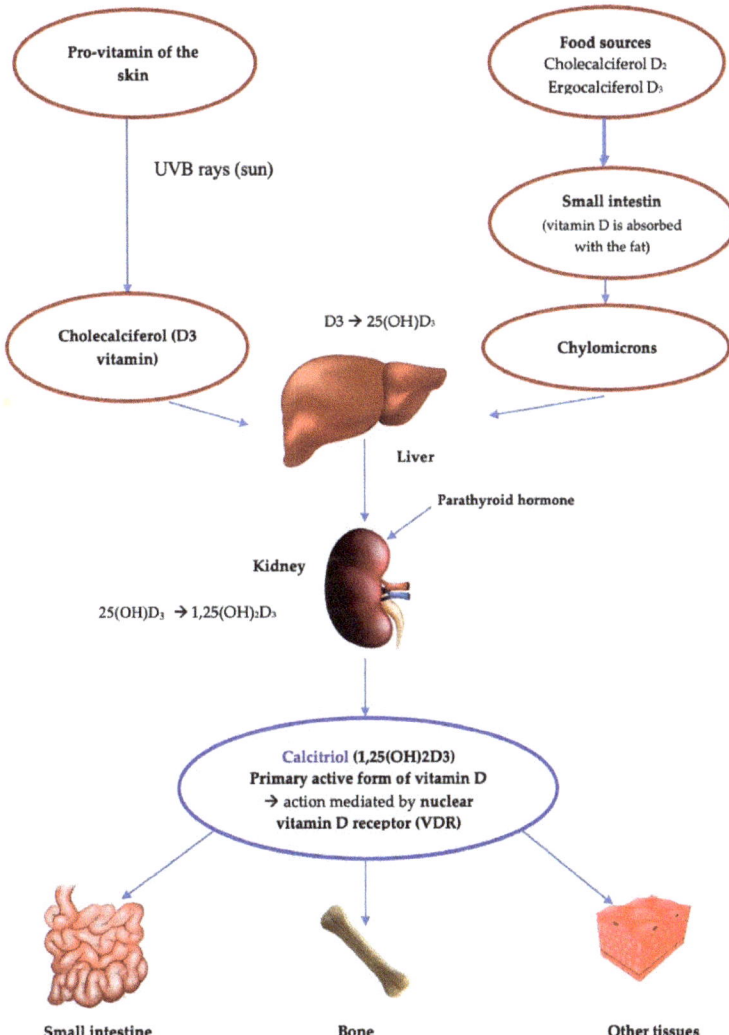

Figure 1. Schematic representation of vitamin D sources and metabolism.

The most common circulating form of vitamin D is 25(OH)D, which is also the best indicator for monitoring vitamin D status. In terms of vitamin D status, most studies have been performed on adults and define severe vitamin D deficiency as 25(OH)D levels < 10 ng/mL, resulting in an increased risk of rickets even when calcium intake is adequate, whereas in the presence of improper calcium intake, a level of 10–15 ng/mL vitamin D also leads to a high chance of developing rickets [10–12]. In adults, a vitamin D level of at least 20 ng/mL prevents the occurrence of rickets in up to 97.5% of the population, whereas levels ≥ 30 ng/mL have been proven sufficient to assure bone health [13,14]. In the pediatric population, the definition of an accurate cutoff level for vitamin D is difficult to establish. Despite the positive association between vitamin D levels, bone mineral density and bone mineral content revealed by pediatric studies, no specific threshold has been identified [15]. Moreover, it has been proven that calcium absorption in children might display an age-related compensatory mechanism that does not rely on vitamin D levels [16–18]. Similarly, a Chinese study performed on pediatric subjects aged between 0 and 7 years underlined that in the setting of 25(OH)D levels >30 ng/mL, the prevalence of decreased tibial bone mineral density plateaued [19]. Nevertheless, vitamin D deficiency and hypovitaminosis D were proven to be extremely common, irrespective of age. The National Health and Nutrition Examination in the US reported a prevalence of vitamin D deficiency of between 9–18% and 51–61% for hypovitaminosis D [20,21]. In Europe, a meta-analysis that involved 14,971 pediatric subjects identified a varying prevalence of vitamin D deficiency depending on age: 4–7% between 1 and 6 years, 1–8% between 7 and 14 years and 12–40% between 15 and 18 years, revealing that the prevalence increases with age [22]. Moreover, the authors found a higher prevalence in subjects living in relatively mid-latitude countries and non-white individuals.

The skin is the most important organ, involved in up to 90% of vitamin D synthesis as a result of sun ultraviolet B radiation exposure, which is influenced by skin pigmentation, altitude, latitude, daily timing of sun exposure, seasonality, atmospheric pollution, type of clothing, percentage of skin area exposed and sunscreen use [23]. Based on their higher body surface-area-to-volume ratio and their augmented capacity to produce vitamin D, children clearly require less sunlight exposure compared to adults in order to produce sufficient amounts of vitamin D for proper bone mineralization and development [24]. Most foods, including breast milk, contain only low amounts of vitamin D and are considered insufficient as sources of vitamin D [25,26]. Thus, experts worldwide agree that vitamin D should be supplemented independent of the dietary habits. In the United Kingdom, the Scientific Advisory Committee on Nutrition recommends a safe vitamin D intake of 340–400 IU/day in infants, 400 IU/day in children aged between 1 and 4 years and 400 IU/day for the population aged 4 years and older [27]. The European Union recommendations differ, suggesting that an intake of 400 IU/day in infants between 7 and 11 months and of 600 IU/day in pediatric subjects aged 1–17 years might be sufficient to prevent further complications due to vitamin D deficiency [28]. Nevertheless, according to both the European Society for Pediatric Gastroenterology, Hepatology and Nutrition [29] and the European Academy of Pediatrics [30], the tolerable upper intake levels of vitamin D are 1000 IU/day in infants, 2000 IU/day for children aged between 1 and 10 years and 4000 IU/day for those aged between 11 and 17 years [31].

Besides the historical skeletal functions of vitamin D, in recent years it has been emphasized that vitamin D is involved, in a direct or indirect manner, in the regulation of up to 1250 genes, implying a wide spectrum of extraskeletal roles [23].

Thus, *the aim* of this review was to assess the role of vitamin D in the development of gastrointestinal disorders.

2. Vitamin D and Gastrointestinal Disorders

Based on the wide spectrum of immune-modulatory properties of vitamin D, its involvement in the development of gastrointestinal disorders is not surprising. Vitamin D deficiency has been proven to result in severe dysfunctions of the intestinal barrier [32], mucosal damage [33] and increased susceptibility to infectious agents, thus altering the development and maintenance of gut homeostasis [34]. On the contrary, adequate levels of vitamin D have been associated with the integrity of junction complexes, therefore protecting the intestine from injury [35,36].

2.1. Vitamin D, Gastritis and Gastroesophageal Reflux

The role of vitamin D in modulating the host's response to pathogens and foreign antigens, along with the properties of vitamin D receptors as regulators of the immune system, attracted considerable attention in the research community during the last century [37]. Several hypotheses were proposed as potential mechanisms to explain the involvement of vitamin D in host defense against infection, such as the ability of immune cells to produce cytochrome P450 family 27 subfamily B member 1 and to convert 25(OH)D into 1,25(OH)2D; the expression of vitamin D receptor by the majority of immune cells; the strong relationship between 1,25(OH)2D production in immune cells and subsequent synthesis of antibacterial products, such as β-defensin and cathelicidin; and the strong evidence that vitamin D deficiency augments the burden of infectious diseases worldwide [38]. Moreover, epidemiologic studies revealed that the altered status of vitamin D is closely involved in mitigating susceptibility to various pathogens [39]. The wide spectrum of vitamin-D-related functions in terms of the immune system includes stimulation of macrophages and activated B and T cells, as well as maturation of dendritic cells; production of neutral antibacterial peptides and proteins, as well as reactive oxygen species; and the expression of inducible nitric oxide synthase [40]. Moreover, children with rickets were found to be at increased risk of developing infections, especially those involving the respiratory tract [41] (Table 1).

A recent study performed on subjects with *Helicobacter Pylori* (*H. pylori*) infection proved higher eradication rates if vitamin D supplements were combined with clarithromycin-based triple therapy [42], suggesting that vitamin D might also exert a protective antimicrobial effect against *H. pylori* infection. These findings were obtained in a study by Yildirim et al., who reported significantly lower eradication rates in deficient individuals [43]. Moreover, another study that included Italian subjects highlighted that patients with *H. pylori*-positive gastritis had lower serum vitamin D concentrations compared to uninfected individuals [44]. Similarly, Guo et al. [45] reported that vitamin D plays a major role in gastric mucosa homeostasis, exerting an antimicrobial effect against *H. pylori* based on its implications in sustaining host defense mechanisms. Thus, in patients with vitamin D deficiency, the infected macrophages no longer produce sufficient amounts of 1,25-(OH)D2, altering the subsequent synthesis of antimicrobial peptides and proteins and eventually disabling their ability to suppress and kill *H. pylori* strains [46]. Another potential explanation for the positive association between vitamin D levels and *H. pylori* eradication was suggested by an in vitro study that proved that the vitamin D3 decomposition product has a selective antibacterial effect against *H. pylori* [47]. In addition, vitamin D deficiency is associated with the augmentation of T-cell aggression in patients with chronic *H. pylori* infection, worsening gastric mucosal injury [44]. A recently reported case in an 18-month-old child underlined that hypovitaminosis D might result in an exacerbation of *H. pylori* gastritis, despite the young age of the patient [48] (Table 1).

As previously mentioned, gut epithelial VDR signaling seems to play a crucial role in regulating mucosal inflammation; although vitamin D is not produced in the stomach, it alters immune regulatory responses through the presence of this receptor within the stomach [45,49]. Studies proved that VDR mRNA expression levels were significantly increased in patients with *H. pylori* infection and were positively correlated with the activity scores of chronic inflammation [45]. Animal studies also revealed out a strong association between VDR and *H. pylori* infection, with VDR knockdown mice experiencing an increased susceptibility to this infection [50] (Table 1).

Chronic atrophic autoimmune gastritis is another pathology worth mentioning in the discussion of vitamin D. In addition to vitamin B12 deficiency and iron malabsorption, which are the most common disturbances in patients with this condition, other deficiencies were also recently described in these patients, including vitamin D deficiency [51] (Table 1).

The relationship between vitamin D and gastroesophageal reflux is less studied than the effect of vitamin D on gastritis. Thus, a recent study with the aim of assessing vitamin D intake and vitamin D levels in children with gastroesophageal reflux disease reported that children with this pathology had a normal level of vitamin D, despite a level of vitamin D intake below the daily recommended intake [52].

Undoubtedly, there is a strong relationship between vitamin D levels in children and *H. pylori*-positive gastritis, and vitamin D most likely also impacts other types of gastritis and even gastroesophageal reflux disease. However, further studies are required to define the precise role of this vitamin in the pathophysiology of these disorders.

2.2. Vitamin D and Celiac Disease

It is well-documented that celiac disease (CD) is an autoimmune disorder of the gastrointestinal tract triggered by an immune response to gluten-containing grains in individuals carrying HLA class II molecules HLA-DQ2 and HLA-DQ-8 [53]. The prevalence of CD in the US and most of European countries is approximately 1% [54]. Early-life vitamin D deficiency might be linked to the development of CD < 15 years of age [55]. The main mechanism implicated in childhood-onset CD involves the dysregulation of the intestinal response in deficient subjects, resulting in a disruption of the epithelial barrier, further increasing gluten permeability [56]. Moreover, the negative effects of vitamin D deficiency might begin during the intrauterine life, several studies have highlighted that low vitamin D concentrations in pregnant women may negatively affect fetal development, increasing the offspring's susceptibility to developing both infections [57,58] and autoimmune disorders [59,60] (Table 1). Nevertheless, the results on this topic remain controversial, as although the authors of some studies have hypothesized the role of maternal vitamin D deficiency in the onset of CD [61,62], a recent study that tested this hypothesis revealed no association between gestational or early-life vitamin D levels and the development of childhood CD [63] (Table 1).

The core of the complex pathophysiology of CD is represented by the intestinal barrier. The gut barrier is a complex structure meant to prevent harmful agents from passing though the gut mucosa and reaching the lamina propria [64]. The proper functioning of this barrier is closely related to epithelial layer integrity, intestinal microbiota homeostasis and gut-associated lymphoid tissue health [65–67]. Although the main trigger of all pathological events in CD is gluten, it seems that early disruption of the intestinal barrier in susceptible individuals and subsequent increased permeability could also contribute to the onset of immune responses triggered by gluten [65,66]. Aside from the positive effect of vitamin D on lymphocyte T and dendritic cells, this vitamin in also involved in the regulation of gut barrier integrity based on its close interaction with tight junctions, enabling the suppression of the zonulin release signaling pathway to upregulate tight junction protein expression and to consequently suppress the increase in gut mucosa permeability [64,66]. Moreover, vitamin D was reported to be involved in regulating inflammatory cytokines, such as tumor necrosis factor α [68], adding to its crucial role regarding gut barrier integrity maintenance (Table 1).

Children with CD are commonly reported to have low vitamin D levels, and it is difficult to establish whether this deficiency is a result of their dietary restrictions or whether vitamin D deficiency is involved in the onset of childhood CD. This phenomenon is most likely a vicious circle in which general trends of hypovitaminosis D during childhood contribute to the onset of CD, and its persistently decreased levels during the clinical course of CD augment disease severity. A recent study indicated that the decreased expression of VDR and epithelial barrier proteins claudin-2 and E-cadherin are positively correlated with histological findings of disease severity [69]. The authors pointed out that this decreased expression of VDR and epithelial barrier proteins is the result of vitamin D deficiency. Similar findings were reported by Zanchi et al., who found that 35% of biopsy-proven CD children included in their study experienced vitamin D deficiency [70]. On the contrary, Villanueva et al. failed to identify a positive association regarding vitamin D levels in healthy children and those with CD [71]. As previously stated, vitamin D deficiency is also common after the initiation of a gluten-free diet, most likely due to imbalances in calcium and vitamin D levels caused by this type of diet [72]. Although gluten-free diet was associated with considerable improvement in bone mineral density after only one year [73], the complete normalization of bone mineral density cannot always be achieved only by excluding dietary gluten [72]. Multiple controversies emerged regarding the supplementation of vitamin D in patients with CD based on the contradictory findings reported in the literature. The authors of a study that assessed children and teenagers with CD reported that a 2-year course of vitamin D (400 UI/day) and calcium (1 g/day) supplementation had a positive impact on bone mineral density [74]. On the contrary, another study proved that a gluten-free diet alone lasting for approximately 6 months was sufficient to resolve hypocalcemia and hyperparathyroidism, as well to normalize vitamin D levels [70]. Therefore, the choice to supplement vitamin D in combination with a gluten-free diet in patients with CD should be judiciously weighed (Table 1).

It has been reported that at the time of diagnosis, low bone mineral density might be present in CD patients, regardless of symptomatic or asymptomatic status [75,76]. Thus, there is a global consensus that vitamin D levels should be assessed upon diagnosis of CD [23,77–79]. Nevertheless, a recent study reported no difference in mean 25-(OH)D in recently diagnosed CD patients compared to healthy controls [80].

Thus, the assessment of vitamin D levels is mandatory in children with CD upon diagnosis and even during the clinical course in order to avoid improper the use of vitamin D supplements.

2.3. Vitamin D and Cystic Fibrosis (CF)

CF is an autosomal recessive disease and one of the most common causes of death related to this type of disorders among Caucasians in the US. The incidence of this disease is of 1 in 3200 live births, accounting for approximately 30,000 patients in the US and approximately 70,000 patients worldwide [81,82]. CF is caused by a mutation in the cystic fibrosis conductance regulator (CFTR) gene, resulting in an absent or dysfunctional CFTR protein-altering chloride transport through the apical epithelial membrane [83]. Several studies reported that the prevalence of vitamin D insufficiency is as high as 90% in the CF population [84,85]. A wide spectrum of factors was incriminated in the etiology of this deficiency, such as pancreatic insufficiency, reduction in body fat and vitamin D binding protein, reduced sunlight exposure and improper hepatic hydroxylation of vitamin D [86]. According to the Cystic Fibrosis Foundation, the serum 25(OH)D concentration should be determined annually, especially at the end of winter, and should be preserved > 30 ng/mL year round [87] (Table 1).

Studies performed on both adults and children revealed that vitamin D deficiency (<10 ng/mL) in adults with advanced CF was positively correlated with low hip and spine bone mineral density as compared to CF patients with higher vitamin D levels, whereas in children, the concentration of the same vitamin was also positively correlated with femoral neck and lumbar spine Z scores [88,89]. Vitamin D may be also be involved in preserving lung function in patients with CF [90], as a positive correlation was identified between vitamin D status and lung function indicators, such as forced expiratory volume in 1 s and forced vital capacity [91]. Several mechanisms were suggested to explain the role of vitamin D in preserving lung function, such as the effect of this vitamin on decreasing airway inflammation, the impact on airway remodeling as a response to various injuries caused by CF and the ability to decrease airway bacterial colonization [92] (Table 1).

Moreover, increased vitamin D levels were proven to be associated with both improved lung function and a reduction in the frequency of pulmonary exacerbation episodes [92]. In terms of lung exacerbations and infections, it was proven that locally produced 1,25(OH)2D enhances interleukin (IL)-37 airway concentrations, which further decrease airway colonization by certain pathogens, such as Pseudomonas aeruginosa and Bordetella bronchiseptica [93]. Vitamin D has the ability to downregulate proinflammatory cytokine synthesis in macrophages, resulting in a reduction in CF airway inflammation [94]. Another beneficial effect of vitamin D is reactive nitrogen and oxygen intermediate production, with a major effect on inducing autophagy to clear infections [95]. The authors of a randomized, controlled, double-blind placebo trial that included 30 CF adults hospitalized for a pulmonary exacerbation concluded that patients who were administered a one-time oral dose of 250,000 IU of vitamin D3 experienced more antibiotic therapy-free days and hospital-free days, as well as 1-year survival rate in comparison to those who received a placebo [96]. In addition, the authors pointed out that the high-dose vitamin D group presented with a significant decrease in inflammatory biomarkers, such as tumor necrosis factor α and IL-6. According to these findings, a high dose of vitamin D might represent a beneficial adjunctive therapy in CF patients with acute airway infections, which was also supported follow-up in a larger multicenter study performed by the CF Foundation [97] (Table 1).

CF-related intestinal microbial dysbiosis has been well-documented to result from both bacterial overgrowth as a result of poor intestinal motility and alterations of bacterial populations due to commonly used antibiotic treatment [98]. Studies on animals revealed that vitamin D exerts strong anti-inflammatory effects in the intestine of CF patients, resulting in decreased synthesis of proinflammatory markers, such as nuclear factor kB and IL-8, as well as reduced eosinophilia levels within the duodenal mucosa and fewer apoptotic cells [99]. Multiple factors can alter the microbial population in CF patients, such as common pulmonary infections, malnutrition and repeated systemic or local antibiotic treatment [100], impairing microbial communities within both the lungs and intestine. A recent study that assessed the influence of vitamin D on the lung and intestinal microbiome of CF patients revealed that vitamin D treatment led to major changes in lung and intestinal microbiome compositions, enhancing the development of healthier intestinal and respiratory microbes [101] (Table 1).

Another emerging topic related to vitamin D and CF is represented by metabolomic studies. A study on CF adult patients hospitalized with lung exacerbations aimed to assess the role of vitamin D in biochemical and metabolomic studies by dividing patients into two groups: a vitamin D group, which received a single 250,000 IU bolus dose of vitamin D, and a placebo group [102]. The authors collected baseline serum samples prior to drug administration and 7 days later for metabolomic analysis and reported that the baseline metabolome of CF patients was mainly catabolic, implying increased markers of lipid and fatty acid metabolism and reduced levels of essential amino acids. The samples collected after drug administration revealed that the placebo group exhibited 15 more catabolic pathways involving carbohydrates, amino acids and lipid metabolism overall compared to the vitamin D group (Table 1).

Based on the aforementioned facts, prescribing daily or weekly supplements of vitamin D in CF patients seems a reasonable choice.

2.4. Vitamin D and Inflammatory Bowel Disease (IBD)

IBD comprises two major clinical entities, Chron's disease (ChD) and ulcerative (UC), represents a chronic, relapsing–remitting systemic disorder with onset usually occurring during young adulthood and lasting throughout life [103]. Remission maintenance through medical therapy represents the cornerstone of management in IBD patients [104]. Vitamin D was proven to induce and maintain remission in IBD patients based on its anti-inflammatory and antibacterial properties, although it might also contribute to the repair of the intestinal mucosal barrier [105,106]. Moreover, vitamin D might also impact the incidence and progression of ChD and UC [107–109], as although controversial, it seems to be involved in the development of IBD and its severity according to several findings revealing common vitamin D deficiency in newly diagnosed IBD patients [104,110,111]. Similar findings were reported by Li et al., who found a significant association between vitamin D levels and IBD [103]. Moreover, previous studies highlighted that this micronutrient might also be involved in IBD-specific complications [112,113]. Studies with the aim of stratifying the impact of vitamin D on either UC or ChD remain controversial. Veit et al. [114] and El-

Matary et al. [115] reported that vitamin D levels were higher in pediatric patients with UC as compared to those with ChD, whereas Li et al. found no significant differences between UC and ChD patients in terms of vitamin D levels [103] (Table 1).

The prevalence of vitamin D deficiency in IBD patients is significantly higher than that in other populations, independent of IBD type [116]. A systematic review and meta-analysis of 14 observational studies including 938 IBD patients underlined a prevalence of vitamin D deficiency of 38.1% in ChD patients and of 31.6% in those with UC [117]. Several studies assessed the predictors of vitamin D deficiency in IBD and reported IBD-related surgery, non-white ethnicity [118,119], African-American ethnicity and body mass index > 30 kg/m^2 as the most common [120] (Table 1).

Vitamin D status also seems to be related to IBD activity. Worldwide studies [121–127] proved a significant association between vitamin D and disease activity, raising a 'chicken or egg' question, calling into doubt whether vitamin D levels are linked to intestinal inflammation or whether intestinal inflammation results in low vitamin D absorption. Nevertheless, more recent evidence suggests that serum vitamin D concentrations are inversely correlated with endoscopic and histologically proven inflammation, mucosal expression of proinflammatory cytokines and disease activity [128,129]. A reverse correlation was also highlighted between vitamin D levels and both fecal calprotectin and erythrocyte sedimentation rate [124]. Some studies have suggested that these findings were accurate only in ChD and not UC patients [126,130]. Other studies suggest that low or insufficient vitamin D levels are related to the increased need for hospitalization and surgery in patients with IBD compared to those with normal serum levels [131,132]. Another important aspect of disease activity in IBD patients is related to the gut microbiota, as it is well-documented that abnormal immune response to intestinal commensal bacteria is a specific feature of IBD, resulting in a less diverse and imbalanced microbial community [133–135]. Several promising effects of vitamin D on IBD gut microbiota modulation were recently reported by Battistini et al., suggesting its crucial positive role in modulating the composition of the gut microbial community [9] (Table 1).

In terms of vitamin D supplementation, IBD patients might require higher doses to achieve the recommended circulating level (>20 ng/mL) due to common nutrient malabsorption issues in these patients [13]. Nevertheless, supplementation has been reported to be beneficial, as it is associated with an improvement in inflammatory biomarkers, such as the erythrocyte sedimentation rate, C-reactive protein and suppression of the Th1 immune response, reducing the clinical disease activity index [136–143] (Table 1). Thus, the complex beneficial implications of vitamin D in the pathophysiology, outcome and disease activity of IBD should increase the awareness in clinical practice regarding the supplementation of this micronutrient in IBD patients.

2.5. Vitamin D and Food Allergies

Recent evidence suggests that the prevalence of vitamin D insufficiency in the population increases in parallel with the prevalence of food allergies [144]. Moreover, the role of vitamin D insufficiency at the age of 12 moths in the development of food allergy was emphasized by a population-based study performed on infants in Melbourne [144]. Nevertheless, the precise mechanisms involved in this relationship remain unclear. It was proven that vitamin D receptor agonists influence Th1 and Th2 cell function by suppressing allergen-specific IgE synthesis, inhibiting the maturation of dendritic cells, inducing tolerogenic dendritic cells and eventually contributing to the induction of regulatory CD4$^+$CD25$^+$Foxp3$^+$ T cells [145]. A potential mechanism described by Vassallo and Camargo implies the negative impact of vitamin D deficiency on the integrity of the gut barrier, resulting in increased permeability due to colonization by pathogenic microbial flora and subsequent inadequate immune system exposure to dietary allergens [146]. Another potential mechanism emphasizes the possibility of transcutaneous sensitization in children with vitamin D deficiency [147]. Thus, reduced antimicrobial factors at the skin level and the lack of effective tight junctions due to this deficiency might lead to inappropriate exposure and stimulation of the immune system, triggering the development of allergic sensitization, eczema and food allergy [147], in addition to worsening the evolution of atopic dermatitis [148]. The genetic aspect of the relationship between vitamin D deficiency and allergic disorders should not be neglected being, proving that certain individuals are more susceptible to developing food allergies, most likely due to differences in the genes involved in vitamin D metabolism and the response to vitamin D supplementation [149].

Recently, a worldwide increase in the prevalence of allergic diseases was reported [150,151]. Vitamin D deficiency was associated with the development of several allergic disorders, such as atopic dermatitis, asthma and food allergy [152]. A study conducted in Australia revealed that vitamin D levels < 50 nmo/L at 1 year of age were associated with an 11-fold increased risk of peanut allergy and a 4-fold increased risk of egg allergy [153]. Nevertheless, the question, 'which came first: the chicken or the egg?' also applies to this topic, as vitamin D deficiency was also reported in patients already diagnosed with food allergies, including cow's milk allergy (CMA), due decreased intake [154]. Children with both IgE- and non-IgE-mediated food allergies were proven to be at increased risk of vitamin D deficiency [155–157]. On the contrary, it was recently suggested that increased levels of vitamin D might increase the likelihood of sensitization and food allergy [158]. Similarly, a recent review revealed no benefit of vitamin D supplementation with respect to primary allergy prevention [159]. A recent Japanese study concluded that the correction of vitamin D deficiency might have a positive impact on food allergy prognosis, emphasizing the domino effect between inadequate sunlight exposure, vitamin D deficiency, altered gut barrier integrity, impaired immune response and food allergies [160].

The contradictory findings reported regarding the role of vitamin D in the development of food allergies represent proof that further studies are required in order to clearly delineate the effect of vitamin D on patients with food allergies and the effect of food allergies on vitamin D status. However, vitamin D status should be closely monitored in children with food allergies in order to assure its appropriate level for the best outcome.

Vitamin D and Cow's Milk Allergy (CMA)

Taking into account that CMA is one of the most common food allergy in infants [161], we considered that it would be useful to briefly discuss certain aspects regarding the relationship between vitamin D and CMA. It is essential to underline that cow's milk composition contributes to normal development and growth, especially during early childhood; its micro- and macronutrients, such as protein, energy, B vitamins and calcium, are particularly important for the proper development of bones and teeth [162]. Several studies revealed that the exclusion of cow's milk from the diet might lead to the impairment of bone health, short stature or weight deficit [151,163,164]. Infants with CMA were reported to have lower levels of vitamin D compared to healthy controls [165]. On the contrary, other authors failed to identify any significant difference regarding vitamin D status between CMA infants and healthy controls [166,167]. The contradictions become even more exacerbated, as a recent study performed on infants with CMA found no correlation between the serum level of vitamin D and eosinophilic cationic protein, an indicator of allergic diseases [161].

All these findings represent a burden for clinical practice in terms of correct workup of infants with CMA. Further studies including larger samples should be performed in order to provide an accurate evidence-based approach to these patients.

2.6. Vitamin D and Diarrhea

Diarrhea represents one of the most common pathologies in children younger than the age of 5 years in developing countries and the second most common cause of morbidity and mortality related to infectious causes in these patients [168,169]. Given that vitamin D deficiency is related to susceptibility to and the severity of acute infections and poor outcomes in several chronic infections [170], it is not surprising that studies have been conducted with the aim of identifying the role of this vitamin in pediatric patients with diarrhea; however, the evidence remains scarce. Several studies from different geographic areas, such as Columbia, Egypt, Pakistan and Saudi Arabia, reported a significant association between low vitamin levels and increased incidence of diarrhea in children [171–174]. A recent study questioned these findings, proving that although children younger than five years were commonly found to be vitamin-D-deficient, this deficiency is not necessarily related to the incidence of diarrhea in this age group [175]. Similarly, Ahmed et al. found no association between vitamin D status and the incidence or severity of diarrhea in children aged 6–24 months [176]. Nevertheless, Wang et al. suggested that low vitamin D levels might be associated with ab increased likelihood of recurrence in patients with *Clostridium difficile*-associated diarrhea [177]. Similar findings were concluded in a study including patients with *Rotavirus* infections, with the authors proving that rotaviral diarrhea was associated with low vitamin D levels [178].

2.7. Vitamin D and Constipation

The relationship between vitamin D and chronic constipation is probably one of the less studied topics and; it remains unclear how vitamin D influences the motility of the gastrointestinal tract. It is well-documented that the presence of VDR on the surface of macrophages, lymphocytes and gut epithelial cells represents the key factor linking vitamin D deficiency, VDR dysfunction and altered gut microbial composition, eventually leading to the onset of several chronic conditions [179–181]. The relationship between vitamin D deficiency and both slow colonic motility and autonomic rectal dysfunction was previously proven in patients with multiple sclerosis [182–185]. Moreover, Panarese et al. recently hypothesized that vitamin D deficiency might be responsible for immunologic/metabolic damage to neuromuscular and epithelial components of the gut [186]. The authors proved that vitamin D levels were independently related to intestinal motility disorders. In addition, the symptoms of patients with functional chronic constipation were reported to worsen in parallel with decreased vitamin D levels. These findings remain to be further validated in larger studies focusing on the effect of vitamin D supplementation in patients with chronic functional constipation.

Table 1. The role of Vitamin D in pediatric digestive disorders.

Disease	Vitamin D Roles
Gastritis and gastroesophageal reflux	• Increased eradication rates of *H. pylori* infection if vitamin D supplementation is combined with clarithromycin-based triple therapy [42] → protective antimicrobial effect against *H. pylori* infection • Patients with *H. pylori*-positive gastritis: lower serum vitamin D concentrations compared to uninfected individuals [44] • Vitamin D plays a major role in gastric mucosa homeostasis [45] • Vitamin D receptor mRNA expression levels were significantly increased in patients with *H. pylori* infection and positively correlated with the activity scores of chronic inflammation [45]
Celiac disease	• Vitamin D deficiency might be linked to the development of CD < 15 years of age [55] • Negative effects of vitamin D deficiency might begin during intrauterine life, with maternal vitamin D deficiency implicated in the onset of CD [61,62] • Positive effect of vitamin D on lymphocytes, as well as T and dendritic cells, which are involved in the regulation of gut barrier integrity, upregulating tight junction protein expression and consequently suppressing the increase in gut mucosa permeability [64,66] • Vitamin D is involved in regulating inflammatory cytokines, such as TNF α, playing a crucial role in the maintenance of gut barrier integrity [68] • Decreased expression of vitamin D receptor and epithelial barrier proteins claudin-2 and E-cadherin is positively correlated with histological findings of disease severity [69] • A gluten-free diet alone lasting for approximately 6 months was sufficient to resolve hypocalcemia and hyperparathyroidism, as well as to normalize vitamin D levels [70] • In teenagers with CD, a 2-year course of vitamin D (400 UI/day) and calcium (1 g/day) supplementation had a positive impact on bone mineral density [74]

Table 1. *Cont.*

Disease	Vitamin D Roles
Cystic fibrosis	• Vitamin D deficiency (<10 ng/mL) in adults with advanced CF was positively correlated with reduced hip and spine bone mineral density compared to CF patients with higher vitamin D levels [88,89] • In children, the concentration of vitamin D was positively correlated with femoral neck and lumbar spine Z scores [88,89] • Vitamin D may be also involved in preserving lung function in patients with CF [90] • In lung exacerbations and infections, locally produced 1,25(OH)2D enhances the IL-37 airway concentrations, further decreasing airway colonization by certain pathogens, such as *Pseudomonas aeruginosa* and *Bordetella bronchiseptica* [93] • Vitamin D downregulates proinflammatory cytokine synthesis in macrophages, resulting in a reduction in CF airway inflammation [94] • High-dose vitamin D supplementation decreases inflammatory biomarkers TNF α and IL-6 [96] • High-dose vitamin D represents an adjunctive therapy in CF patients with acute airway infections [97] • Vitamin D exerts anti-inflammatory effects in the intestine of CF patients, resulting in decreased synthesis of proinflammatory markers, reduced eosinophilia levels within the duodenal mucosa and fewer apoptotic cells [99] • Vitamin D contributes to the development of healthier intestinal and respiratory microbes [101] • Vitamin D exerted an anticatabolic effect in CF patients [102]
Inflammatory bowel disease	• Vitamin D induces and maintains remission in IBD patients based on its anti-inflammatory and antibacterial properties [105,106] • Vitamin D might also impact the incidence and progression of CD and UC [107–109] • Vitamin D is involved in IBD-specific complications [112,113] • Vitamin D levels might be higher in pediatric patients with UC compared to those with CD [114,115] • Predictors of vitamin D deficiency in IBD include IBD-related surgery, non-white ethnicity [118,119], African-American ethnicity and body mass index > 30 kg/m^2 [120] • Serum vitamin D concentrations are inversely correlated with endoscopic and histologically proven inflammation, mucosal expression of proinflammatory cytokines and disease activity [128,129] • Low or insufficient vitamin D levels are related to increased need for hospitalization and surgery in patients with IBD compared to those with normal serum levels [131,132] • Promising effects of vitamin D on IBD gut microbiota modulation [9] • Supplementation of vitamin D in IBD is associated with an improvement in inflammatory biomarkers, suppression of Th1 immune response and reduced clinical disease activity index [136–143]
Food allergy	• Vitamin D insufficiency supports the development of food allergies [144] • Vitamin D receptor agonists influence Th1 and Th2 cell function, inhibiting the maturation of dendritic cells and inducing tolerogenic dendritic cells, as well as contributing to the induction of regulatory CD4$^+$CD25$^+$Foxp3$^+$ T cells [145] • Vitamin D deficiency increases gut permeability due to colonization by pathogenic microbial flora, resulting in inadequate immune system exposure to dietary allergens [146], allergic sensitization, eczema and food allergies [147] • Vitamin D deficiency is associated with the development of atopic dermatitis, asthma and food allergies [152] • IgE- and non-IgE-mediated food allergies are associated with increased risk of vitamin D deficiency [155–157] • Higher levels of vitamin D might increase the likelihood of sensitization and food allergies [158] • The correction of vitamin D deficiency has a positive impact on food allergy prognosis, with a domino effect between inadequate sunlight exposure, vitamin D deficiency, altered gut barrier integrity, impaired immune response and food allergies [160] • Infants with CMA present with lower levels of vitamin D compared to healthy controls [165] • No correlation between the serum level of vitamin D and eosinophilic cationic protein, which is an indicator of allergic diseases [161]

Table 1. *Cont.*

Disease	Vitamin D Roles
Diarrhea	• Significant association between low vitamin levels and the increased incidence of diarrhea in children [171–174] • No association between vitamin D status and incidence or severity of diarrhea in children aged 6–24 months [176] • Low vitamin D levels associated with increased likelihood of recurrence in patients with *Clostridium difficile*-associated diarrhea [177]
Constipation	• Vitamin D deficiency might be responsible for immunologic/metabolic damage to neuromuscular and epithelial components of the gut [186] • Vitamin D levels are related to intestinal motility disorders [186] • The symptoms of patients with functional chronic constipation worsened in association with a decrease in vitamin D levels [186]

3. Conclusions

Vitamin D plays a crucial role in terms of gastrointestinal health. Thus, besides the classical role of vitamin D in calcium metabolism and bone health, emerging evidence indicates a wide spectrum of other multisystemic implications. The antimicrobial effect is extremely useful in enhancing *H. pylori* eradication. Studies of pediatric patients proved that supplementation of vitamin D in combination with standard eradication regimens increases *H. pylori* eradication rates. In terms of gastroesophageal reflux, the evidence in pediatric ages remains scarce, suggested that these children have normal levels of vitamin D despite their low intake. Moreover, this beneficial micronutrient acts as an immunomodulator of both innate and adaptive immune responses at the level of the gastrointestinal tract. In terms of CD, vitamin D deficiency is involved not only in the onset of CD, but it might also aggravate its clinical course. Therefore, early disruption of the intestinal barrier in susceptible individuals and subsequently increased permeability triggered by vitamin D deficiency could contribute to the onset of immune responses triggered by gluten. Maternal vitamin D status might also be involved in the early onset of CD in genetically susceptible offspring. The impact of vitamin D on CF is complex, as it was proven to exert antimicrobial, modulatory and anticatabolic effects. Moreover, vitamin D deficiency in CF children was proven to be positively correlated with reduced bone mineral density. Vitamin D may be also involved in preserving lung function in patients with CF. The supplementation of vitamin D in CF patients might enhance the development of healthier intestinal and respiratory microbes, improving the composition of the lung and gut microbiome. The role of vitamin D on maintaining gut barrier integrity was demonstrated to be of considerable importance in IBD patients. Moreover, based on its immunomodulatory properties, this vitamin seems to decrease disease activity in these patients, preventing IBD-related complications. Pediatric patients with ChD were proven to have lower vitamin D levels compared to those with UC. Children with food allergies were reported to have lower levels of vitamin D, and vitamin D was found to increase the risk of developing food allergies in the pediatric population. CMA infants were found to have lower levels of vitamin D levels compared to controls, although the reported findings remain controversial. Several studies worldwide have reported that low vitamin D levels are associated with increased incidence of diarrhea in children; however, other authors found no association between vitamin D status and increased likelihood of diarrhea. Vitamin D was recently linked to the development of intestinal motility dysfunctions, proving that vitamin D deficiency might increase the risk of chronic constipation, worsening its associated symptoms. Nevertheless, further studies including larger samples should be performed in order to define the precise systemic role of vitamin D and to elucidate the related 'chicken or egg' controversies.

Author Contributions: Conceptualization, C.O.M., L.E.M. and A.M.V.; methodology, C.O.M., L.E.M., A.M.V. and T.F.; validation, C.O.M. and L.E.M.; investigation, A.M.V., R.B.B. and T.F.; writing—original draft preparation, C.O.M. and L.E.M.; writing—review and editing, C.O.M., L.E.M., A.M.V. and R.B.B.; supervision, C.O.M., L.E.M. and A.M.V. All authors approved the final manuscript as submitted and agree to be accountable for all aspects of the work. All authors have read and agreed to the published version of the manuscript.

Funding: This research received no external funding.

Institutional Review Board Statement: Not applicable.

Informed Consent Statement: Not applicable.

Data Availability Statement: Not applicable.

Conflicts of Interest: The authors declare no conflict of interest.

Abbreviations

CD	celiac disease
CF	cystic fibrosis
CFTR	cystic fibrosis conductance regulator
ChD	Crohn's disease
CMA	cow's milk allergy
H. pylori	*Helicobacter Pylori*
IBD	inflammatory bowel disease
IL	interleukin
RXR	retinoic acid receptor
UC	ulcerative colitis
VDR	vitamin D receptor
VDRE	vitamin D response element

References

1. Holick, M.F. The Vitamin D Deficiency Pandemic: Approaches for Diagnosis, Treatment and Prevention. *Rev. Endocr. Metab. Disord.* **2017**, *18*, 153–165. [CrossRef]
2. Bakke, D.; Chatterjee, I.; Agrawal, A.; Dai, Y.; Sun, J. Regulation of Microbiota by Vitamin D Receptor: A Nuclear Weapon in Metabolic Diseases. *Nucl. Receptor. Res.* **2018**, *5*, 101377. [CrossRef]
3. Haussler, M.R.; Jurutka, P.W.; Mizwicki, M.; Norman, A.W. Vitamin D Receptor (VDR)-Mediated Actions of $1\alpha,25(OH)_2$ vitamin D_3: Genomic and Non-Genomic Mechanisms. *Best Pract. Res. Clin. Endocrinol. Metab.* **2011**, *25*, 543–559. [CrossRef]
4. Wu, S.; Zhang, Y.-G.; Lu, R.; Xia, Y.; Zhou, D.; Petrof, E.O.; Claud, E.C.; Chen, D.; Chang, E.B.; Carmeliet, G.; et al. Intestinal Epithelial Vitamin D Receptor Deletion Leads to Defective Autophagy in Colitis. *Gut* **2015**, *64*, 1082–1094. [CrossRef]
5. Wang, J.; Thingholm, L.B.; Skiecevičienė, J.; Rausch, P.; Kummen, M.; Hov, J.R.; Degenhardt, F.; Heinsen, F.-A.; Rühlemann, M.C.; Szymczak, S.; et al. Genome-Wide Association Analysis Identifies Variation in Vitamin D Receptor and Other Host Factors Influencing the Gut Microbiota. *Nat. Genet.* **2016**, *48*, 1396–1406. [CrossRef]
6. Zhang, Y.-G.; Lu, R.; Wu, S.; Chatterjee, I.; Zhou, D.; Xia, Y.; Sun, J. Vitamin D Receptor Protects Against Dysbiosis and Tumorigenesis via the JAK/STAT Pathway in Intestine. *Cell Mol. Gastroenterol. Hepatol.* **2020**, *10*, 729–746. [CrossRef]
7. Jin, D.; Zhang, Y.-G.; Wu, S.; Lu, R.; Lin, Z.; Zheng, Y.; Chen, H.; Cs-Szabo, G.; Sun, J. Vitamin D Receptor Is a Novel Transcriptional Regulator for Axin1. *J. Steroid. Biochem. Mol. Biol.* **2017**, *165*, 430–437. [CrossRef]
8. Bashir, M.; Prietl, B.; Tauschmann, M.; Mautner, S.I.; Kump, P.K.; Treiber, G.; Wurm, P.; Gorkiewicz, G.; Högenauer, C.; Pieber, T.R. Effects of High Doses of Vitamin D3 on Mucosa-Associated Gut Microbiome Vary between Regions of the Human Gastrointestinal Tract. *Eur J. Nutr.* **2016**, *55*, 1479–1489. [CrossRef]
9. Battistini, C.; Ballan, R.; Herkenhoff, M.E.; Saad, S.M.I.; Sun, J. Vitamin D Modulates Intestinal Microbiota in Inflammatory Bowel Diseases. *Int. J. Mol. Sci.* **2020**, *22*, E362. [CrossRef]
10. Thacher, T.D.; Fischer, P.R.; Pettifor, J.M.; Lawson, J.O.; Isichei, C.O.; Chan, G.M. Case-Control Study of Factors Associated with Nutritional Rickets in Nigerian Children. *J. Pediatr.* **2000**, *137*, 367–373. [CrossRef]
11. Atapattu, N.; Shaw, N.; Högler, W. Relationship between Serum 25-Hydroxyvitamin D and Parathyroid Hormone in the Search for a Biochemical Definition of Vitamin D Deficiency in Children. *Pediatr. Res.* **2013**, *74*, 552–556. [CrossRef]
12. Pettifor, J.M. Nutritional Rickets: Pathogenesis and Prevention. *Pediatr. Endocrinol. Rev.* **2013**, *10* (Suppl. S2), 347–353.
13. Institute of Medicine (US) Committee to Review Dietary Reference Intakes for Vitamin D and Calcium. *Dietary Reference Intakes for Calcium and Vitamin D*; Ross, A.C., Taylor, C.L., Yaktine, A.L., Del Valle, H.B., Eds.; The National Academies Collection: Reports Funded by National Institutes of Health; National Academies Press (US): Washington, DC, USA, 2011.

14. Holick, M.F.; Binkley, N.C.; Bischoff-Ferrari, H.A.; Gordon, C.M.; Hanley, D.A.; Heaney, R.P.; Murad, M.H.; Weaver, C.M. Endocrine Society Evaluation, Treatment, and Prevention of Vitamin D Deficiency: An Endocrine Society Clinical Practice Guideline. *J. Clin. Endocrinol. Metab.* **2011**, *96*, 1911–1930. [CrossRef]
15. Winzenberg, T.; Jones, G. Vitamin D and Bone Health in Childhood and Adolescence. *Calcif. Tissue Int.* **2013**, *92*, 140–150. [CrossRef]
16. Abrams, S.A.; Griffin, I.J.; Hawthorne, K.M.; Gunn, S.K.; Gundberg, C.M.; Carpenter, T.O. Relationships among Vitamin D Levels, Parathyroid Hormone, and Calcium Absorption in Young Adolescents. *J. Clin. Endocrinol. Metab.* **2005**, *90*, 5576–5581. [CrossRef]
17. Abrams, S.A.; Hicks, P.D.; Hawthorne, K.M. Higher Serum 25-Hydroxyvitamin D Levels in School-Age Children Are Inconsistently Associated with Increased Calcium Absorption. *J. Clin. Endocrinol. Metab.* **2009**, *94*, 2421–2427. [CrossRef]
18. Abrams, S.A.; Hawthorne, K.M.; Rogers, S.P.; Hicks, P.D.; Carpenter, T.O. Effects of Ethnicity and Vitamin D Supplementation on Vitamin D Status and Changes in Bone Mineral Content in Infants. *BMC Pediatr.* **2012**, *12*, 6. [CrossRef]
19. Fu, Y.; Hu, Y.; Qin, Z.; Zhao, Y.; Yang, Z.; Li, Y.; Liang, G.; Lv, H.; Hong, H.; Song, Y.; et al. Association of Serum 25-Hydroxyvitamin D Status with Bone Mineral Density in 0–7 Year Old Children. *Oncotarget* **2016**, *7*, 80811–80819. [CrossRef]
20. Kumar, J.; Muntner, P.; Kaskel, F.J.; Hailpern, S.M.; Melamed, M.L. Prevalence and Associations of 25-Hydroxyvitamin D Deficiency in US Children: NHANES 2001–2004. *Pediatrics* **2009**, *124*, e362–e370. [CrossRef]
21. Mansbach, J.M.; Ginde, A.A.; Camargo, C.A. Serum 25-Hydroxyvitamin D Levels among US Children Aged 1 to 11 Years: Do Children Need More Vitamin D? *Pediatrics* **2009**, *124*, 1404–1410. [CrossRef]
22. Cashman, K.D.; Dowling, K.G.; Škrabáková, Z.; Gonzalez-Gross, M.; Valtueña, J.; De Henauw, S.; Moreno, L.; Damsgaard, C.T.; Michaelsen, K.F.; Mølgaard, C.; et al. Vitamin D Deficiency in Europe: Pandemic? *Am. J. Clin. Nutr.* **2016**, *103*, 1033–1044. [CrossRef]
23. Saggese, G.; Vierucci, F.; Prodam, F.; Cardinale, F.; Cetin, I.; Chiappini, E.; De' Angelis, G.L.; Massari, M.; Miraglia Del Giudice, E.; Miraglia Del Giudice, M.; et al. Vitamin D in Pediatric Age: Consensus of the Italian Pediatric Society and the Italian Society of Preventive and Social Pediatrics, Jointly with the Italian Federation of Pediatricians. *Ital. J. Pediatr.* **2018**, *44*, 51. [CrossRef]
24. Paller, A.S.; Hawk, J.L.M.; Honig, P.; Giam, Y.C.; Hoath, S.; Mack, M.C.; Stamatas, G.N. New Insights about Infant and Toddler Skin: Implications for Sun Protection. *Pediatrics* **2011**, *128*, 92–102. [CrossRef]
25. Misra, M.; Pacaud, D.; Petryk, A.; Collett-Solberg, P.F.; Kappy, M. Drug and Therapeutics Committee of the Lawson Wilkins Pediatric Endocrine Society Vitamin D Deficiency in Children and Its Management: Review of Current Knowledge and Recommendations. *Pediatrics* **2008**, *122*, 398–417. [CrossRef]
26. Holick, M.F. Vitamin D Deficiency. *N. Engl. J. Med.* **2007**, *357*, 266–281. [CrossRef]
27. SACN Vitamin D and Health Report. Available online: https://www.gov.uk/government/publications/sacn-vitamin-d-and-health-report (accessed on 31 July 2022).
28. Dietary Reference Values for Vitamin D | EFSA. Available online: https://www.efsa.europa.eu/en/efsajournal/pub/4547 (accessed on 31 July 2022).
29. Braegger, C.; Campoy, C.; Colomb, V.; Decsi, T.; Domellof, M.; Fewtrell, M.; Hojsak, I.; Mihatsch, W.; Molgaard, C.; Shamir, R.; et al. Vitamin D in the Healthy European Paediatric Population. *J. Pediatr. Gastroenterol. Nutr.* **2013**, *56*, 692–701. [CrossRef]
30. Grossman, Z.; Hadjipanayis, A.; Stiris, T.; Del Torso, S.; Mercier, J.-C.; Valiulis, A.; Shamir, R. Vitamin D in European Children-Statement from the European Academy of Paediatrics (EAP). *Eur. J. Pediatr.* **2017**, *176*, 829–831. [CrossRef]
31. Scientific Opinion on the Tolerable Upper Intake Level of Vitamin D | EFSA. Available online: https://www.efsa.europa.eu/en/efsajournal/pub/2813 (accessed on 31 July 2022).
32. Assa, A.; Vong, L.; Pinnell, L.J.; Avitzur, N.; Johnson-Henry, K.C.; Sherman, P.M. Vitamin D Deficiency Promotes Epithelial Barrier Dysfunction and Intestinal Inflammation. *J. Infect. Dis.* **2014**, *210*, 1296–1305. [CrossRef]
33. Kong, J.; Zhang, Z.; Musch, M.W.; Ning, G.; Sun, J.; Hart, J.; Bissonnette, M.; Li, Y.C. Novel Role of the Vitamin D Receptor in Maintaining the Integrity of the Intestinal Mucosal Barrier. *Am. J. Physiol. Gastrointest Liver Physiol.* **2008**, *294*, G208–G216. [CrossRef]
34. Torki, M.; Gholamrezaei, A.; Mirbagher, L.; Danesh, M.; Kheiri, S.; Emami, M.H. Vitamin D Deficiency Associated with Disease Activity in Patients with Inflammatory Bowel Diseases. *Dig. Dis. Sci.* **2015**, *60*, 3085–3091. [CrossRef]
35. Lu, R.; Wu, S.; Xia, Y.; Sun, J. The Vitamin D Receptor, Inflammatory Bowel Diseases, and Colon Cancer. *Curr. Colorectal. Cancer Rep.* **2012**, *8*, 57–65. [CrossRef] [PubMed]
36. Shang, M.; Sun, J. Vitamin D/VDR, Probiotics, and Gastrointestinal Diseases. *Curr. Med. Chem.* **2017**, *24*, 876–887. [CrossRef] [PubMed]
37. White, J.H. Vitamin D Metabolism and Signaling in the Immune System. *Rev. Endocr. Metab. Disord.* **2012**, *13*, 21–29. [CrossRef] [PubMed]
38. Huang, S.-J.; Wang, X.-H.; Liu, Z.-D.; Cao, W.-L.; Han, Y.; Ma, A.-G.; Xu, S.-F. Vitamin D Deficiency and the Risk of Tuberculosis: A Meta-Analysis. *Drug Des. Devel Ther.* **2017**, *11*, 91–102. [CrossRef] [PubMed]
39. Coussens, A.K. The Role of UV Radiation and Vitamin D in the Seasonality and Outcomes of Infectious Disease. *Photochem. Photobiol. Sci.* **2017**, *16*, 314–338. [CrossRef]
40. Lang, P.O.; Samaras, N.; Samaras, D.; Aspinall, R. How Important Is Vitamin D in Preventing Infections? *Osteoporos Int.* **2013**, *24*, 1537–1553. [CrossRef]

41. Khajavi, A.; Amirhakimi, G.H. The Rachitic Lung. Pulmonary Findings in 30 Infants and Children with Malnutritional Rickets. *Clin. Pediatr.* **1977**, *16*, 36–38. [CrossRef]
42. El Shahawy, M.S.; Shady, Z.M.; Gaafar, A. Influence of Adding Vitamin D3 to Standard Clarithromycin-Based Triple Therapy on the Eradication Rates of *Helicobacter Pylori* Infection. *Arab J. Gastroenterol.* **2021**, *22*, 209–214. [CrossRef]
43. Yildirim, O.; Yildirim, T.; Seckin, Y.; Osanmaz, P.; Bilgic, Y.; Mete, R. The Influence of Vitamin D Deficiency on Eradication Rates of *Helicobacter Pylori*. *Adv. Clin. Exp. Med.* **2017**, *26*, 1377–1381. [CrossRef]
44. Antico, A.; Tozzoli, R.; Giavarina, D.; Tonutti, E.; Bizzaro, N. Hypovitaminosis D as Predisposing Factor for Atrophic Type A Gastritis: A Case-Control Study and Review of the Literature on the Interaction of Vitamin D with the Immune System. *Clin. Rev. Allergy Immunol.* **2012**, *42*, 355–364. [CrossRef]
45. Guo, L.; Chen, W.; Zhu, H.; Chen, Y.; Wan, X.; Yang, N.; Xu, S.; Yu, C.; Chen, L. *Helicobacter Pylori* Induces Increased Expression of the Vitamin d Receptor in Immune Responses. *Helicobacter* **2014**, *19*, 37–47. [CrossRef]
46. Danai, P.A.; Sinha, S.; Moss, M.; Haber, M.J.; Martin, G.S. Seasonal Variation in the Epidemiology of Sepsis. *Crit. Care Med.* **2007**, *35*, 410–415. [CrossRef] [PubMed]
47. Hosoda, K.; Shimomura, H.; Wanibuchi, K.; Masui, H.; Amgalanbaatar, A.; Hayashi, S.; Takahashi, T.; Hirai, Y. Identification and Characterization of a Vitamin D$_3$ Decomposition Product Bactericidal against *Helicobacter Pylori*. *Sci. Rep.* **2015**, *5*, 8860. [CrossRef]
48. Bharwani, S.S.; Shaukat, Q.; Balhaj, G.; Ashari, M. A Failing to Thrive 18 Month Old with Vitamin D Deficiency Rickets and *Helicobacter Pylori* Gastritis. *BMJ Case Rep.* **2011**, *2011*, bcr0420114160. [CrossRef]
49. Bao, A.; Li, Y.; Tong, Y.; Zheng, H.; Wu, W.; Wei, C. Tumor-Suppressive Effects of 1, 25-Dihydroxyvitamin D3 in Gastric Cancer Cells. *Hepatogastroenterology* **2013**, *60*, 943–948. [CrossRef] [PubMed]
50. Zhou, A.; Li, L.; Zhao, G.; Min, L.; Liu, S.; Zhu, S.; Guo, Q.; Liu, C.; Zhang, S.; Li, P. Vitamin D3 Inhibits *Helicobacter Pylori* Infection by Activating the VitD3/VDR-CAMP Pathway in Mice. *Front. Cell Infect. Microbiol.* **2020**, *10*, 566730. [CrossRef] [PubMed]
51. Cavalcoli, F.; Zilli, A.; Conte, D.; Massironi, S. Micronutrient Deficiencies in Patients with Chronic Atrophic Autoimmune Gastritis: A Review. *World J. Gastroenterol.* **2017**, *23*, 563–572. [CrossRef] [PubMed]
52. Mehta, P.; Furuta, G.T.; Brennan, T.; Henry, M.L.; Maune, N.C.; Sundaram, S.S.; Menard-Katcher, C.; Atkins, D.; Takurukura, F.; Giffen, S.; et al. Nutritional State and Feeding Behaviors of Children With Eosinophilic Esophagitis and Gastroesophageal Reflux Disease. *J. Pediatr. Gastroenterol. Nutr.* **2018**, *66*, 603–608. [CrossRef]
53. Giustina, A.; Adler, R.A.; Binkley, N.; Bollerslev, J.; Bouillon, R.; Dawson-Hughes, B.; Ebeling, P.R.; Feldman, D.; Formenti, A.M.; Lazaretti-Castro, M.; et al. Consensus Statement from 2nd International Conference on Controversies in Vitamin D. *Rev. Endocr. Metab. Disord.* **2020**, *21*, 89–116. [CrossRef]
54. Hill, I.D. Celiac Disease–a Never-Ending Story? *J. Pediatr.* **2003**, *143*, 289–291. [CrossRef]
55. Tanpowpong, P.; Camargo, C.A. Early-Life Vitamin D Deficiency and Childhood-Onset Coeliac Disease. *Public Health Nutr.* **2014**, *17*, 823–826. [CrossRef] [PubMed]
56. Ahlawat, R.; Weinstein, T.; Pettei, M.J. Vitamin D in Pediatric Gastrointestinal Disease. *Curr. Opin Pediatr.* **2017**, *29*, 122–127. [CrossRef] [PubMed]
57. Magnus, M.C.; Stene, L.C.; Håberg, S.E.; Nafstad, P.; Stigum, H.; London, S.J.; Nystad, W. Prospective Study of Maternal Mid-Pregnancy 25-Hydroxyvitamin D Level and Early Childhood Respiratory Disorders. *Paediatr. Perinat. Epidemiol.* **2013**, *27*, 532–541. [CrossRef]
58. Aghajafari, F.; Nagulesapillai, T.; Ronksley, P.E.; Tough, S.C.; O'Beirne, M.; Rabi, D.M. Association between Maternal Serum 25-Hydroxyvitamin D Level and Pregnancy and Neonatal Outcomes: Systematic Review and Meta-Analysis of Observational Studies. *BMJ* **2013**, *346*, f1169. [CrossRef] [PubMed]
59. Munger, K.L.; Åivo, J.; Hongell, K.; Soilu-Hänninen, M.; Surcel, H.-M.; Ascherio, A. Vitamin D Status During Pregnancy and Risk of Multiple Sclerosis in Offspring of Women in the Finnish Maternity Cohort. *JAMA Neurol.* **2016**, *73*, 515–519. [CrossRef] [PubMed]
60. Sørensen, I.M.; Joner, G.; Jenum, P.A.; Eskild, A.; Torjesen, P.A.; Stene, L.C. Maternal Serum Levels of 25-Hydroxy-Vitamin D during Pregnancy and Risk of Type 1 Diabetes in the Offspring. *Diabetes* **2012**, *61*, 175–178. [CrossRef] [PubMed]
61. Lebwohl, B.; Green, P.H.R.; Murray, J.A.; Ludvigsson, J.F. Season of Birth in a Nationwide Cohort of Coeliac Disease Patients. *Arch. Dis. Child.* **2013**, *98*, 48–51. [CrossRef]
62. Tanpowpong, P.; Obuch, J.C.; Jiang, H.; McCarty, C.E.; Katz, A.J.; Leffler, D.A.; Kelly, C.P.; Weir, D.C.; Leichtner, A.M.; Camargo, C.A. Multicenter Study on Season of Birth and Celiac Disease: Evidence for a New Theoretical Model of Pathogenesis. *J. Pediatr.* **2013**, *162*, 501–504. [CrossRef]
63. Mårild, K.; Tapia, G.; Haugen, M.; Dahl, S.R.; Cohen, A.S.; Lundqvist, M.; Lie, B.A.; Stene, L.C.; Størdal, K. Maternal and Neonatal Vitamin D Status, Genotype and Childhood Celiac Disease. *PLoS ONE* **2017**, *12*, e0179080. [CrossRef]
64. Vici, G.; Camilletti, D.; Polzonetti, V. Possible Role of Vitamin D in Celiac Disease Onset. *Nutrients* **2020**, *12*, E1051. [CrossRef]
65. Cukrowska, B.; Sowińska, A.; Bierła, J.B.; Czarnowska, E.; Rybak, A.; Grzybowska-Chlebowczyk, U. Intestinal Epithelium, Intraepithelial Lymphocytes and the Gut Microbiota—Key Players in the Pathogenesis of Celiac Disease. *World J. Gastroenterol.* **2017**, *23*, 7505–7518. [CrossRef] [PubMed]
66. Dong, S.; Singh, T.P.; Wei, X.; Yao, H.; Wang, H. Protective Effect of 1,25-Dihydroxy Vitamin D3 on Pepsin-Trypsin-Resistant Gliadin-Induced Tight Junction Injuries. *Dig. Dis. Sci.* **2018**, *63*, 92–104. [CrossRef]

67. Fasano, A. All Disease Begins in the (Leaky) Gut: Role of Zonulin-Mediated Gut Permeability in the Pathogenesis of Some Chronic Inflammatory Diseases. *F1000Res* **2020**, *9*, F1000 Faculty Rev-69. [CrossRef] [PubMed]
68. Chen, S.; Zhu, J.; Chen, G.; Zuo, S.; Zhang, J.; Chen, Z.; Wang, X.; Li, J.; Liu, Y.; Wang, P. 1,25-Dihydroxyvitamin D3 Preserves Intestinal Epithelial Barrier Function from TNF-α Induced Injury via Suppression of NF-KB P65 Mediated MLCK-P-MLC Signaling Pathway. *Biochem. Biophys. Res. Commun.* **2015**, *460*, 873–878. [CrossRef] [PubMed]
69. Aydemir, Y.; Erdogan, B.; Türkeli, A. Vitamin D Deficiency Negatively Affects Both the Intestinal Epithelial Integrity and Bone Metabolism in Children with Celiac Disease. *Clin. Res. Hepatol. Gastroenterol.* **2021**, *45*, 101523. [CrossRef]
70. Zanchi, C.; Di Leo, G.; Ronfani, L.; Martelossi, S.; Not, T.; Ventura, A. Bone Metabolism in Celiac Disease. *J. Pediatr.* **2008**, *153*, 262–265. [CrossRef]
71. Villanueva, J.; Maranda, L.; Nwosu, B.U. Is Vitamin D Deficiency a Feature of Pediatric Celiac Disease? *J. Pediatr. Endocrinol. Metab* **2012**, *25*, 607–610. [CrossRef]
72. Caruso, R.; Pallone, F.; Stasi, E.; Romeo, S.; Monteleone, G. Appropriate Nutrient Supplementation in Celiac Disease. *Ann. Med.* **2013**, *45*, 522–531. [CrossRef]
73. Sdepanian, V.L.; de Miranda Carvalho, C.N.; de Morais, M.B.; Colugnati, F.A.B.; Fagundes-Neto, U. Bone Mineral Density of the Lumbar Spine in Children and Adolescents with Celiac Disease on a Gluten-Free Diet in São Paulo, Brazil. *J. Pediatr. Gastroenterol. Nutr.* **2003**, *37*, 571–576. [CrossRef]
74. Shepherd, S.J.; Gibson, P.R. Nutritional Inadequacies of the Gluten-Free Diet in Both Recently-Diagnosed and Long-Term Patients with Coeliac Disease. *J. Hum. Nutr. Diet.* **2013**, *26*, 349–358. [CrossRef]
75. Jansen, M.A.E.; Kiefte-de Jong, J.C.; Gaillard, R.; Escher, J.C.; Hofman, A.; Jaddoe, V.W.V.; Hooijkaas, H.; Moll, H.A. Growth Trajectories and Bone Mineral Density in Anti-Tissue Transglutaminase Antibody-Positive Children: The Generation R Study. *Clin. Gastroenterol. Hepatol.* **2015**, *13*, 913–920.e5. [CrossRef] [PubMed]
76. Mager, D.R.; Qiao, J.; Turner, J. Vitamin D and K Status Influences Bone Mineral Density and Bone Accrual in Children and Adolescents with Celiac Disease. *Eur. J. Clin. Nutr.* **2012**, *66*, 488–495. [CrossRef] [PubMed]
77. Hill, I.D.; Fasano, A.; Guandalini, S.; Hoffenberg, E.; Levy, J.; Reilly, N.; Verma, R. NASPGHAN Clinical Report on the Diagnosis and Treatment of Gluten-Related Disorders. *J. Pediatr. Gastroenterol. Nutr.* **2016**, *63*, 156–165. [CrossRef] [PubMed]
78. Rubio-Tapia, A.; Hill, I.D.; Kelly, C.P.; Calderwood, A.H.; Murray, J.A. American College of Gastroenterology ACG Clinical Guidelines: Diagnosis and Management of Celiac Disease. *Am. J. Gastroenterol.* **2013**, *108*, 656–676, quiz 677. [CrossRef]
79. Ludvigsson, J.F.; Bai, J.C.; Biagi, F.; Card, T.R.; Ciacci, C.; Ciclitira, P.J.; Green, P.H.R.; Hadjivassiliou, M.; Holdoway, A.; van Heel, D.A.; et al. Diagnosis and Management of Adult Coeliac Disease: Guidelines from the British Society of Gastroenterology. *Gut* **2014**, *63*, 1210–1228. [CrossRef]
80. Ahlawat, R.; Weinstein, T.; Markowitz, J.; Kohn, N.; Pettei, M.J. Should We Assess Vitamin D Status in Pediatric Patients With Celiac Disease? *J. Pediatr. Gastroenterol. Nutr.* **2019**, *69*, 449–454. [CrossRef]
81. Strausbaugh, S.D.; Davis, P.B. Cystic Fibrosis: A Review of Epidemiology and Pathobiology. *Clin. Chest Med.* **2007**, *28*, 279–288. [CrossRef]
82. Salvatore, D.; Buzzetti, R.; Baldo, E.; Forneris, M.P.; Lucidi, V.; Manunza, D.; Marinelli, I.; Messore, B.; Neri, A.S.; Raia, V.; et al. An Overview of International Literature from Cystic Fibrosis Registries. Part 3. Disease Incidence, Genotype/Phenotype Correlation, Microbiology, Pregnancy, Clinical Complications, Lung Transplantation, and Miscellanea. *J. Cyst. Fibros* **2011**, *10*, 71–85. [CrossRef]
83. Collawn, J.F.; Matalon, S. CFTR and Lung Homeostasis. *Am. J. Physiol Lung Cell Mol. Physiol.* **2014**, *307*, L917–L923. [CrossRef]
84. Wolfenden, L.L.; Judd, S.E.; Shah, R.; Sanyal, R.; Ziegler, T.R.; Tangpricha, V. Vitamin D and Bone Health in Adults with Cystic Fibrosis. *Clin. Endocrinol. (Oxf)* **2008**, *69*, 374–381. [CrossRef]
85. Rovner, A.J.; Stallings, V.A.; Schall, J.I.; Leonard, M.B.; Zemel, B.S. Vitamin D Insufficiency in Children, Adolescents, and Young Adults with Cystic Fibrosis despite Routine Oral Supplementation. *Am. J. Clin. Nutr.* **2007**, *86*, 1694–1699. [CrossRef] [PubMed]
86. Hall, W.B.; Sparks, A.A.; Aris, R.M. Vitamin d Deficiency in Cystic Fibrosis. *Int. J. Endocrinol* **2010**, *2010*, 218691. [CrossRef] [PubMed]
87. Tangpricha, V.; Kelly, A.; Stephenson, A.; Maguiness, K.; Enders, J.; Robinson, K.A.; Marshall, B.C.; Borowitz, D. Cystic Fibrosis Foundation Vitamin D Evidence-Based Review Committee An Update on the Screening, Diagnosis, Management, and Treatment of Vitamin D Deficiency in Individuals with Cystic Fibrosis: Evidence-Based Recommendations from the Cystic Fibrosis Foundation. *J. Clin. Endocrinol. Metab.* **2012**, *97*, 1082–1093. [CrossRef]
88. Cemlyn-Jones, J.; Gamboa, F.; Teixeira, L.; Bernardo, J.; Robalo Cordeiro, C. Sarcoidosis: A Less Common Presentation. *Rev. Port. Pneumol.* **2009**, *15*, 543–552. [CrossRef]
89. Douros, K.; Loukou, I.; Nicolaidou, P.; Tzonou, A.; Doudounakis, S. Bone Mass Density and Associated Factors in Cystic Fibrosis Patients of Young Age. *J. Paediatr. Child. Health* **2008**, *44*, 681–685. [CrossRef] [PubMed]
90. Finklea, J.D.; Grossmann, R.E.; Tangpricha, V. Vitamin D and Chronic Lung Disease: A Review of Molecular Mechanisms and Clinical Studies. *Adv. Nutr.* **2011**, *2*, 244–253. [CrossRef]
91. Black, P.N.; Scragg, R. Relationship between Serum 25-Hydroxyvitamin d and Pulmonary Function in the Third National Health and Nutrition Examination Survey. *Chest* **2005**, *128*, 3792–3798. [CrossRef]
92. Chesdachai, S.; Tangpricha, V. Treatment of Vitamin D Deficiency in Cystic Fibrosis. *J. Steroid. Biochem. Mol. Biol.* **2016**, *164*, 36–39. [CrossRef]

93. Yim, S.; Dhawan, P.; Ragunath, C.; Christakos, S.; Diamond, G. Induction of Cathelicidin in Normal and CF Bronchial Epithelial Cells by 1,25-Dihydroxyvitamin D(3). *J. Cyst. Fibros* **2007**, *6*, 403–410. [CrossRef]
94. Herscovitch, K.; Dauletbaev, N.; Lands, L.C. Vitamin D as an Anti-Microbial and Anti-Inflammatory Therapy for Cystic Fibrosis. *Paediatr. Respir. Rev.* **2014**, *15*, 154–162. [CrossRef]
95. Korf, H.; Decallonne, B.; Mathieu, C. Vitamin D for Infections. *Curr. Opin. Endocrinol. Diabetes Obes.* **2014**, *21*, 431–436. [CrossRef] [PubMed]
96. Grossmann, R.E.; Zughaier, S.M.; Kumari, M.; Seydafkan, S.; Lyles, R.H.; Liu, S.; Sueblinvong, V.; Schechter, M.S.; Stecenko, A.A.; Ziegler, T.R.; et al. Pilot Study of Vitamin D Supplementation in Adults with Cystic Fibrosis Pulmonary Exacerbation: A Randomized, Controlled Trial. *Dermatoendocrinol* **2012**, *4*, 191–197. [CrossRef] [PubMed]
97. Lee, M.J.; Alvarez, J.A.; Smith, E.M.; Killilea, D.W.; Chmiel, J.F.; Joseph, P.M.; Grossmann, R.E.; Gaggar, A.; Ziegler, T.R.; Tangpricha, V.; et al. Changes in Mineral Micronutrient Status During and After Pulmonary Exacerbation in Adults With Cystic Fibrosis. *Nutr. Clin. Pract.* **2015**, *30*, 838–843. [CrossRef] [PubMed]
98. Dorsey, J.; Gonska, T. Bacterial Overgrowth, Dysbiosis, Inflammation, and Dysmotility in the Cystic Fibrosis Intestine. *J. Cyst. Fibros* **2017**, *16* (Suppl. S2), S14–S23. [CrossRef]
99. Morin, G.; Orlando, V.; St-Martin Crites, K.; Patey, N.; Mailhot, G. Vitamin D Attenuates Inflammation in CFTR Knockdown Intestinal Epithelial Cells but Has No Effect in Cells with Intact CFTR. *Am. J. Physiol. Gastrointest Liver Physiol.* **2016**, *310*, G539–G549. [CrossRef]
100. Le, T.N. Updates in Vitamin D Therapy in Cystic Fibrosis. *Curr. Opin. Endocrinol. Diabetes Obes.* **2018**, *25*, 361–365. [CrossRef]
101. Kanhere, M.; He, J.; Chassaing, B.; Ziegler, T.R.; Alvarez, J.A.; Ivie, E.A.; Hao, L.; Hanfelt, J.; Gewirtz, A.T.; Tangpricha, V. Bolus Weekly Vitamin D3 Supplementation Impacts Gut and Airway Microbiota in Adults With Cystic Fibrosis: A Double-Blind, Randomized, Placebo-Controlled Clinical Trial. *J. Clin. Endocrinol. Metab.* **2018**, *103*, 564–574. [CrossRef]
102. Alvarez, J.A.; Chong, E.Y.; Walker, D.I.; Chandler, J.D.; Michalski, E.S.; Grossmann, R.E.; Uppal, K.; Li, S.; Frediani, J.K.; Tirouvanziam, R.; et al. Plasma Metabolomics in Adults with Cystic Fibrosis during a Pulmonary Exacerbation: A Pilot Randomized Study of High-Dose Vitamin D3 Administration. *Metabolism* **2017**, *70*, 31–41. [CrossRef]
103. Li, X.-X.; Liu, Y.; Luo, J.; Huang, Z.-D.; Zhang, C.; Fu, Y. Vitamin D Deficiency Associated with Crohn's Disease and Ulcerative Colitis: A Meta-Analysis of 55 Observational Studies. *J. Transl. Med.* **2019**, *17*, 323. [CrossRef]
104. Garg, M.; Lubel, J.S.; Sparrow, M.P.; Holt, S.G.; Gibson, P.R. Review Article: Vitamin D and Inflammatory Bowel Disease—Established Concepts and Future Directions. *Aliment. Pharmacol. Ther.* **2012**, *36*, 324–344. [CrossRef]
105. Zhao, H.; Zhang, H.; Wu, H.; Li, H.; Liu, L.; Guo, J.; Li, C.; Shih, D.Q.; Zhang, X. Protective Role of 1,25(OH)2 Vitamin D3 in the Mucosal Injury and Epithelial Barrier Disruption in DSS-Induced Acute Colitis in Mice. *BMC Gastroenterol.* **2012**, *12*, 57. [CrossRef] [PubMed]
106. Gombart, A.F.; Borregaard, N.; Koeffler, H.P. Human Cathelicidin Antimicrobial Peptide (CAMP) Gene Is a Direct Target of the Vitamin D Receptor and Is Strongly up-Regulated in Myeloid Cells by 1,25-Dihydroxyvitamin D3. *FASEB J.* **2005**, *19*, 1067–1077. [CrossRef] [PubMed]
107. Bora, S.; Cantorna, M.T. The Role of UVR and Vitamin D on T Cells and Inflammatory Bowel Disease. *Photochem. Photobiol. Sci.* **2017**, *16*, 347–353. [CrossRef]
108. Barbalho, S.M.; Goulart, R.d.A.; Gasparini, R.G. Associations between Inflammatory Bowel Diseases and Vitamin D. *Crit. Rev. Food Sci Nutr* **2019**, *59*, 1347–1356. [CrossRef] [PubMed]
109. Ananthakrishnan, A.N. Epidemiology and Risk Factors for IBD. *Nat. Rev. Gastroenterol. Hepatol.* **2015**, *12*, 205–217. [CrossRef] [PubMed]
110. Lim, W.-C.; Hanauer, S.B.; Li, Y.C. Mechanisms of Disease: Vitamin D and Inflammatory Bowel Disease. *Nat. Clin. Pract. Gastroenterol Hepatol* **2005**, *2*, 308–315. [CrossRef] [PubMed]
111. Farraye, F.A.; Nimitphong, H.; Stucchi, A.; Dendrinos, K.; Boulanger, A.B.; Vijjeswarapu, A.; Tanennbaum, A.; Biancuzzo, R.; Chen, T.C.; Holick, M.F. Use of a Novel Vitamin D Bioavailability Test Demonstrates That Vitamin D Absorption Is Decreased in Patients with Quiescent Crohn's Disease. *Inflamm. Bowel. Dis.* **2011**, *17*, 2116–2121. [CrossRef]
112. Gorham, E.D.; Garland, C.F.; Garland, F.C.; Grant, W.B.; Mohr, S.B.; Lipkin, M.; Newmark, H.L.; Giovannucci, E.; Wei, M.; Holick, M.F. Vitamin D and Prevention of Colorectal Cancer. *J. Steroid. Biochem. Mol. Biol.* **2005**, *97*, 179–194. [CrossRef]
113. Wilkins, C.H.; Sheline, Y.I.; Roe, C.M.; Birge, S.J.; Morris, J.C. Vitamin D Deficiency Is Associated with Low Mood and Worse Cognitive Performance in Older Adults. *Am. J. Geriatr. Psychiatry* **2006**, *14*, 1032–1040. [CrossRef]
114. Raffner Basson, A.; Swart, R.; Jordaan, E.; Mazinu, M.; Watermeyer, G. Vitamin D Deficiency Increases the Risk for Moderate to Severe Disease Activity in Crohn's Disease Patients in South Africa, Measured by the Harvey Bradshaw Index. *J. Am. Coll Nutr.* **2016**, *35*, 163–174. [CrossRef]
115. El-Matary, W.; Sikora, S.; Spady, D. Bone Mineral Density, Vitamin D, and Disease Activity in Children Newly Diagnosed with Inflammatory Bowel Disease. *Dig. Dis. Sci.* **2011**, *56*, 825–829. [CrossRef] [PubMed]
116. Gubatan, J.; Moss, A.C. Vitamin D in Inflammatory Bowel Disease: More than Just a Supplement. *Curr. Opin. Gastroenterol.* **2018**, *34*, 217–225. [CrossRef] [PubMed]
117. Del Pinto, R.; Pietropaoli, D.; Chandar, A.K.; Ferri, C.; Cominelli, F. Association between Inflammatory Bowel Disease and Vitamin D Deficiency: A Systematic Review and Meta-Analysis. *Inflamm. Bowel. Dis.* **2015**, *21*, 2708–2717. [CrossRef] [PubMed]

118. Chatu, S.; Chhaya, V.; Holmes, R.; Neild, P.; Kang, J.-Y.; Pollok, R.C.; Poullis, A. Factors Associated with Vitamin D Deficiency in a Multicultural Inflammatory Bowel Disease Cohort. *Frontline Gastroenterol.* **2013**, *4*, 51–56. [CrossRef]
119. Zullow, S.; Jambaulikar, G.; Rustgi, A.; Quezada, S.; Cross, R.K. Risk Factors for Vitamin D Deficiency and Impact of Repletion in a Tertiary Care Inflammatory Bowel Disease Population. *Dig. Dis. Sci.* **2017**, *62*, 2072–2078. [CrossRef]
120. Lee, S.; Metcalfe, A.; Raman, M.; Leung, Y.; Aghajafari, F.; Letourneau, N.; Panaccione, R.; Kaplan, G.G.; Seow, C.H. Pregnant Women with Inflammatory Bowel Disease Are at Increased Risk of Vitamin D Insufficiency: A Cross-Sectional Study. *J. Crohns Colitis* **2018**, *12*, 702–709. [CrossRef]
121. Blanck, S.; Aberra, F. Vitamin d Deficiency Is Associated with Ulcerative Colitis Disease Activity. *Dig. Dis. Sci.* **2013**, *58*, 1698–1702. [CrossRef]
122. Ulitsky, A.; Ananthakrishnan, A.N.; Naik, A.; Skaros, S.; Zadvornova, Y.; Binion, D.G.; Issa, M. Vitamin D Deficiency in Patients with Inflammatory Bowel Disease: Association with Disease Activity and Quality of Life. *JPEN J. Parenter. Enteral. Nutr.* **2011**, *35*, 308–316. [CrossRef]
123. Dolatshahi, S.; Pishgar, E.; Jamali, R. Does Serum 25 Hydroxy Vitamin D Level Predict Disease Activity in Ulcerative Colitis Patients? *Acta Clin. Belg.* **2016**, *71*, 46–50. [CrossRef]
124. Scolaro, B.L.; Barretta, C.; Matos, C.H.; Malluta, E.F.; de Almeida, I.B.T.; Braggio, L.D.; Bobato, S.; Specht, C.M. Deficiency of Vitamin D and Its Relation with Clinical and Laboratory Activity of Inflammatory Bowel Diseases. *J. Coloproctol. (Rio J.)* **2018**, *38*, 99–104. [CrossRef]
125. Schäffler, H.; Schmidt, M.; Huth, A.; Reiner, J.; Glass, Ä.; Lamprecht, G. Clinical Factors Are Associated with Vitamin D Levels in IBD Patients: A Retrospective Analysis. *J. Dig. Dis.* **2018**, *19*, 24–32. [CrossRef]
126. Frigstad, S.O.; Høivik, M.; Jahnsen, J.; Dahl, S.R.; Cvancarova, M.; Grimstad, T.; Berset, I.P.; Huppertz-Hauss, G.; Hovde, Ø.; Torp, R.; et al. Vitamin D Deficiency in Inflammatory Bowel Disease: Prevalence and Predictors in a Norwegian Outpatient Population. *Scand. J. Gastroenterol.* **2017**, *52*, 100–106. [CrossRef] [PubMed]
127. Alrefai, D.; Jones, J.; El-Matary, W.; Whiting, S.J.; Aljebreen, A.; Mirhosseini, N.; Vatanparast, H. The Association of Vitamin D Status with Disease Activity in a Cohort of Crohn's Disease Patients in Canada. *Nutrients* **2017**, *9*, E1112. [CrossRef] [PubMed]
128. Meckel, K.; Li, Y.C.; Lim, J.; Kocherginsky, M.; Weber, C.; Almoghrabi, A.; Chen, X.; Kaboff, A.; Sadiq, F.; Hanauer, S.B.; et al. Serum 25-Hydroxyvitamin D Concentration Is Inversely Associated with Mucosal Inflammation in Patients with Ulcerative Colitis. *Am. J. Clin. Nutr.* **2016**, *104*, 113–120. [CrossRef]
129. Ye, L.; Lin, Z.; Liu, J.; Cao, Q. Vitamin D Deficiency Is Associated with Endoscopic Severity in Patients with Crohn's Disease. *Gastroenterol. Res. Pract.* **2017**, *2017*, 4869718. [CrossRef] [PubMed]
130. Ko, K.H.; Kim, Y.S.; Lee, B.K.; Choi, J.H.; Woo, Y.M.; Kim, J.Y.; Moon, J.S. Vitamin D Deficiency Is Associated with Disease Activity in Patients with Crohn's Disease. *Intest. Res.* **2019**, *17*, 70–77. [CrossRef]
131. Ananthakrishnan, A.N.; Cagan, A.; Gainer, V.S.; Cai, T.; Cheng, S.-C.; Savova, G.; Chen, P.; Szolovits, P.; Xia, Z.; De Jager, P.L.; et al. Normalization of Plasma 25-Hydroxy Vitamin D Is Associated with Reduced Risk of Surgery in Crohn's Disease. *Inflamm. Bowel Dis.* **2013**, *19*, 1921–1927. [CrossRef]
132. Kabbani, T.A.; Koutroubakis, I.E.; Schoen, R.E.; Ramos-Rivers, C.; Shah, N.; Swoger, J.; Regueiro, M.; Barrie, A.; Schwartz, M.; Hashash, J.G.; et al. Association of Vitamin D Level With Clinical Status in Inflammatory Bowel Disease: A 5-Year Longitudinal Study. *Am. J. Gastroenterol.* **2016**, *111*, 712–719. [CrossRef]
133. Ryan, F.J.; Ahern, A.M.; Fitzgerald, R.S.; Laserna-Mendieta, E.J.; Power, E.M.; Clooney, A.G.; O'Donoghue, K.W.; McMurdie, P.J.; Iwai, S.; Crits-Christoph, A.; et al. Colonic Microbiota Is Associated with Inflammation and Host Epigenomic Alterations in Inflammatory Bowel Disease. *Nat. Commun.* **2020**, *11*, 1512. [CrossRef]
134. Schirmer, M.; Garner, A.; Vlamakis, H.; Xavier, R.J. Microbial Genes and Pathways in Inflammatory Bowel Disease. *Nat. Rev. Microbiol.* **2019**, *17*, 497–511. [CrossRef]
135. Stange, E.F.; Schroeder, B.O. Microbiota and Mucosal Defense in IBD: An Update. *Expert Rev. Gastroenterol. Hepatol.* **2019**, *13*, 963–976. [CrossRef]
136. Gubatan, J.; Chou, N.D.; Nielsen, O.H.; Moss, A.C. Systematic Review with Meta-Analysis: Association of Vitamin D Status with Clinical Outcomes in Adult Patients with Inflammatory Bowel Disease. *Aliment. Pharmacol. Ther.* **2019**, *50*, 1146–1158. [CrossRef]
137. Garg, M.; Hendy, P.; Ding, J.N.; Shaw, S.; Hold, G.; Hart, A. The Effect of Vitamin D on Intestinal Inflammation and Faecal Microbiota in Patients with Ulcerative Colitis. *J. Crohns Colitis* **2018**, *12*, 963–972. [CrossRef]
138. Garg, M.; Rosella, O.; Rosella, G.; Wu, Y.; Lubel, J.S.; Gibson, P.R. Evaluation of a 12-Week Targeted Vitamin D Supplementation Regimen in Patients with Active Inflammatory Bowel Disease. *Clin. Nutr.* **2018**, *37*, 1375–1382. [CrossRef]
139. Guzman-Prado, Y.; Samson, O.; Segal, J.P.; Limdi, J.K.; Hayee, B. Vitamin D Therapy in Adults With Inflammatory Bowel Disease: A Systematic Review and Meta-Analysis. *Inflamm. Bowel Dis.* **2020**, *26*, 1819–1830. [CrossRef]
140. Mechie, N.-C.; Mavropoulou, E.; Ellenrieder, V.; Petzold, G.; Kunsch, S.; Neesse, A.; Amanzada, A. Serum Vitamin D but Not Zinc Levels Are Associated with Different Disease Activity Status in Patients with Inflammatory Bowel Disease. *Medicine* **2019**, *98*, e15172. [CrossRef]
141. Mentella, M.C.; Scaldaferri, F.; Pizzoferrato, M.; Gasbarrini, A.; Miggiano, G.A.D. The Association of Disease Activity, BMI and Phase Angle with Vitamin D Deficiency in Patients with IBD. *Nutrients* **2019**, *11*, E2583. [CrossRef]
142. Sharifi, A.; Hosseinzadeh-Attar, M.J.; Vahedi, H.; Nedjat, S. A Randomized Controlled Trial on the Effect of Vitamin D3 on Inflammation and Cathelicidin Gene Expression in Ulcerative Colitis Patients. *Saudi J. Gastroenterol.* **2016**, *22*, 316–323. [CrossRef]

143. Sharifi, A.; Vahedi, H.; Nedjat, S.; Rafiei, H.; Hosseinzadeh-Attar, M.J. Effect of Single-Dose Injection of Vitamin D on Immune Cytokines in Ulcerative Colitis Patients: A Randomized Placebo-Controlled Trial. *APMIS* **2019**, *127*, 681–687. [CrossRef]
144. Allen, K.J.; Koplin, J.J.; Ponsonby, A.-L.; Gurrin, L.C.; Wake, M.; Vuillermin, P.; Martin, P.; Matheson, M.; Lowe, A.; Robinson, M.; et al. Vitamin D Insufficiency Is Associated with Challenge-Proven Food Allergy in Infants. *J. Allergy Clin. Immunol.* **2013**, *131*, 1109–1116, 1116.e1-6. [CrossRef]
145. Peroni, D.G.; Boner, A.L. Food Allergy: The Perspectives of Prevention Using Vitamin D. *Curr. Opin. Allergy Clin. Immunol.* **2013**, *13*, 287–292. [CrossRef]
146. Vassallo, M.F.; Camargo, C.A. Potential Mechanisms for the Hypothesized Link between Sunshine, Vitamin D, and Food Allergy in Children. *J. Allergy Clin. Immunol.* **2010**, *126*, 217–222. [CrossRef]
147. Lack, G. Clinical Practice. Food Allergy. *N. Engl. J. Med.* **2008**, *359*, 1252–1260. [CrossRef]
148. Peroni, D.G.; Piacentini, G.L.; Cametti, E.; Chinellato, I.; Boner, A.L. Correlation between Serum 25-Hydroxyvitamin D Levels and Severity of Atopic Dermatitis in Children. *Br. J. Dermatol.* **2011**, *164*, 1078–1082. [CrossRef]
149. Poole, A.; Song, Y.; Brown, H.; Hart, P.H.; Zhang, G.B. Cellular and Molecular Mechanisms of Vitamin D in Food Allergy. *J. Cell Mol. Med.* **2018**, *22*, 3270–3277. [CrossRef]
150. Koplin, J.J.; Peters, R.L.; Allen, K.J. Prevention of Food Allergies. *Immunol. Allergy Clin. N. Am.* **2018**, *38*, 1–11. [CrossRef]
151. Berry, M.J.; Adams, J.; Voutilainen, H.; Feustel, P.J.; Celestin, J.; Järvinen, K.M. Impact of Elimination Diets on Growth and Nutritional Status in Children with Multiple Food Allergies. *Pediatr. Allergy Immunol.* **2015**, *26*, 133–138. [CrossRef]
152. Miraglia Del Giudice, M.; Allegorico, A. The Role of Vitamin D in Allergic Diseases in Children. *J. Clin. Gastroenterol.* **2016**, *50* (Suppl. S2), S133–S135. [CrossRef]
153. Allen, K.J.; Koplin, J.J. Why Does Australia Appear to Have the Highest Rates of Food Allergy? *Pediatr. Clin. N. Am.* **2015**, *62*, 1441–1451. [CrossRef]
154. Nowak, S.; Wang, H.; Schmidt, B.; Jarvinen, K.M. Vitamin D and Iron Status in Children with Food Allergy. *Ann. Allergy Asthma Immunol* **2021**, *127*, 57–63. [CrossRef]
155. Silva, C.M.; da Silva, S.A.; Antunes, M.M.d.C.; da Silva, G.A.P.; Sarinho, E.S.C.; Brandt, K.G. Do Infants with Cow's Milk Protein Allergy Have Inadequate Levels of Vitamin D? *J. Pediatr. (Rio J.)* **2017**, *93*, 632–638. [CrossRef] [PubMed]
156. Shaker, M.; Venter, C. The Ins and Outs of Managing Avoidance Diets for Food Allergies. *Curr. Opin. Pediatr.* **2016**, *28*, 567–572. [CrossRef] [PubMed]
157. Foong, R.-X.; Meyer, R.; Dziubak, R.; Lozinsky, A.C.; Godwin, H.; Reeve, K.; Hussain, S.T.; Nourzaie, R.; Shah, N. Establishing the Prevalence of Low Vitamin D in Non-Immunoglobulin-E Mediated Gastrointestinal Food Allergic Children in a Tertiary Centre. *World Allergy Organ. J.* **2017**, *10*, 4. [CrossRef] [PubMed]
158. Giannetti, A.; Bernardini, L.; Cangemi, J.; Gallucci, M.; Masetti, R.; Ricci, G. Role of Vitamin D in Prevention of Food Allergy in Infants. *Front. Pediatr.* **2020**, *8*, 447. [CrossRef] [PubMed]
159. Yepes-Nuñez, J.J.; Brożek, J.L.; Fiocchi, A.; Pawankar, R.; Cuello-García, C.; Zhang, Y.; Morgano, G.P.; Agarwal, A.; Gandhi, S.; Terracciano, L.; et al. Vitamin D Supplementation in Primary Allergy Prevention: Systematic Review of Randomized and Non-Randomized Studies. *Allergy* **2018**, *73*, 37–49. [CrossRef]
160. Matsui, T.; Tanaka, K.; Yamashita, H.; Saneyasu, K.-I.; Tanaka, H.; Takasato, Y.; Sugiura, S.; Inagaki, N.; Ito, K. Food Allergy Is Linked to Season of Birth, Sun Exposure, and Vitamin D Deficiency. *Allergol. Int.* **2019**, *68*, 172–177. [CrossRef] [PubMed]
161. Dogan, E.; Sevinc, E. The Vitamin D Status and Serum Eosinophilic Cationic Protein Levels in Infants with Cow's Milk Protein Allergy. *Am. J. Transl Res.* **2020**, *12*, 8208–8215.
162. Venter, C.; Groetch, M.; Netting, M.; Meyer, R. A Patient-Specific Approach to Develop an Exclusion Diet to Manage Food Allergy in Infants and Children. *Clin. Exp. Allergy* **2018**, *48*, 121–137. [CrossRef]
163. Rozenberg, S.; Body, J.-J.; Bruyère, O.; Bergmann, P.; Brandi, M.L.; Cooper, C.; Devogelaer, J.-P.; Gielen, E.; Goemaere, S.; Kaufman, J.-M.; et al. Effects of Dairy Products Consumption on Health: Benefits and Beliefs—A Commentary from the Belgian Bone Club and the European Society for Clinical and Economic Aspects of Osteoporosis, Osteoarthritis and Musculoskeletal Diseases. *Calcif. Tissue Int.* **2016**, *98*, 1–17. [CrossRef]
164. Mehta, H.; Ramesh, M.; Feuille, E.; Groetch, M.; Wang, J. Growth Comparison in Children with and without Food Allergies in 2 Different Demographic Populations. *J. Pediatr.* **2014**, *165*, 842–848. [CrossRef]
165. Sardecka-Milewska, I.; Łoś-Rycharska, E.; Gawryjołek, J.; Toporowska-Kowalska, E.; Krogulska, A. Role of FOXP3 Expression and Serum Vitamin D and C Concentrations When Predicting Acquisition of Tolerance in Infants With Cow's Milk Allergy. *J. Investig. Allergol. Clin. Immunol.* **2020**, *30*, 182–190. [CrossRef] [PubMed]
166. Li, J.; Mei, X.; Cai, X.; Zhuo, Y.; Zhang, L.; Guo, H.; Yang, H.; Yang, G. Association of Blood Eosinophilia and Vitamin D Insufficiency in Young Infants with Cow Milk Allergy. *Asia Pac. J. Clin. Nutr.* **2019**, *28*, 550–557. [CrossRef] [PubMed]
167. Ercan, N.; Bostanci, İ.B.; Ozmen, S.; Tekindal, M.A. Is There an Association between Vitamin D Levels and Cow's Milk Protein Allergy at Infancy? *Arch. Argent. Pediatr.* **2019**, *117*, 306–313. [CrossRef] [PubMed]
168. Kosek, M.; Bern, C.; Guerrant, R.L. The Global Burden of Diarrhoeal Disease, as Estimated from Studies Published between 1992 and 2000. *Bull. World Health Organ.* **2003**, *81*, 197–204. [PubMed]
169. Liu, L.; Johnson, H.L.; Cousens, S.; Perin, J.; Scott, S.; Lawn, J.E.; Rudan, I.; Campbell, H.; Cibulskis, R.; Li, M.; et al. Global, Regional, and National Causes of Child Mortality: An Updated Systematic Analysis for 2010 with Time Trends since 2000. *Lancet* **2012**, *379*, 2151–2161. [CrossRef]

170. Yin, K.; Agrawal, D.K. Vitamin D and Inflammatory Diseases. *J. Inflamm. Res.* **2014**, *7*, 69–87. [CrossRef]
171. Thornton, K.A.; Marín, C.; Mora-Plazas, M.; Villamor, E. Vitamin D Deficiency Associated with Increased Incidence of Gastrointestinal and Ear Infections in School-Age Children. *Pediatr. Infect. Dis. J.* **2013**, *32*, 585–593. [CrossRef]
172. Abed, N.; Shaban, N.; Aly, M.; Abdel-gawad, E. Vitamin D Status in Children with Re-Current Acute Diarrhea. *Int. J. Curr. Microbiol. Appl. Sci.* **2014**, *3*, 856–868.
173. Bahijri, S.M. Serum 25-Hydroxy Cholecalciferol in Infants and Preschool Children in the Western Region of Saudi Arabia. Etiological Factors. *Saudi Med. J.* **2001**, *22*, 973–979.
174. Siddiqui, T.S.; Rai, M.I. Presentation and Predisposing Factors of Nutritional Rickets in Children of Hazara Division. *J. Ayub Med. Coll Abbottabad* **2005**, *17*, 29–32.
175. Hassam, I.; Kisenge, R.; Aboud, S.; Manji, K. Association of Vitamin D and Diarrhoea in Children Aged Less than Five Years at Muhimbili National Hospital, Dar Es Salaam: An Unmatched Case Control Study. *BMC Pediatr.* **2019**, *19*, 237. [CrossRef] [PubMed]
176. Ahmed, A.M.S.; Magalhaes, R.J.S.; Ahmed, T.; Long, K.Z.; Hossain, M.; Islam, M.M.; Mahfuz, M.; Gaffar, S.M.A.; Sharmeen, A.; Haque, R.; et al. Vitamin-D Status Is Not a Confounder of the Relationship between Zinc and Diarrhoea: A Study in 6-24-Month-Old Underweight and Normal-Weight Children of Urban Bangladesh. *Eur. J. Clin. Nutr.* **2016**, *70*, 620–628. [CrossRef] [PubMed]
177. Wang, W.J.; Gray, S.; Sison, C.; Arramraju, S.; John, B.K.; Hussain, S.A.; Kim, S.H.; Mehta, P.; Rubin, M. Low Vitamin D Level Is an Independent Predictor of Poor Outcomes in Clostridium Difficile-Associated Diarrhea. *Therap. Adv. Gastroenterol.* **2014**, *7*, 14–19. [CrossRef] [PubMed]
178. Bucak, I.H.; Ozturk, A.B.; Almis, H.; Cevik, M.Ö.; Tekin, M.; Konca, Ç.; Turgut, M.; Bulbul, M. Is There a Relationship between Low Vitamin D and Rotaviral Diarrhea? *Pediatr. Int.* **2016**, *58*, 270–273. [CrossRef] [PubMed]
179. Clark, A.; Mach, N. Role of Vitamin D in the Hygiene Hypothesis: The Interplay between Vitamin D, Vitamin D Receptors, Gut Microbiota, and Immune Response. *Front. Immunol.* **2016**, *7*, 627. [CrossRef] [PubMed]
180. He, L.; Liu, T.; Shi, Y.; Tian, F.; Hu, H.; Deb, D.K.; Chen, Y.; Bissonnette, M.; Li, Y.C. Gut Epithelial Vitamin D Receptor Regulates Microbiota-Dependent Mucosal Inflammation by Suppressing Intestinal Epithelial Cell Apoptosis. *Endocrinology* **2018**, *159*, 967–979. [CrossRef]
181. Shahini, E.; Iannone, A.; Romagno, D.; Armandi, A.; Carparelli, S.; Principi, M.; Viggiani, M.T.; Ierardi, E.; Di Leo, A.; Barone, M. Clinical Relevance of Serum Non-Organ-Specific Antibodies in Patients with HCV Infection Receiving Direct-Acting Antiviral Therapy. *Aliment. Pharmacol. Ther.* **2018**, *48*, 1138–1145. [CrossRef]
182. Thompson, A.J.; Baranzini, S.E.; Geurts, J.; Hemmer, B.; Ciccarelli, O. Multiple Sclerosis. *Lancet* **2018**, *391*, 1622–1636. [CrossRef]
183. Spear, E.T.; Holt, E.A.; Joyce, E.J.; Haag, M.M.; Mawe, S.M.; Hennig, G.W.; Lavoie, B.; Applebee, A.M.; Teuscher, C.; Mawe, G.M. Altered Gastrointestinal Motility Involving Autoantibodies in the Experimental Autoimmune Encephalomyelitis Model of Multiple Sclerosis. *Neurogastroenterol. Motil.* **2018**, *30*, e13349. [CrossRef]
184. Chia, Y.W.; Gill, K.P.; Jameson, J.S.; Forti, A.D.; Henry, M.M.; Swash, M.; Shorvon, P.J. Paradoxical Puborectalis Contraction Is a Feature of Constipation in Patients with Multiple Sclerosis. *J. Neurol. Neurosurg. Psychiatry* **1996**, *60*, 31–35. [CrossRef]
185. Li, Q.; Michel, K.; Annahazi, A.; Demir, I.E.; Ceyhan, G.O.; Zeller, F.; Komorowski, L.; Stöcker, W.; Beyak, M.J.; Grundy, D.; et al. Anti-Hu Antibodies Activate Enteric and Sensory Neurons. *Sci. Rep.* **2016**, *6*, 38216. [CrossRef] [PubMed]
186. Panarese, A.; Pesce, F.; Porcelli, P.; Riezzo, G.; Iacovazzi, P.A.; Leone, C.M.; De Carne, M.; Rinaldi, C.M.; Shahini, E. Chronic Functional Constipation Is Strongly Linked to Vitamin D Deficiency. *World J. Gastroenterol.* **2019**, *25*, 1729–1740. [CrossRef] [PubMed]

MDPI AG
Grosspeteranlage 5
4052 Basel
Switzerland
Tel.: +41 61 683 77 34

Diagnostics Editorial Office
E-mail: diagnostics@mdpi.com
www.mdpi.com/journal/diagnostics

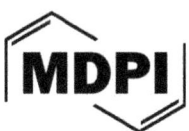

Disclaimer/Publisher's Note: The title and front matter of this reprint are at the discretion of the . The publisher is not responsible for their content or any associated concerns. The statements, opinions and data contained in all individual articles are solely those of the individual Editor and contributors and not of MDPI. MDPI disclaims responsibility for any injury to people or property resulting from any ideas, methods, instructions or products referred to in the content.

www.ingramcontent.com/pod-product-compliance
Lightning Source LLC
LaVergne TN
LVHW070617100526
838202LV00012B/671